Risk Factors in
Coronary
Artery
Disease

Fundamental and Clinical Cardiology

Editor-in-Chief

Samuel Z. Goldhaber, M.D.
Harvard Medical School
and Brigham and Women's Hospital
Boston, Massachusetts, U.S.A.

Risk Factors in
Coronary
Artery
Disease

edited by
P. K. Shah
Cedars-Sinai Medical Center
Los Angeles, California, U.S.A.

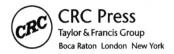
CRC Press
Taylor & Francis Group
Boca Raton London New York

CRC Press is an imprint of the
Taylor & Francis Group, an **informa** business
A TAYLOR & FRANCIS BOOK

First published 2006 by Taylor & Francis

Published 2019 by CRC Press
Taylor & Francis Group
6000 Broken Sound Parkway NW, Suite 300
Boca Raton, FL 33487-2742

© 2006 by Taylor & Francis Group, LLC
CRC Press is an imprint of Taylor & Francis Group, an Informa business

First issued in paperback 2019

No claim to original U.S. Government works

ISBN 13: 978-0-367-45371-8 (pbk)
ISBN 13: 978-0-8247-4095-5 (hbk)

Visit the Taylor & Francis Web site at
http://www.taylorandfrancis.com

and the CRC Press Web site at
http://www.crcpress.com

Library of Congress Cataloging-in-Publication Data

Risk factors in coronary artery disease / edited by P.K. Shah.
     p. ; cm. -- (Fundamental and clinical cardiology ; v. 59)
  Includes bibliographical references and index.
  ISBN-13: 978-0-8247-4095-5 (hardcover : alk. paper)
  ISBN-10: 0-8247-4095-5 (hardcover : alk. paper)
  1. Coronary heart disease--Risk factors. I. Shah, P. K. II. Series.
  [DNLM: 1. Coronary Arteriosclerosis. 2. Risk Factors. WG 300 R5952 2006]

RC685.C6R56 2006
616.1'23--dc22   2006040409

Library of Congress Card Number 2006040409

Series Introduction

Taylor & Francis Group has developed various series of beautifully produced books in different branches of medicine. These series have facilitated the integration of rapidly advancing information for both the clinical specialist and the researcher.

My goal as Editor-in-Chief of the Fundamental and Clinical Cardiology Series is to assemble the talents of world-renowned authorities to discuss virtually every area of cardiovascular medicine. In the current monograph, Dr. Prediman K. Shah has written and edited a much-needed and timely book which addresses those risk factors for coronary artery disease that have until now received insufficient emphasis. Dr. Shah has selected several risk factors for special emphasis, including, hemostatic risk factors, chronic infections, psychosocial factors, and clinical application of genotyping to risk stratification.

Future contributions to this series will include books on molecular biology, interventional cardiology, and clinical management of such problems as coronary artery disease and ventricular arrhythmias.

Samuel Z. Goldhaber, MD
Professor of Medicine
Harvard Medical School
Boston, Massachusetts, U.S.A.

Preface

Coronary artery disease (CAD), resulting from atherosclerosis and thrombosis (atherothrombosis), is the leading cause of death and morbidity in much of the industrialized world and is rapidly achieving the same dubious distinction in developing nations as well. In the cardiovascular field, prevention of CAD and its effective treatment remain paramount objectives of clinical practice as well as targets of ongoing research. The precise etiology and mechanism(s) leading to the development of CAD remain incompletely understood although a number of risk factors have been identified over the past several decades. These include abnormal levels of circulating cholesterol with elevated levels of LDL and reduced levels of HDL cholesterol, hypertension, cigarette smoking, diabetes, male gender, post-menopausal state, advancing age, sedentary lifestyle, obesity, and a positive family history of premature vascular disease. Increasing recognition that many patients (as many as 30–50%) with established CAD lack these traditional risk factors has led to a search for additional new risk factors that may predispose individuals to CAD. Over the past several years, observational and epidemiologic studies have identified a host of new and potential risk factors for atherothrombotic vascular disease. Of this growing list of new and emerging risk factors, elevated blood levels of homocysteine, fibrinogen, inflammation and infection, atherogenic lipoprotein phenotype associated with small LDL cholesterol particles and elevated triglycerides, elevated levels of lipoprotein(a) (Lpa), insulin resistance syndrome (syndrome X or Reaven's syndrome or deadly quartet), psychosocial factors and a number of genetic polymorphisms are of particular interest. The goal of this monograph is to bring to our readers the latest update on these new and emerging risk factors that could open up new opportunities for diagnosis, risk prediction, prevention, and treatment of atherothrombotic vascular disease.

P. K. Shah

Contents

Contributors

Bojan Cercek   Atherosclerosis Research Center, Division of Cardiology and Department of Medicine, Cedars-Sinai Medical Center and David Geffen School of Medicine, University of California, Los Angeles, California, U.S.A.

Prakash C. Deedwania   University of California San Francisco-Fresno, Fresno, California, U.S.A.

James Dwyer[‡]   Department of Preventive Medicine, University of Southern California School of Medicine, Los Angeles, California, U.S.A.

Sanjay Kaul   Division of Cardiology, Cedars-Sinai Medical Center and the David Geffen School of Medicine, University of California, Los Angeles, California, U.S.A.

Spencer King III   Fuqua Heart Center/Piedmont Hospital, Cholesterol, Genetics, and Heart Disease Institute, Atlanta, Georgia, U.S.A.

Willem J. Kop   Uniformed Services University of the Health Sciences, Bethesda, Maryland, U.S.A.

David S. Krantz   Uniformed Services University of the Health Sciences, Bethesda, Maryland, U.S.A.

[‡]Deceased.

C. Noel Bairey Merz   Preventive and Rehabilitative Cardiac Center, Cedars-Sinai Medical Center, Los Angeles, California, U.S.A.

Jan Nilsson   Department of Clinical Sciences, Malmö University Hospital, Lund University, Lund, Sweden

Cheryl K. Nordstrom   Department of Preventive Medicine, University of Southern California School of Medicine, Los Angeles, California, U.S.A.

Donna M. Polk   Division of Cardiology, Department of Medicine, Cedars-Sinai Research Institute, Cedars-Sinai Medical Center, and Department of Medicine, University of California at Los Angeles School of Medicine, Los Angeles, California, U.S.A.

Mathew J. Price   Division of Cardiovascular Diseases, Scripps Clinic, La Jolla, California, U.S.A.

Maren T. Scheuner   UCLA School of Public Health, Department of Health Services, RAND Corporation, Santa Monica, California, U.S.A.

P. K. Shah   Atherosclerosis Research Center, Division of Cardiology and Department of Medicine, Cedars-Sinai Medical Center and David Geffen School of Medicine, University of California, Los Angeles, California, U.S.A.

H. Robert Superko   Fuqua Heart Center/Piedmont Hospital, Cholesterol, Genetics, and Heart Disease Institute, Atlanta, Georgia, U.S.A.

Natalia Volkova   University of California San Francisco-Fresno, Fresno, California, U.S.A.

Szilard Voros   Fuqua Heart Center/Piedmont Hospital, Cholesterol, Genetics, and Heart Disease Institute, Atlanta, Georgia, U.S.A.

Andrew A. Zadeh   Department of Medicine, Cedars-Sinai Medical Center and the David Geffen School of Medicine, University of California, Los Angeles, California, U.S.A.

Metabolic Syndrome and Cardiovascular Disease: Epidemiology, Pathophysiology, and Therapeutic Considerations

Prakash C. Deedwania and Natalia Volkova

University of California San Francisco-Fresno, Fresno, California, U.S.A.

INTRODUCTION

Metabolic syndrome and diabetes mellitus are as much vascular conditions as they are metabolic disorders. It is now well established that a majority (as high as 80%) of diabetic patients die of cardiovascular complications. Current evidence also suggest that, on average, diabetic patients have evidence of insulin resistance for approximately 5 to 6 years before the onset of clinical hyperglycemia. This prediabetic state can manifest itself as metabolic syndrome, which is a constellation of several cardiovascular risk factors including obesity (especially truncal), hypertension, dyslipidemia, glycemic abnormalities, and other metabolic perturbations, which are caused primarily by insulin resistance (1,2). The final products of this syndrome, affecting the cardiovascular system, are endothelial dysfunction, atherosclerosis, and cardiovascular disease (Fig. 1) (3).

Recent studies suggest that changes leading to metabolic syndrome may originate in utero and continue to progress during childhood and adolescence, reaching almost 50% in prevalence in severely obese youngsters (4–8). It is estimated that about 47 million U.S. residents have metabolic syndrome (including those with diabetes), corresponding to 22% of men and 24% of women age 20 years and above, and it rises to more than 40% in patients older than 60 years

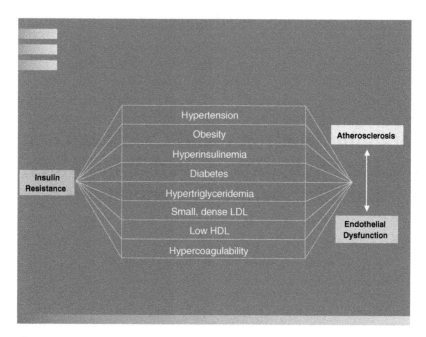

Figure 1 The role of insulin resistance as a key event in metabolic syndrome. *Source*: From Ref. 3.

of age (9). The prevalence of metabolic syndrome in the Hypertension Genetic Epidemiology Network study was found to be 34% in blacks and 39% in whites with compound phenotype with separate domains for obesity, blood pressure, and lipids (10). In this genetic study the dominant factor for metabolic syndrome was obesity and its relationship to lipids and insulin (10).

The growth in prevalence of metabolic syndrome parallels the dramatic rise in prevalence of obesity (11–14).

Individuals with metabolic syndrome are at a three-fold greater risk of coronary heart disease and stroke and more than a four-fold greater risk of cardiovascular mortality (11,15).

The contribution of metabolic syndrome to atherosclerotic disease can be best illustrated by the relationship of diabetes to atherosclerotic disease. Cardiovascular events account for approximately 80% of all diabetic mortality and cardiovascular disorders account for more than 75% of all hospitalizations for diabetic patients (16).

This chapter will review current evidence linking metabolic syndrome with cardiovascular morbidity and mortality and discuss the various available management strategies.

METABOLIC SYNDROME AND CARDIOVASCULAR DISEASE MORBIDITY AND MORTALITY

A number of studies have shown a strong association between metabolic syndrome and CVD morbidity and mortality. One of the first studies, which demonstrated the relationship between cardiovascular diseases and metabolic syndrome, was based on the large population in Italy, which included 22,256 men and 18,495 women. These individuals were participants in a series of epidemiologic investigations of cardiovascular disease conducted in Italy between 1978 and 1987. They were followed for an average of 7 years, during which time a total of 1218 deaths occurred (1003 in men and 215 in women). The risk of death from all causes and cardiovascular disease increased with increased numbers of metabolic abnormalities in both men and women. The majority of individuals who died from cardiovascular disease in this study presented with one or more of the metabolic abnormalities (high blood glucose level, high blood pressure, low HDL-cholesterol level, and high triglyceride level) (17). The Framingham Offspring Study also provided data regarding evaluation of common metabolic coronary disease risk factors in a community sample of 2406 men and 2569 women aged 18 to 74 years. After adjustment for age and weight, a 2.25-kg (5-lb) weight increase over 16 years was associated with an increased prevalence and clustering of metabolic risk factors in both men and women, and a 2.25 kg weight loss was associated with a lower prevalence of the risk factors. Clusters of three or more risk factors were associated with a 2.39 and 5.90 times greater risk of coronary heart disease in men and women, respectively (Fig. 2) (18).

The prevalence of the cardiovascular risks associated with the metabolic syndrome using the definition proposed by the World Health Organization (WHO) was evaluated in 4483 subjects aged 35–70 years participating in a large family study of type 2 diabetes in Finland and Sweden (the Botnia study). Cardiovascular

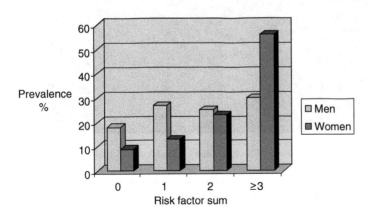

Figure 2   Age-adjusted risk factor sum in correlation with 16 year coronary heart disease risk. *Source*: From Ref. 18.

mortality was assessed in 3606 subjects with a median follow-up of 6.9 years. In women and men, respectively, the metabolic syndrome was seen in 10% and 15% of subjects with normal glucose tolerance, 42% and 64% of those with impaired glucose tolerance, and 78% and 84% of those with type 2 diabetes. The risk for coronary heart disease and stroke was increased three-fold and there was also increased cardiovascular mortality in subjects with the metabolic syndrome (12.0 vs. 2.2%). Of the individual components of the metabolic syndrome, microalbuminuria conferred the strongest risk of cardiovascular death (11). Kuopio Ischemic Heart Disease Study is a population-based, prospective cohort study of 1209 Finnish men aged 42 to 60 years at baseline (1984–1989) who were initially without cardiovascular disease, cancer, or diabetes and were followed for 11.4 years. Using both ATP III (Third Report of the Expert Panel on Detection, Evaluation, and Treatment of High Blood Cholesterol in Adults-Adult Treatment Panel III) and WHO definitions of metabolic syndrome, this study demonstrated that even in the absence of diabetes or prior cardiovascular disease, the presence of metabolic syndrome was associated with a significant increase in the risk of cardiovascular disease and overall mortality (Fig. 3) (15). A recently published

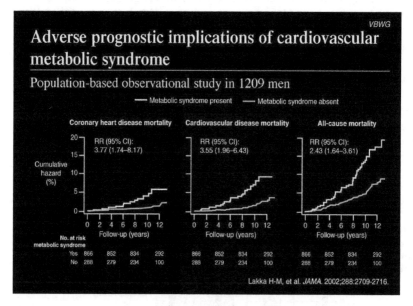

Figure 3 Kuopio Ischemic Heart Disease Study Unadjusted Kaplan-Meier Hazard Curves. Curves for men with versus without the metabolic syndrome based on factor analysis (men in the highest quarter of the distribution of the metabolic syndrome factor were considered to have the metabolic syndrome). Median follow-up (range) for survivors was 11.6 (9.1–13.7) years. Relative risks were determined by age-adjusted Cox proportional hazards regression analysis. *Abbreviations*: RR, relative risk; CI, confidence interval. *Source*: From Ref. 15.

study based on 11 prospective European cohort studies included 6156 men and 5356 women without diabetes, aged 30 to 89 years with 8.8 years follow-up. Based on modified WHO definition, the prevalence of metabolic syndrome was slightly higher in men (15.7%), than in women (14.2%). This study also demonstrated that non-diabetic patients with metabolic syndrome had an increased risk of cardiovascular mortality (19). The Strong Heart Study examined 2283 non-diabetic American Indians who were free of cardiovascular disease at the baseline examination. Based on ATP III definition, metabolic syndrome was present in 798 individuals (35%), and 181 participants (7.9%) developed cardiovascular disease over 7.6+/−1.8 years of follow-up (20).

The Third National Health and Nutrition Examination Survey (NHANES III) was used to categorize adults over 50 years of age by presence of metabolic syndrome (National Cholesterol Education Program definition) with or without diabetes. Demographic and risk factor information was determined for each group, as well as the proportion of each group meeting specific criteria for metabolic syndrome. A subset of adults ≥50 years of age representing 76.1 million Americans was used for this adult in-home questionnaire analysis and 3510 patients underwent physical examination. Older Americans over 50 years of age without metabolic syndrome regardless of diabetes status had the lowest cardiovascular disease prevalence (8.7% without diabetes, 7.5% with diabetes). Compared with those with metabolic syndrome, patients with diabetes without metabolic syndrome did not have an increase in prevalence of cardiovascular disease. Those with metabolic syndrome without diabetes had relatively higher cardiovascular disease prevalence (13.9%), and those with both metabolic syndrome and diabetes had the highest prevalence of cardiovascular disease (19.2%) compared to those with neither. Based on these data, metabolic syndrome was considered to be the factor associated with increased prevalence of cardiovascular disease (Fig. 4) (21). Another analysis from the NHANES III database of 10,357 patients revealed that the prevalence of metabolic syndrome was significantly higher in the group of patients with myocardial infarction, stroke, or myocardial infarction and stroke together, compared with subjects with no history of myocardial infarction or stroke (22). Metabolic syndrome was found to be a major predictor of cardiovascular risk in women in the Women's Ischemia Syndrome Evaluations (WISE) study, which evaluated 755 women who were referred for coronary angiography to evaluate for suspected myocardial ischemia (23). A cross-sectional study of 3770 women aged 60–79 years randomly selected from 23 British towns demonstrated that the prevalence of metabolic syndrome is high in older British women and is associated with cardiovascular disease. This study also demonstrated that association was similar when patients were stratified using WHO definition versus ATP III definition of metabolic syndrome (24). The strong association between metabolic syndrome and cardiovascular disease emphasizes the need for better understanding of the pathophysiological mechanisms responsible for this relationship. In the following

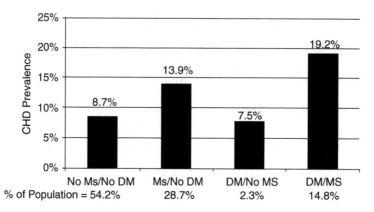

Figure 4 Age-adjusted prevalence of CHD in the U.S. population over 50 years of age categorized by presence of metabolic syndrome and diabetes. Combinations of metabolic syndrome (MS) and diabetes mellitus (DM) status are shown. *Source*: From Ref. 21.

section we will discuss the current concepts regarding the significance of each component of the metabolic syndrome.

VISCERAL OBESITY

Visceral or abdominal obesity is the form of obesity most strongly associated with metabolic syndrome and cardiovascular risk factors. It presents clinically as increased waist circumference (Table 1). However, the absolute waist circumference criteria may not be applicable for certain populations, such as South Asians and other immigrant groups. In these individuals, WHO criteria, which utilize the waist-to-hip ratio might be more suitable in identifying patients with metabolic syndrome (Table 2). Waist circumference was shown to independently predict obesity-related cardiovascular disease even in patients with normal weight (25). ATP III considered the "obesity epidemic" as mainly responsible for the rising prevalence of metabolic syndrome (26).

Increased visceral adipose tissue is considered to be a major factor responsible for many of the abnormalities associated with metabolic syndrome including insulin resistance. Adipocyte is now recognized as an important secretory organ (Fig. 5) (27). Adipocyte-secreted molecules are called "adipokines." Adiponectin is one of the adipokines, which is considered to be an important mediator of insulin sensitivity (28). Adiponectin works via activation of the adenosine monophosphate-activated protein kinase in skeletal muscle and liver, leading to phosphorylation of acetyl coenzyme A carboxylase, increased fatty acid oxidation and glucose uptake, reduced fatty acid synthesis, and reduction of molecules involved in gluconeogenesis (29–36). In the absence

Table 1 Modified Clinical Identification of Metabolic Syndrome

Risk factor	Characteristic
Waist circumference	Men > 102 cm (>40 inches)
	Women >88 cm (>35 inches)
Triglycerides	≥150 mg/dL (≥1.69 mmol/L)
HDL-cholesterol	Men <40 mg/dL (<1.03 mmol/L)
	Women <50 mg/dL (<1.29 mmol/L)
Blood pressure	≥130/≥85 mm Hg
Fasting glucose	≥100 mg/dl (≥5.55 mmol/L)

The diagnosis of metabolic syndrome is made when three or more of these risk factors are present. Information from the Executive summary of the third report of the National Cholesterol Education Program (NCEP) Expert Panel on Detection, Evaluation, and Treatment of High Blood Cholesterol in Adults (Adult Treatment Panel III).

of metabolic syndrome, these effects result in reduction in triglyceride content in the liver and skeletal muscle and suppression of hepatic glucose production and increase in high density lipoprotein levels (28,36–39).

Adiponectin may also lower C-reactive protein and other inflammatory cytokines (40). An injection of an adiponectin-producing adenovirus was shown to reverse the significantly increased adipose tissue tumor necrosis factor (TNF-α) messenger RNA and plasma TNF-α levels in adiponectin knockout mice (41). Human studies found negative correlation between adiponectin and the inflammatory markers TNF-α, interleukin 6, and C-reactive protein (42–46). Patients with coronary artery disease were found to have lower adiponectin levels compared to those without coronary artery disease (30). Another recent study found that high plasma adiponectin levels were associated with lower risk of myocardial infarction independent of hypertension, diabetes, glycohemoglobin levels, and C-reactive protein. The relationship between adiponectin level and

Table 2 The WHO Metabolic Syndrome

Risk factor	Characteristic
Central obesity	Waist-to-hip ratio (men >0.90; women >0.85)
	and/or Body mass index >30 kg/m^2
Triglycerides	>150 mg/dL (≥1.69 mmol/L)
HDL-cholesterol	Men <35 mg/dL (<0.9 mmol/L)
	Women <39 mg/dL (<1.0 mmol/L)
Blood pressure	≥140/≥90 mm Hg
Fasting glucose	≥110 mg/dl (≥6.1 mmol/L)
Microalbuminuria	Urinary albumin excretion rate ≥20 mg/min
	or
	Albumin/creatinine ratio ≥ 30 mg/g

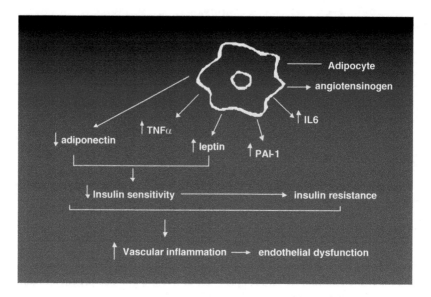

Figure 5   Adipocyte role in visceral obesity and metabolic syndrome.

myocardial infarction was only partly explained by differences in blood lipid levels (36).

Current evidence suggests that adiponectin is not only a marker of cardiovascular risk but also a significant contributor to the pathophysiological process involving atherosclerosis. Previously published animal and human data suggest that adiponectin can lower the risk of cardiovascular disease by improving insulin sensitivity and blood lipid levels (28,34,36,37–46). Adiponectin suppresses lipid accumulation and class A scavenger receptor expression in macrophages and, consequently, the transformation of macrophages to foam cells, which plays an important role in the atherogenic process (36,47,48).

It was also demonstrated that adiponectin binds to subendothelial collagens and suppresses proliferation and migration of human aortic smooth muscle cells (36,48,49).

In apolipoprotien E-deficient mice, adiponectin significantly reduced the development of atherosclerosis that usually occurs in these animals. These findings might help explain the observation in humans showing low adiponectin levels in patients with coronary artery disease (30,50–54).

Modest weight reduction of 10% can lead to significant increase in serum adiponectin levels in overweight diabetic and nondiabetic patients (30). Similar results were observed in another study evaluating obese patients undergoing gastric bypass surgery (30,35). However, the removal of subcutaneous fat by liposuction did not significantly improve obesity-related metabolic abnormalities and could not achieve the metabolic benefits of weight loss (55). This emphasizes the pivotal role of visceral adipose tissue in the pathophysiology of insulin resistance and related cytokines abnormalities.

Adiponectin is not the only cytokine released by the adipose tissue. Adipose tissue also produces other cytokines, such as resistin, interleukin-6, TNF-α, PAI-1, and angiotensin II. These cytokines seem to have opposite effects compared to adiponectin. Therefore, the overall effects of adipokines on insulin sensitivity and other cardiovascular risk factors depend on the net balance of their production by adipose tissue (Fig. 5) (54).

Based on the above discussion, it is apparent that reduction in visceral adiposity would be beneficial. It has been shown that with a 10% decrease in total body weight there can be as much as 40% loss of visceral adipose tissue. Therapeutic lifestyle changes (TLC) are a crucial part of the obesity treatment. Current evidence suggests that the longer the behavior therapy program, the better the long-term weight loss outcome compared with standard treatment. One of the recently suggested models of TLC, which could be utilized in metabolic syndrome, describes visit intervals and goals for follow up (Fig. 6) (56). Structured meal plans, which provide adequate nutrition with portion size restriction for at least two meals a day, may improve the risk factors for metabolic syndrome and assist with healthy meal choices. Sustained dietary changes will require continued physician counseling and nutritionist support to maintain the weight loss without compromising electrolyte balance and adequate vitamin intake.

A number of studies have shown the benefit of regular physical activity in patients with metabolic syndrome (57–59). A structured exercise program is necessary for successful long-term maintenance of weight loss, although the effect of exercise alone on weight loss is not as powerful as caloric restriction. Although

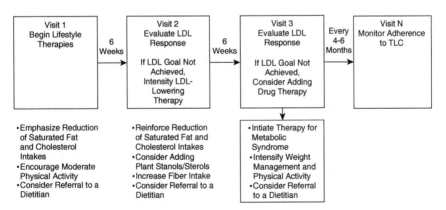

Figure 6 Steps in therapeutic lifestyle changes (TLC). *Abbreviation*: LDL, low-density lipoprotein. *Source*: From Ref. 56.

30 minutes of physical activity a day five times a week was previously considered adequate, the recent multidisciplinary expert panel, after reviewing the data and the results of epidemiologic studies, recommends for adults and children 60 minutes of daily physical activity (59). Every patient needs individual readiness evaluation by his/her primary care physician and obstacles to daily exercise should be discussed and eliminated. Patients need to be advised regarding the importance of the warm-up and cool-down periods and the incorporation of the exercise into daily life. Exercise recommendations should include setting certain goals such, as improving cardiovascular fitness, increasing strength with resistance training, and enhancing flexibility through a wide range of motion.

Medications for treatment of obesity are currently recommended for patients who have a body mass index of 27 kg/m^2 or higher with complications of obesity, or patients with a body mass index of 30 kg/m^2 without complications. The U.S. Food and Drug Administration approved two medications for long-term weight loss—sibutramine (Meredia®) and orlistat (Xenical®). Patients who were treated with sibutramine demonstrated three times more likely to achieve between 5 to 10% weight loss and also maintain their initial weight loss better 90 than placebo patients with the same diet and exercise. Orlistat is an inhibitor of pancreatic lipase, which leads to decreased fat absorption in the intestine. With this medication the weight loss of approximately 10% can be achieved. Steatorrhea is a common side effect, as well as reduction in fat-soluble vitamins (vitamins D and E), leading to the need to supplement these vitamins while on orlistat. A recently published study done in Greece confirmed in 6 months follow-up that orlistat and a hypocaloric diet had modifying effects on cardiovascular risk factors in patients with metabolic syndrome and type 2 diabetes (60).

In addition, there is now considerable interest and emerging evidence regarding the role of drugs that modify the endocannabinoid system in the treatment of obesity and metabolic syndrome. These drugs not only help in achieving sustained weight reduction, but they are also associated with favorable changes in dyslipidemia. The recent data from RIO-EUROPE and RIO-USA presented at the American Hearth Association and American College of Cardiology meetings have provided good evidence in support of the beneficial effects of rimonabant, selective CB1 endocannabinoid receptor antagonist, in the treatment of obesity. It was particularly interesting to note in these studies that there was substantially greater reduction in visceral adiposity in patients receiving rimonabant.

In morbidly obese patients who are unable to achieve appropriate weight reduction, a surgical approach can achieve the most profound and long-lasting weight loss, leading to improvement in the comorbidities related to obesity including hypertension, hyperlipidemia, and insulin resistance. Gastric bypass surgery is considered the best bariatric operation and may help to achieve permanent weight loss of more than 50% of excess body weight in the majority of patients. After bariatric surgery, patients need to be managed with the help of a nutritionist as well as physical and occupational therapists. Although frequently used for cosmetic reasons liposuction, which predominantly removes subcutaneous fat, is not associated with significant improvement in various hormonal and cytokine abnormalities that have been linked with adverse cardiovascular consequences of obesity (55).

INSULIN RESISTANCE

The primary abnormality responsible for the most features of metabolic syndrome-related cardiovascular complications is insulin resistance. Insulin resistance can be defined as inability to respond appropriately to the various actions of insulin. Insulin resistance and metabolic syndrome are not synonymous. In the insulin resistance state, cells are deprived from glucose, which is critical for metabolic activity. The fasting plasma glucose concentration is the variable with the greatest positive predictive value for insulin resistance and hyperinsulinemia, especially when between 110 and 126 mg/dL. Despite the above, fasting plasma glucose concentration cannot be used as a sensitive indicator due to the fact that the majority of insulin resistant individuals will have glucose concentrations less than 110 mg/dL (61). Due to these limitations, a recent American Diabetic Association statement defines plasma glucose concentration higher than 100 mg/dL as the new criteria for metabolic syndrome (Table 1).

The Collaborative Analysis of Diagnostic Criteria in Europe (DECODE) study, which summarized the results of 22 large, European population-based studies, revealed that increasing fasting plasma glucose and 2-hour post-challenge glucose were associated with increasing risk of cardiovascular death. In this study insulin resistance, which was indicated by increased 2-hour post-challenge glucose, was a better predictor of cardiovascular mortality in subjects without diabetes, than elevated fasting plasma glucose (62). The importance of postprandial hyperglycemia was supported by another study, which revealed a reduction in the risk of cardiovascular disease in insulin resistant patients who were taking an α-glucosidase inhibitor (acarbose), decreasing postprandial hyperglycemia (63).

A recently published study on mice exhibiting a type 2 diabetes phenotype revealed that lipid accumulation in the liver leads to subacute hepatic "inflammation" through NF-kappaB activation and downstream cytokine production. This causes insulin resistance both locally in the liver and systemically (64). Also, IKK-beta acts locally in the liver and systemically in myeloid cells, where NF-kappaB activation induces inflammatory mediators that cause insulin resistance. These findings demonstrate the importance of liver cell IKK-beta in hepatic insulin resistance and the central role of myeloid cells in development of systemic insulin resistance. It was proposed that inhibition of IKK-beta, especially in myeloid cells, may be used to treat insulin resistance (65).

Insulin has multiple other roles besides glucose metabolism. It promotes protein and amino acid metabolism and the storage and utilization of fatty acids; therefore, in cases of insulin resistance, fatty acids and amino acids are not being metabolized normally. Insulin also plays a role in vascular disorders, especially endothelial dysfunction. The abnormalities of fatty acid metabolism leads to accelerated atherosclerosis, increased risk of myocardial infarction, peripheral artery disease, and stroke (66).

The association between insulin resistance, hyperinsulinemia, and coronary disease is supported by a number of observational studies (67–69). Despite the fact that the strength of insulin resistance as a predictor of cardiovascular disease is substantially attenuated after adjustment for risk factors, which was reflected in review of studies examining both fasting and stimulated insulin concentrations, most recent trials revealed that it could be an independent risk factor for coronary artery disease and stroke (Fig. 7) (69–74).

Although exercise and weight loss ameliorate insulin resistance and may in some cases prevent or delay onset of the metabolic syndrome or diabetes, pharmacologic intervention that improves insulin resistance is often needed in those who fail to respond to TLC. Presently there is no single pharmacologic approach that is effective in improving all of the consequences of insulin resistance, which include hyperglycemia, dyslipidemia, abnormal coagulation and fibrinolysis, and hypertension. Thus, currently, treatment of individual

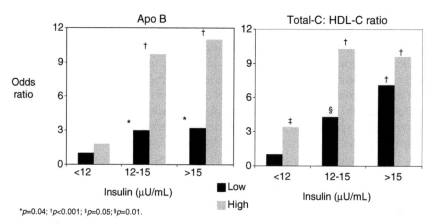

$*p=0.04; \dagger p<0.001; \ddagger p=0.05; \S p=0.01.$

Figure 7 Odds ratios for ischemic heart disease according to plasma insulin and triglyceride concentrations, total:HDL cholesterol ratios, and apolipoprotein B Concentrations. Insulin was measured after subjects had fasted for 12 hours. The median triglyceride concentration [150 mg per deciliter (1.7 mmol per liter)], total:HDL cholesterol ratio (6.0), and apolipoprotein B concentration (119 mg per deciliter) were used to define men with either low levels (below the 50th percentile) or high levels (at or above the 50th percentile) for these variables. The results of tests for multiplicative interactions did not reach significance at the 0.05 level for any of the combinations. P values are for comparisons with the reference group, which was assigned an odds ratio of 1.0. To convert values for insulin to pi-comoles per liter, multiply by 6. *Source*: From Ref. 69.

components of metabolic syndrome is the best available approach. However, the development of drugs targeted to reverse insulin resistance is important. The insulin-sensitizing agents thiazolidinediones, which are selective ligands of the nuclear transcription factor peroxisome-proliferator-activated receptor (PPAR), are the first drugs to address the basic problem of insulin resistance in patients with metabolic syndrome and type 2 diabetes (75). The two currently available PPAR agonists, rosiglitazone and pioglitizone, consistently lower fasting and postprandial glucose levels, as well as insulin and free fatty acid levels. Thiazolidinediones also improve dyslipidemias, though no studies are available to explain the precise mechanisms (71). Although nonalcoholic fatty liver disease is not a component of the metabolic syndrome diagnostic criteria, it is frequently present in obese individuals. Thiazolidinediones can improve not only laboratory markers of the liver disease but also a histological picture in these patients (76). Weight gain is an undesirable consequence of thiazolidinediones therapy, though the underlying mechanism is not clear. For example, patients with type 2 diabetes will gain 2 to 3 kg for every percent decrease in glycosylated hemoglobin values (75). The Food and Drug Administration has also included a warning in the prescription information for rosiglitazone (Avandia®) and pioglitazone (Actos®) regarding the possibility of developing anemia and edema.

The PPARα agonists, such as fenofibrate and gemfibrozil, which have cardioprotective effect due to the lipid lowering action, and the glucose-lowering effects of thiazolidinediones have led to a search for dual PPAR agonists (compounds with the combined effects of PPARα and PPAR) (75). According to the Food, Drug, and Cosmetic Act reports of new drug applications, as many as eight dual PPAR agonists are currently under clinical development, including two in phase 3 trials (75). An additional pathophysiological mechanism related to insulin resistance is artherosclerosis leading to cardiovascular disease.

DYSLIPIDEMIA

Atherogenic dyslipedemia (Table 1) is an integral component of metabolic syndrome and is a major contributor to the cardiovascular risks in these patients. Combination of various risk factors seen in metabolic syndrome can lead to a significant increase in the risks of cardiovascular disease. For example, it was demonstrated that addition of dyslipidemia to the presence of diabetes or hypertension results in an increased risk of myocardial infarction by nineteen-fold (77). It is also important to note that an abnormal lipid profile was found to be a more significant risk factor than either hypertension or diabetes alone (77).

The typical lipid abnormalities defined in patients with metabolic syndrome consist of a triad: increased triglycerides, decreased high density lipoprotein-cholesterol, and increased small, dense low density lipoprotein-cholesterol (LDL). The role of LDL in the development of cardiovascular disease is indisputable, but it is necessary to emphasize that patients with metabolic syndrome have far more complex lipid abnormalities. The atherogenic lipid abnormalities associated with metabolic syndrome are comparable to dyslipidemia found in patients with type 2 diabetes. In patients with metabolic syndrome, the suppression of free fatty acid release from adipose tissue is impaired, secondary to insulin resistance (78). This translates into increased influx of free fatty acids into the liver, the consequences of which are an increase in hepatic production and release of VLDL and triglycerides associated with decreased clearance of these substances, resulting in increase in VLDL and triglycerides levels. Transportation of cholesterol and triglyceride ester between HDL, LDL, and VLDL leads to formation of triglyceride-rich LDL and HDL particles, which become the preferred substrate for hepatic triglyceride lipase. Due to the lack of hepatic lipase, there is poor clearance of small, dense particles of LDL-cholesterol, which are more atherogenic and have higher susceptibility to oxidation. Elevated levels of triglyceride-rich lipoproteins lower HDL-cholesterol by inducing cholesterol exchange from HDL to VLDL via cholesteryl-ester transfer protein. A high proportion of small, dense LDL particles has been classified as a LDL subclass B, or atherogenic lipoprotein phenotype (79).

The atherogenic dyslipidemia of metabolic syndrome is similar to combined hyperlipidemia, and there appears to be an overlap of these two phenotypes (80). The cardiovascular outcomes associated with atherogenic form of dyslipidemia typical in metabolic syndrome patients are much worse, compared to clinical outcomes in patients with isolated elevation of LDL-cholesterol (81). Also, patients having this triad are more likely to have other features of the metabolic syndrome, which puts them at greater risk for cardiovascular events (82).

Another lipid abnormality of interest, which may contribute to an increased risk of cardiovascular disease in patients with metabolic syndrome, is postprandial hyperlipemia. After food digestion, plasma concentration of chylomicrones increases and these triglyceride-rich remnant particles struggle to be cleared by the liver with endogenous triglyceride-rich proteins, for example VLDL-triglyceride. Due to high levels of VLDL-triglyceride, clearance of chylomycrones is affected and leads to postprandial lipemia. It is known that postprandial hyperlipidemia is associated with endothelial dysfunction and this increase in triglyceride-rich remnant particles in the postprandial state in patients with metabolic syndrome could play a major role in development of atherosclerosis and subsequent development cardiovascular disease (83).

Despite complex pathophysiology of the lipid abnormalities in metabolic syndrome, it is crucial for clinicians to recognize and manage them effectively in an attempt to reduce increased risks of cardiovascular disease.

The current ATP guidelines recommend the use of 3-hydroxy-3-methylglutaryl coenzyme A reductase inhibitors (statins) in the treatment of metabolic syndrome patients, who have concomitant increase in LDL-C. The statins have been found to have multiple indirect effects on the vasculature, besides the direct cholesterol lowering effect. These positive actions are commonly referred to as pleotropic effects, which include effects on inflammation, coagulability, and adhesion of cells to the vascular endothelium and effects on nitric oxide metabolism. Statins also can improve endothelial function, reduce vascular inflammation, reduce oxidative stress, decrease thrombosis and platelet aggregation and adhesion of platelets and white cells to the vascular endothelium, stabilize vulnerable plaques, and promote new vessel formation (84). These properties of statins might prove to be clinically useful in reducing the risk of cardiovascular events in patients with metabolic syndrome and diabetes.

Because of the significant increased risk of cardiovasclular event in patients with diabetes and metabolic syndrome, it is important to set aggressive LDL-C goals with an effort to reduce the risk of cardiovascular events. Recent trial data suggest that coronary plaque progression is delayed and the incidence of coronary events is reduced when LDL-C levels are lowered to approximately 70 mg/dl in high-risk patients (85).

The selection of the statin should be primarily based on its effect in reducing the LDL-C. It is important to note that the currently available statins have different effects not only on LDL-C, but also on triglycerides and HDL-C (Table 3) (86,87).

Gastrointestinal upset, muscle aches, and hepatitis are among the most common adverse effects of statins. Hepatotoxicity is very rare in patients taking high doses (approximately 1%) and myotoxicity is even more uncommon (86). Some patients can develop insomnia, bad or vivid dreams, and difficulty sleeping or concentrating. For these patients statin with low penetration in central nervous system should be used for example pravastatin (86).

Combination therapy may often be necessary to combat all lipid abnormalities in metabolic syndrome (88). In the past, lipid-lowering therapy was preferred; bile acid-binding resins are now largely used as adjuncts to statin therapy, especially in patients for whom additional reduction in LDL-C by 10–20% is desired and level of triglycerides is not elevated. Currently available bile acid resins include cholestyramine, colesevelam, and colestipol. These medications are usually given in doses of 4–10 grams twice a day with meals as a suspension in juice or water. The increase in triglyceride concentrations induced by bile acid resins can be a problem, especially in patients prone to hypertrigly-ceridemia. Due to their mechanism of action based on binding to bile acids in the small intestine and leading to interruption of the enterohepatic circulation of bile acids and increasing the conversion of cholesterol to bile in the liver, these agents can inhibit the intestinal absorption of fat soluble vitamins, including vitamin D, warfarin, digoxin, levothyroxin, thiazide diuretics, folic acid, and statins as well. Also, up to 30% of patients will develop abdominal fullness, gas, and constipation while taking bile acid resins, which could be corrected with dose adjustment and the use of fiber or prune juice in daily diet (89).

Based on the current evidence, the European Consensus Panel recommends that the minimum target for HDL-C should be 40 mg/dL in patients with metabolic syndrome (84).

Nicotinic acid inhibits the mobilization of free fatty acids from peripheral tissue, thereby reducing hepatic synthesis of trigylycerides and secretion of VLDL-C and its conversion to LDL-C. Nicotinic acid has a unique ability to

Table 3 Mean ± SD Percent Changes in Lipids, Apolipoproteins, and Total Cholesterol/HDL Cholesterol and Apolipoprotein Ratios in Patients with and without the Metabolic Syndrome (MS) Pooled Across Doses for Each Drug

	Rosuvastatin 10, 20, 40 mg		Atorvastatin 10, 20, 40, 80 mg		Simvastatin 10, 20, 40, 80 mg		Pravastatin 10, 20, 40 mg	
	MS (n = 165)	No MS (n = 308)	MS (n = 220)	No MS (n = 414)	MS (n = 227)	No MS (n = 421)	MS (n = 186)	No MS (n = 299)
LDL cholesterol	−51 ± 15	−51 ± 13	−44 ± 13	−45 ± 14	−38 ± 13	−36 ± 15	−24 ± 12	−25 ± 12
Triglycerides	−27 ± 19	−21 ± 25	−28 ± 19	−22 ± 26	−21 ± 21	−13 ± 26	−14 ± 22	−7 ± 26
HDL cholesterol	+10 ± 12	+9 ± 11	+7 ± 12	+3 ± 11	+9 ± 10	+4 ± 10	+6 ± 11	+4 ± 10
Non-HDL cholesterol	−47 ± 13	−47 ± 13	−42 ± 12	−42 ± 14	−35 ± 12	−33 ± 14	−22 ± 10	−23 ± 12
Total cholesterol/HDL cholesterol ratio	−43 ± 12	−41 ± 11	−38 ± 11	−35 ± 12	−34 ± 11	−29 ± 12	−22 ± 11	−20 ± 11
Apolipoprotein B	−41 ± 13	−41 ± 13	−37 ± 13	−37 ± 13	−30 ± 13	−28 ± 14	−19 ± 11	−19 ± 13
Apolipoprotein A-I	+8 ± 13	+8 ± 13	+3 ± 13	+4 ± 12	+8 ± 13	+6 ± 11	+6 ± 12	+5 ± 11
Apolipoprotein ratio	−45 ± 13	−45 ± 14	−39 ± 13	−39 ± 14	−34 ± 14	−32 ± 14	−22 ± 13	−23 ± 13

Source: From Ref. 87.

decrease the triglycerides level by up to 30%. The majority of effects of nicotinic acid on triglycerides and HDL-C occur in the low doses. The administration of aspirin (325 mg 30 to 60 minutes before each dose of nicotinic acid for a few days), and taking nicotinic acid at the end of a meal and not taking it with hot liquids can minimize the flushing of the skin, which 10% of patients find intolerable (82). Starting dose is 250 to 500 mg and should be increased monthly by 500 to 1000 mg to a maximum of 3000 mg a day. Hepatitis is more frequent in patients on nicotinic acid than in those who are taking statins, especially in doses of 2000 to 3000 mg. Other side effects include conjunctivitis, nasal stuffiness, loose bowel movements or diarrhea, acanthosis nigricans, and ichthyosis (86).

The agonistic mechanism of actions of the fibric acid derivates (gemfibrozil, clofibrate, fenofibrate) on PPARα was described above in approaches to insulin resistance. The firbrates are considered the most effective triglyceride-lowering drugs, producing as much as 50% reduction. Clofibrate and fenofibrate cause fewer gastrointestinal symptoms than gemfibrozil. Clofibrate can cause erectile dysfunction. Currently fenofibrate is the preferred agent. All fibrates are renally excreted and can accumulate in the serum in patients with renal failure and lead to myositis. Ezetimibe is the first of a new class of lipid-lowering drugs known as intestinal cholesterol absorption inhibitors. It could be administered in once daily doses of 10 mg. The co-administration of ezetimibe with statins offers a well-tolerated and efficacious treatment of lower LDL-C in patients with metabolic syndrome and diabetes (89). The combination of statin and ezetimibe and statin may result in a small increase in the incidence of elevated liver enzyme levels, although cases of severe hepatotoxicity have not been demonstrated (90).

HYPERTENSION

An integral component of metabolic syndrome is a blood pressure of greater than 130/85 mm Hg (Table 1). The relationship between hypertension and metabolic syndrome is emphasized by the fact that even lean hypertensive patients can manifest insulin resistance. Patients with hypertension are several-fold more likely to develop diabetes and cardiovascular disease over a 3- to 5-year period than are normotensive persons (53,86–89). It is also evident that insulin resistance and hyperinsulinemia contribute to the increase propensity for development of hypertension (91–93). It has been postulated that the direct effect of elevated insulin on sympathetic nervous system activity can lead to elevated blood pressure (54).

Impaired insulin signaling through its phosphoinositol 3-kinase and downstream protein kinase B pathways is increasingly recognized as being important for generation of nirtric oxide and other vasodilatory factors with increased insulin-induced renal sodium retention, which contributes to hypertension (53). The generation of nitric oxide is important for insulin mediated glucose utilization and vasodilatation (94–99).

Activation of the tissue renin-angiotensin system seems also to contribute to impaired insulin use in skeletal muscle and adipose tissue and decreases vasorelaxation (54). Angiotensin II can also be produced by adipose tissue and has potent vasoconstictive potential. In the vasculature, angiotensin II results in increased production of reactive oxygen species by stimulation of the NAD(P)H oxidase enzyme, which is expressed in endothelial cells, vascular smooth muscle cells, and vascular adventitial cells (54,99–102). Increased production of reactive oxygen species in turn results in increased nitric oxide turnover by its conversion to peroxynitrite, which also blocks vasodilation (54,103). In hypertensive patients, increased local formation of anigotensin II in adipose tissue was noted and appears to be of considerable interest, given the close relationship between angiotensin II and insulin resistance (104).

There is evidence confirming that insulin resistance and resulting hyperinsulinemia relate with hypertension and coronary artery disease. Untreated hypertensive patients often have higher fasting and postprandial insulin levels than normotensive persons regardless of body mass, as well as direct correlation between plasma insulin concentrations and blood pressure levels (54,86,87).

Genetic predisposition most likely contributes to coexistence of insulin resistance and hyperinsulinemia with hypertension. Changes in glucose metabolism in normotensive offspring of hypertensive parents could support the concept of genetic predisposition for this coexistence (105,106). The fact of increased plasma insulin levels predicting elevated blood pressures in healthy children also supports this concept (107).

Based on the recommendations of the Seventh Report of the Joint National Committee on Prevention, Detection, Evaluation, and Treatment of High Blood Pressure, the goal for blood pressure in patients with diabetes and other high risk individuals (such as those with metabolic syndrome) should be below 120 mm Hg systolic and 80 mm Hg diastolic. Lifestyle modifications described above and dietary changes would be initial steps to control blood pressure. There is some evidence that a low sodium diet helps to maintain lower blood pressure following withdrawal of antihypertensive medications (108). It was also demonstrated that patients who consumed a diet low in saturated fat and high in carbohydrates experienced a significant reduction in blood pressure, even without weight reduction. This diet called DASH (The Dietary Approaches to Stop Hypertension) emphasizes fruits, vegetables, low-fat dairy foods, whole grains, poultry, fish, and nuts, while reducing saturated fats, red meat, sweets, and sugar-containing beverages (109).

In hypertensive patients, increased local formation of anigotensin II in adipose tissue was noted and appears to be of considerable interest, given the close relationship between angiotensin II and insulin resistance (110). Activation of the tissue renin-angiotensin system seems also to contribute to impaired insulin action in skeletal muscle cells and adipose tissue as well as endothelial dysfunction (54).

There is emerging evidence, that insulin resistance and resulting hyperinsulinemia relate to hypertension and coronary artery disease. Untreated hypertensive patients often have higher fasting and postprandial insulin levels than normotensive persons regardless of body mass; as well, a direct correlation exists between plasma insulin concentrations and blood pressure levels (54).

The beneficial effects of renin-angiotensin system blockade by angiotensin enzyme inhibitor or angiontensin receptor blocker on insulin sensitivity and the development of type 2 diabetes in several clinical trials further support a pathopysiological role of the renin-angiotensin system in metabolic syndrome and its cardiovascular complications (Fig. 5) (51,111–113). In addition, treatment with angiotensin-converting enzyme inhibitor with ramipril over 4.5 years was associated with a 25% reduction in the primary outcome of myocardial infarction, stroke, or a cardiovascular death among 3577 diabetic patients (114). It was also demonstrated that angiotensin receptor blockers have benefit in patients with diabetes, reducing morbidity and mortality (115,116).

β-Blocker therapy in patients with metabolic syndrome can also lead to reduction in cardiovascular mortality. Despite the fact that historically β-blockers were withheld from diabetic patients due to the possibility of masking hypoglycemia and increasing insulin resistance, the cardioselective β-blockers should be considered as preferred agents for treatment of hypertension in patients with ischemic heart disease who have metabolic syndrome.

The importance of blood pressure control in reduction of cardiovascular mortality and morbidity, irrespective of the class of drugs used, has been confirmed in a number of large prospective randomized clinical trials (117). Therefore it is of paramount importance that the hypertensive component of metabolic syndrome should be aggressively treated because of the increased risk of cardiovascular events.

FIBRINOLYTIC DYSFUNCTION, ENDOTHELIAL DYSFUNCTION, C-REACTIVE PROTEIN

Patients with metabolic syndrome also have multiple abnormalities, which lead to increased risk of thrombosis. Some of these abnormalities are considered to be driven by adipokines (118–120). Various associated coagulation abnormalities include increased platelet aggregation and activation and elevation of procoagulants, such as fibrinogen and von Willebrand's factor. Defects of fibrinolysis include increased production and activity of plasminogen activator inhibitor-1 (PAI-1) with low levels of tissue plasminogen activator (t-PA) (54,93). PAI-1 has been found to be elevated in patients with type 2 diabetes. The increase in PAI-1 is related to complex interaction between glucose, insulin, and angiotesnisin II and endothelial cell. Increased levels of PAI-1 have been also associated with visceral obesity and hyperinsulinemia (121). Studies of the promoter region of the PAI-1 gene have shown that hyperglycemia stimulates

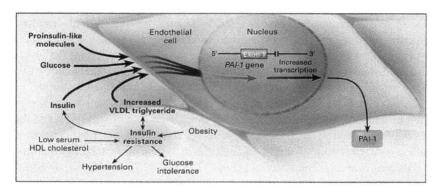

Figure 8 Relation between the synthesis of plasminogen-activator inhibitor type 1 (PAI-1) and the insulin resistance syndrome. The main feature of the insulin resistance syndrome is insulin resistance accompanied by hyperinsulinemia, abnormalities of glucose metabolism, hypertriglyceridemia with low serum high-density lipoprotein (HDL) cholesterol concentrations, hypertension, and obesity. Insulin, proinsulin-like molecules, glucose, and very-low-density lipoprotein (VLDL) triglyceride directly stimulate PAI-1 transcription and secretion in endothelial cells. *Source*: From Ref. 126.

transcription of the gene and reduction of blood glucose usually results in lower PAI-1 levels (Fig. 8) (122).

Increased levels of PAI-1 correlate with increased risk of myocardial infarction (123,124). Firbrinolytic dysfunction increases the propensity to develop arterial thrombosis, which leads to increased incidence in cardiovascular events in patients with metabolic syndrome (125). Plasma concentrations of PAI-1 are highest at night and early morning hours and it has been proposed that the higher incidence of myocardial infarction in the early morning hours could be due to higher plasma PAI-1 concentrations, leading to lower fibrinolytic activity and thrombosis at night (126).

Diabetes and abdominal obesity are risk predictors of both venous thrombosis and an occlusive arterial disease most likely due to existence of an atherothrombotic syndrome secondary to insulin resistance and defective fibrinolysis. Patients with metabolic syndrome were found to have significantly more atherosclerosis compared with patients without metabolic syndrome, independent of their diabetes status (123). These data suggest that the higher risk of cardiovascular events among patients with metabolic syndrome could be related to impaired fibrinolysis and more advanced artherosclerosis (123).

Current evidence also emphasizes that endothelial function is compromised in patients with metabolic syndrome. Endothelial dysfunction has been documented to occur in association with all of the factors that predispose to the development of atherosclerosis and is the initial step in the development of vascular pathology. For clinical evaluation, endothelial cell function can be estimated by measuring changes in blood flow in response to physical or pharmacologic stimuli using invasive or non-invasive techniques. It has been demonstrated that increase of blood flow in the legs in response to metacholine, which is a stimulator of nitric oxide release, is impaired in nondiabetic insulin-resistant individuals (125).

In patients with insulin resistance, nitric oxide synthesis, which is partially mediated by insulin, is blunted and nitric oxide mediated vasodilation is adversely affected (104). Nitric oxide also inhibits platelet aggregation, leukocytes migration and cellular adhesion to the endothelium, and attenuates vascular smooth muscle cell proliferation and migration. Additional effects of nitric oxide include inhibition of release of cell adhesion molecules and reduced production of superoxide anions. Flow mediated dilatation of the brachial artery, which is nitric oxide dependent, was found to be impaired in metabolic syndrome patients with elevated and normal blood pressure (126,127). It was also found that plasma adhesion molecules are increased in proportion to the degree of insulin resistance in healthy volunteers, which could be related to the decreased nitric oxide production associated with insulin resistance (128).

The degree of endothelial dysfunction was found to be greater in patients with type 2 diabetes compared to type 1 diabetes, suggesting, that besides hyperglycemia, and hyperinsulinemia, the associated dyslipidemia might play an important role (129).

Hyperglycemia was shown to be responsible for endothelial dysfunction in metabolic syndrome. Acute or chronic hyperglycemia can produce impairment of endothelial-dependent vasodilatation (130).

Hyperglycemia-induced activation of protein kinase C (PKC) via increases in the synthesis of diacylglycerol (DAG), followed by activation of phospholipase A2, results in increased production of arachidonic acid metabolites, which have potent oxidizing effects. Reduced nitric oxide synthesis can result from activation of the polyol pathway, which increases the utilization of nicotinamidadenine dinucleotide phosphate (NADPH), an important cofactor in the biosynthesis of nitric oxide (131). Depletion of NADPH, which is essential for the regeneration of antioxidant molecules (such as glutathione, tocopherol, and ascorbate) and cofactor of endothelial nitric oxide synthase (eNOS), leads to depletion of nitric oxide.

Hyperglycemia is also associated with a variety of other molecular changes, including production of advanced glycation end products (AGE), which can increase susceptibility of LDL-cholesterol to oxidation as well as activate the receptors responsible for the release of interleukin-1, tumor-necrosis factor-α and growth factors that can stimulate the migration and proliferation of smooth muscle cells (132).

Endothelial dysfunction plays a role in the development of coronary heart disease and is associated with vascular inflammation and thrombosis, especially in situations with elevated PAI-1 and tPA, which is typical for patients with metabolic syndrome.

The role of inflammation in the process of atherosclerosis is well now established.

C-Reactive protein is an acute-phase reactant, which is clinically used as a marker of inflammation in the body. Mild chronic elevations of CRP concentrations, even when within normal limits, are independently predictive of future cardiovascular events (133,134).

CRP also correlates with every parameter of the metabolic syndrome, including adiposity, hyperinsulinemia, insulin resistance, hypertriglyceridemia, and low HDL cholesterol (119,121).

It was demonstrated that high levels of CRP are related to increased accumulation of visceral and subcutaneous fat deposits measured by computed tomography scan (135).

In postmenopausal women and elderly patients, CRP can be used as a predictor of development of diabetes and accordingly as a predictor of premature coronary artery disease (118,135–138).

It also has been proposed that metabolic syndrome and diabetes mellitus are inflammatory conditions. For example, the risk of developing diabetes and metabolic syndrome in relation to baseline CRP levels in 515 men and 729 women from the Mexico City Diabetes Study revealed that CRP was not a significant predictor of the development of the metabolic syndrome in men, but inflammation was important in pathogenesis of diabetes and metabolic disorders in women, which explains the correlation between CRP and cardiovascular disease (139). West of Scotland Coronary Prevention Study based on the evaluation of 6447 participants concluded that high concentrations of CRP among men with metabolic syndrome can be an independent predictor of both coronary heart disease and diabetes (140). CRP was found to add prognostic information on cardiovascular events when 14,719 initially healthy American women were followed for 8 years in the Women's Health Study (120).

These observations again confirm the role of inflammation in the processes critical to the development of atherothrombosis leading to cardiovascular events.

Furthermore, recent data from the Atherosclerosis Risk in Communities Study (ARIC) also showed that the levels of CRP increase with increasing number of the component risk factors for metabolic syndrome, suggesting that the vascular inflammation in patients with metabolic syndrome is a complex process affected by the number of established risk factors (139).

Based on the current understanding of pathophysiological mechanisms of metabolic syndrome, management of obesity, insulin resistance, and dyslipidemia as described above is crucial in modifying additional cardiovascular risk factors. Although evidence of the benefit of aspirin therapy in primary prevention is not as strong compared to secondary preventions and only limited data is available on protective benefits in individuals with insulin resistance syndrome without diabetes or previously established coronary disease, treatment with aspirin should be strongly considered in patients diagnosed with metabolic syndrome. American Heart Association recommends use of aspirin as prophylaxis in most patients with metabolic syndrome whose 10-year risk for coronary heart disease is $\geq 10\%$ as determined by the global Framingham risk score (140). The decision to recommend aspirin prophylaxis should rely on individual clinical judgment, taking into account the patient's cardiovascular risk profile, the demonstrated benefits of aspirin on reducing risk of first myocardial infraction, and the side effects that can occur. Clopidogrel is an effective alternative in the approximately 5% of the patients who cannot tolerate aspirin. In addition to antipaltelet activity, aspirin may have other beneficial effects in patients with metabolic syndrome. C-reactive protein can be an independent predictor of both coronary heart disease and diabetes and add prognostic information on cardiovascular events in metabolic syndrome patients (141). It was demonstrated that proinflammatory cytokines and C-reactive protein were significantly reduced after only 6 weeks of aspirin therapy (142).

MICROALBUMINURIA

Vasculature and renal glomerulus have a lot in common structurally and functionally. They are derived from the same progenitor cell line. Vascular smooth muscle cells and mesangial cells produce growth factors (angiotensin II, insulin-like growth facor-1, and cytokines), as well as prostaglandins and nitric oxide to counterbalance many of the effects of growth factors. Microalbuminuria occurs due to pathophysiological changes of glomerulosclerosis, which are very similar to those of atherosclerosis, and include mesangial cell proliferation and hypertrophy, foam cell accumulation, build-up of extracellular matrix, and amorphous materials and evolving sclerosis. All of these would lead to matrix expansion, basement membrane abnormalities, and loss of basement membrane permoselectivity resulting in proteinuria. As a parallel process glomerulosclerosis and atherosclerosis associated with enhanced oxidative stress increase inflammation, impair fibrinolysis and endothelial cell dysfunction, and elevate systolic blood pressure and cause lipid abnormalities (54).

The association between microalbuminuria and cardiovascular risk has been extensively studied in diabetics and non-diabetic hypertensive patients. For example, the large study of 11,343 non-diabetic hypertensive patients with mean age 57 years old from a general population sample in Germany, revealed that 51% were men and mean duration of hypertension was 69 months. Twenty-five percent had coronary artery disease, 17% had left ventricular hypertrophy, 5% had had a stroke, and 6% had peripheral vascular disease. Microalbuminuria was present in 32% of men and 28% of women. When patients, with microalbuminuria were compared with normoalbuminuric patients, the increase in coronary artery disease, left ventricular hypertrophy, stroke, and peripheral vascular disease was demonstrated (143). Further, in patients with coronary artery disease, left ventricular hypertrophy, stroke, and peripheral vascular disease, microalbuminuria was significantly greater than in patients who did not have these complications. It was also shown in this study that microalbuminuria increased with age, severity, and duration of hypertension and hyperlipidemia, and it was associated with higher plasma creatinine values (143).

It is well known that microalbuminuria frequently occurs in patients with diabetes and is a marker of early stage nephropathy. It has been shown to be a strong predictor of cardiovascular events. A systematic review of the literature was done to evaluate the role of this phenomenon and included 264 citations, in which 11 cohort studies were selected for inclusion in the overview, and a total of 2138 non-insulin dependent diabetic patients with mean of 6.4 years of follow-up. This study confirmed that microalbuminuria is a strong predictor of total and cardiovascular mortality and cardiovascular morbidity in patients with non-insulin dependent diabetes mellitus, with the overall odds ratio for all cause mortality being 2.4, and for cardiovascular morbidity or mortality being 2.0 (Fig. 9) (144).

WHO definition of metabolic syndrome has included microalbuminuria as one of the criteria (Table 2). Microalbuminuria in association with obesity can also occur due to the fact that high intake of food rich in protein, may lead to renal hyperfiltration, renal impairment, and finally to microalbuminuria, which also correlates with body mass index, waist-to-hip ratio, and insulin levels, and becomes another cardiovascular risk factor in metabolic syndrome patients (144).

Accelerated atherosclerosis and endothelial dysfunction can be recognized earlier if proteinuria is used as a marker. It was noticed that patients with proteinuria have greater left ventricular mass, greater carotid medial thickening, and endothelial dysfunction, which leads to greater risk of myocardial infarction and mortality (Fig. 9) (145,146).

ABNORMAL URIC ACID METABOLISM

Raised uric acid can be seen in patients who have metabolic syndrome. The major component of metabolic syndrome is insulin resistance, which influences protein metabolism and uric acid as protein metabolism becomes elevated. In patients

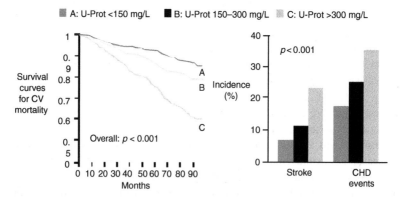

Figure 9 Proteinuria predicts stroke and coronary heart disease in type 2 diabetes patients. *Abbreviation*: U-Prot, urinary protein concentration. *Source*: Ref. 148.

with metabolic syndrome the excretion of uric acid via kidneys is also impaired. The precise role of hyperuricemia in coronary artery disease is controversial. The Framingham Heart Study demonstrated that uric acid does not have a causal role in the development of coronary artery disease or death from cardiovascular disease (147). Contrary to the Framingham data, a cross-sectional population-based study in the First National Health and Nutrition Examination Survey (NHANES I) from 1971–1975 (baseline) and the data from NHANES I Epidemiologic Follow-up Study (NHEFS) suggest that increased serum uric acid levels are independently and significantly associated with risk of cardiovascular mortality (148). In patients with essential hypertension, elevated uric acid levels were associated with increased cardiovascular disease and all causes of mortality (149). Despite the fact that no clear data exist reflecting the relationship between uric acid levels and cardiovascular risks in patients with metabolic syndrome, elevated serum uric acid levels could have a role in increasing these risks.

SUMMARY

The metabolic syndrome represents a clustering of several risk factors linked with marked increase in cardiovascular disease and can be considered a coronary artery disease equivalent. Insulin resistance has been linked to each of the ATP III criteria needed for diagnosis of metabolic syndrome (Table 1). Despite the fact that insulin resistance makes up only one of five criteria for diagnosis of metabolic sydnrome used by WHO (Table 2), the available data indicate that insulin resistance and hyperinsulinemia, even in the absence of overt abnormalities of glucose tolerance, lead to increased cardiovascular disease. Insulin resistance is considered to be a continuous process in which progressive defects in insulin action and insulin release lead to more overt abnormalities of glucose homeostasis. Insulin resistance is an independent risk factor for cardiovascular disease and its presence has been related to macrovascular complications that can occur long before the development of clinical diabetes ("the ticking clock hypothesis") (150).

Obesity is an important component of metabolic syndrome. Visceral adipose tissue has been proposed as the major site of fat deposition associated with the metabolic consequences of obesity that have been related to the cytokine release by the adipocytes (151). Currently, visceral or central adiposity is considered to be the initial physical finding associated with insulin resistance and metabolic syndrome. Increases in visceral adipose tissue lead to increases in free fatty acid flux in portal and systemic circulations, which initiates the cascade of events that are thought to be responsible for insulin resistance and atherogenic dyslipidemia. Visceral adipose tissue may also contribute to other causes of increased atherosclerotic risk, including inflammatory (C-reactive protein), prothrombotic, and fibrinolytic factors. Future assessment of adipose tissue hormonal activity might be helpful in predicting cardiovascular risks. Adiponectin is one of the hormones that is being intensively investigated in this area. Hypertension is also most likely related to adipocytes production of cytokines, including angiotensin II leading to elevated blood pressure.

Atherogenic dyslipedemia is the central player in developing athero-sclerosis, and specific features of lipid disorder in metabolic syndrome put these patients at higher risks. The characteristic lipid disorders seen in this syndrome are hypertriglyceridemia, low levels of high-density lipoprotein cholesterol (HDL-C) and, often, normal levels of low-density lipoprotein cholesterol (LDL-C), which is smaller and more dense than usual.

The evidence described in this chapter from epidemiological and observational studies highlights not only the importance of increasing awareness among clinicians regarding the strong relationship between metabolic syndrome and cardiovascular disease, but also the urgency to intervene and modify the fatal cascade of events in these patients leading to significant increase in mortality and morbidity, which will have a major public health impact worldwide in the coming years (152–154).

REFERENCES

1. Reaven GM. Banting Lecture1988: role of insulin resistance in human disease. Diabetes 1988; 37:1595–1607.
2. Park Y, Shankuan Z, Palaniappan L, et al. The metabolic syndrome. Arch Intern Med 2003; 163:427–436.
3. Fagan TC, Deedwania PC. The cardiovascular dysmetabolic syndrome. Am J Med 1998; 105:S77–S82.
4. Caprio S. Insulin resistance in childhood obesity. J Pediat Endocrinol Metab 2002; 15:487–492.
5. Goran MI, Gower BA. Abdominal obesity and cardiovascular risk in children. Coron Artery Dis 1998; 9:427–436.
6. Weiss R, Dziura J, Burgert T, et al. Obesity and metabolic syndrome in children adolescents. N Engl J Med 2004; 350:2362–2374.
7. Sinha R, Fisch G, Teague B, et al. Prevalence of impaired glucose tolerance among children and adolescents with marked obesity. N Engl J Med 2002; 346:802–810.
8. Strauss RS, Pollack HA. Epidemic increase in childhood overweight, 1986–1998. JAMA 2001; 286:2845–2848.
9. Ford ES, Giles WH, Dietz WH. Prevalence of metabolic syndrome among U.S. Adults: findings from the third National Health and Nutrition Examination Survey. JAMA 2002; 287:356–359.
10. Kraja AT, Hunt SC, Pankow JS, et al. An evaluation of the metabolic syndrome in HyperGen Study. Nutr Metab 2005; 2:1–9.
11. Isomaa B, Almgren P, Tuomi T, et al. Cardiovascular morbidity and mortality associated with the metabolic syndrome. Diabet Care 2001; 24:683–689.
12. Fontaine KR, Redden DT, Wang C, et al. Years of life lost due to obesity. JAMA 2003; 289:187–193.
13. Cook S, Witzman M, Auinger P, et al. Prevalence of a metabolic syndrome phenotype in adolescents. Arch Pediat Adolesc Med 2003; 157:821–827.

14. Malina R, Katzarzyk T. Validity of the body mass index as an indicator of the risk and presence of overweight in adolescents. Am J Clin Nutr 1999; 70:131S–136S.

15. Lakka HM, Laaksonen DE, Lakka TA, et al. The metabolic syndrome and total and cardiovasdculalr disease mortality in middle-aged men. JAMA 2002; 25:2709–2716.

16. National diabetes Data Group Diabetes in America., 2nd ed. Washington, DC: National Institues of Health, 1995.

17. Trevisan M, Liu J, Bahsas FB, et al. Syndrome X and mortality: a population-based study: risk factor and life expectancy research group. Am J Epidemiol 1998; 148:958–966.

18. Wilson PW, Kannel WB, Silberschatz H, et al. Clustering of metabolic factors and coronary heart disease. Arch Intern Med 1999; 159:1104–1109.

19. Hu G, Qiao Q, Tuomilehto J, et al. Prevalence of the metabolic syndrome and it's relation to all-cause and cardiovascular morality in nondiabetic European men and women. Arch Intern Med 2004; 164:1066–1076.

20. Resnick HE, Jones K, Ruotolo G, et al. Insulin resistance, the metabolic syndrome, and risk of incident cardiovascular disease in nondiabetic American Indians. The Strong Heart Study. Diabetes Care 2003; 26:861–867.

21. Alexander CM, Landsman PB, Teutsch S, et al. NCEP-defind metabolic syndrome, diabetes, and prevalence of coronary heart disease among NHANES III participants age 50 or older. Diabetes 2003; 52:1210–1214.

22. Ninomiya JK, L'Itaien G, Criqui MH, et al. Association of the metabolic syndrome with history of myocardial infarction and stroke in the Third National Health and Nutrition Examination Survey. Circulation 2004; 109:42–46.

23. Kip KE, Marroquin OC, Kelley DE, et al. Clinical importance of obesity versus metabolic syndrome in cardiovascular risk in women. A report from the Women's Ischemia Syndrome Study Evaluation (WISE) study. Ciruclation 2004; 109:706–713.

24. Lawlor DA, Ebrahim S, Smith DG. The metabolic syndrome and coronary heart disease in older women: findings from the British Women's Heart and Health Study. Diabet Med 2004; 21:906–913.

25. Janssen I, Katzmarzyk PT, Ross R. Body mass index, waist circumference and health risk. Arch Intern Med 2002; 162:2074–2079.

26. Grundy SM, Brewer HB, Cleeman JI, et al. Definition of metabolic syndrome. Criculation 2004; 109:433–438.

27. Frayn KN. Adipose tissue and the insulin resistance syndrome. Proc Nutr Soc 2001; 60:375–380.

28. Yamauchi T, Kamon J, Waki H, et al. The fat-derived hormone adiponectin reverses insulin resistance associated with both lipoatrophy and obesity. Nat Med 2001; 7:941–946.

29. Combs TP, Berg AH, Obici T, et al. Endogenous glucose production is inhibited by the adipose-derived protein Acrp30. J Clin Invest 2002; 108:1875–1881.

30. Hotta K, Funahashi T, Arita Y, et al. Plasma concentrations of novel, adiopose-specific protein, adiponectin, in type 2 diabetic patients. Arterioscler Thromb Vasc Biol 2000; 20:1595–1599.

31. Weyer C, Funahashi T, Tanaka S, et al. Hypoadiponectinemia in obesity and type 2 diabetes: close association with insulin resistance and hyperinsulinemia. J Clin Endocrionol Metab 2001; 86:1930–1935.

32. Yamauchi T, Kamon J, Minakoshi Y, et al. Adiponectin stimulates glucose utilization and fatty acid oxidation by activating AMP activated protein kinase. Nat Med 2002; 8:1288–1295.

33. Stephan N, Vozarons B, Funahashi T, et al. Plasma adiponectin is associated with skeletal muscle insulin receptor tyrosin phosphorylation, and low plasma concentrations precedes a decrease in whole body insulin sensitivity in humans. Diabetes 2002; 51:564–569.

34. Lindsay RS, Funahashi T, Hanson RL, et al. Adiponectin and development of type 2 diabetes in the pima Indian population. Lancet 2002; 360:57–58.

35. Yang W-S, Lee W-J, Funahashi T, et al. Weight reduction increases plasma levels of adipose-derived antiinflammatory protein, adiponectin. J Clin Endocrinol Metab 2001; 86:2815–2819.

36. Pischon T, Girman CJ, Hotamisligil GS, et al. Plasma adiponectin levels and risk of myocardial infarction in men. JAMA 2004; 291:1730–1737.

37. Berg AH, Combs TP, Du X, et al. The adipocyte-secreted protein Acrp30 enhances hepatic insulin action. Nat Med 2001; 7:947–953.

38. Fruebis J, Tsao TS, Javorschi S, et al. Proteolytic cleavage product of 30-kDa adipocyte complement-related protein increases fatty acid oxidation in muscle and causes weight loss in mice. Proc Natl Acad Sci USA 2001; 98:2005–2010.

39. Combs TP, Berg AH, Obici S, et al. Endogenous glucose production is inhibited by the adipose-derived protein Acrp30. J Clin Invest 2001; 108:1875–1881.

40. Spranger J, Kroke A, Mohlig M, et al. Adiponectin and protection against type 2 diabetes mellitus. Lancet 2003; 361:226–228.

41. Maeda N, Shimomura I, Kishida K, et al. Diet-induced insulin resistance in mice lacking adiponectin/ACRP30. Nat Med 2002; 8:731–737.

42. Engeli S, Feldpausch M, Gorzelniak K, et al. Association between adiponectin and mediators of inflammation in obese women. Diabetes 2003; 52:942–947.

43. Ouchi N, Kihara S, Funahashi T, et al. Reciprocal association of C-reactive protein with adiponectin in blood stream and adipose tissue. Circulation 2003; 107:671–674.

44. Krakoff J, Funahashi T, Stehouwer CD, et al. Infammatory markers, adiponcetin, and risk of type 2 diabetes in Pima Indian. Diabet Care 2003; 26:1745–1751.

45. Matsubara M, Namioka K, Katayose S. Decreased plams adiponectin concentrations in women with low-grade C-reactive protein elevation. Eur J Endocrinol 2003; 148:657–662.

46. Kern PA, Di Gregorio GB, Lu T, et al. Adiponcetin expression from human adipose tissue: relation to obesity, insulin resisitanc, and tumor necrosis factor-alpha expression. Diabetes 2003; 52:1779–1785.

47. Ouchi N, Hihara S, Arita Y, et al. Adipocyte derived plasma protein, adiponcectin, suppresses lipid accumulation and class a scavenger receptor expression in human monocyte-derived macrophages. Circulation 2002; 103:1057–1063.

48. Arita Y, Kihara S, Ouchi N, et al. Adipocyte-derived plasma protein adiponcetin acts as platelet-derived growth factor—BB-binding protein and regulates growth factor—induced common postereceptor signal in vascular smooth muscle cell. Circulation 2002; 105:2893–2898.

49. Okamoto Y, Arita Y, Nishida M, et al. An adipocyte-derived plasma protein, adiponcectin, adheres to injured vascular walls. Horm Metab Res 2000; 32:47–50.

50. Kumada M, Kihara S, Sumitsuji S, et al. Association of hypoadiponectinemia with coronary artery disease in men. Arterioscler Thromb Vasc Biol 2003; 23:85–89.

51. Zoccali C, Mallamaci F, Tripepi G, et al. Adiponectin, metabolic risk factors, and cardiovascular events among patients with end-stage renal disease. J Am Soc Nephrol 2002; 13:134–141.

52. Okamoto Y, Kihara S, Ouchi N, et al. Adioncetin reduces atherosclerosis in apolipoptroein E-deficient mice. Circulation 2002; 106:2767–2770.

53. Yamauchi T, Kamon J, Waki H, et al. Globular adiopnectin protected ob/ob mice from diabetes and ApoE-deficient mice from atherosclerosis. J Biol Chem 2003; 278:2461–2468.

54. Sowers JR, Frohlich ED. Insulin and insulin resistance: impact on blood pressure and cardiovascular disease. Med Clin North Am 2004; 88:63–82.

55. Klein S, Fontana L, Young L, et al. Absence of an effect of liposcutionon insulin action and risk factors for coronary heart disease. N Engl J Med 2004; 350:2549–2557.

56. Grundy SM, Cleeman JI, Merz CNB, et al. Implications of recent clinical trials for the National Cholesterol Education Program Adult Treatment Panel III Guidelines. Endorsed by the National Heart, Lung, and Blood Institute, American College of Cardiology Foundation and American Heart Association. Circulation 2004; 110:227–239.

57. Tuomilehto J, Lindstrom J, Eriksson J, et al. Prevention of type 2 diabetes mellitus by changes in lifestyle among sunjects with impaired glucose tolerance. N Engl J Med 2001; 344:1343–1350.

58. Diabetes Prevention Program Research Group. Reduction in the incidence of type 2 diabetes with lifestyle intervention or metformin. N Engl J Med 2002; 346:393–403.

59. Brooks GA, Butte NF, Rand WM, et al. Chronicle of the Institute of Medicine physical activity recommendation: how a physical activity recommendation came to be among dietary recommendations. Am J Clin Nutr 2004; 79:921S–930S.

60. Didangelos T, Thanopoulou A, Bousboulas, et al. The orlistat and cardiovascular risk profile inpatient swith metabolic syndrome and type 2 diabetes (ORLI-CARDIA) study. Curr Med Res Opin 2004; 20:1393–1401.

61. Reaven G. Metabolic syndrome: pathophysiology and implications for management of cardiovascular disease. Circulation 2002; 106:286–288.

62. The DECODE Study Group on Behalf of the European Diabetes Epidemiology Group. Current definition for diabetes relevant to mortality risk from all causes and cardiovascular and noncardiovascular diseases? Diabetes Care 2003; 26:688–696.

63. Chiasson JL, Josse RG, Gomis R, et al. Acarbose treatment and the risk of cardiovascular disease and hypertension in patients with impaired glucose tolerance. The Stop-NIDDM trial. JAMA 2003; 290:486–494.

64. Cai D, Yuan M, Frantz DF, et al. Local and systemic insulin resistance resulting from hepatic activation of IKK-beta and NF-kappaB. Nat Med 2005; 11:183–191.

65. Arkan MC, Hevener AL, Greten FR, et al. IKK-beta links inflammation to obesity-induced insulin resistance. Nat Med 2005; 11:191–198.

66. Coulston AM, Peragallo-Dittko V. Insulin resistance syndrome: a potent culprit in cardiovascular disease. J Am Diet Assos 2004; 104:176–179.

67. Ducimentiere P, Eschwege E, Papoz L, et al. Relationship of plasma insulin level to the incidence of myocardial infarction and coronary heart disease. Diabetologia 1980; 19:205–210.

68. Fontbonne A, Charles MA, Thibult N, et al. Hyperinsulinemia as a predictor of coronary heart disease mortality in healthy population: The Paris Prospective Study, 15-year follow-up. Diabetologia 1991; 34:356–361.
69. Desperés J-P, Lamarche B, Mauriege P, et al. Hyperinsulinemia is an independent risk factor for ischemic heart disease. N Engl J Med 1996; 334:952–957.
70. Howard BV, Gray RS. Insulin resistance and cardiovascular disease. Diabetes Annu 1999:305–316.
71. Bonora E, Formentine G, Calcaterra F. HOMA-estimated insulin resistance is an independent predictor of cardiovascular disease in type 2 diabetic subjects. Diabetes Care 2002; 25:1135–1141.
72. Salonaa V, Riley W, Kaark JD, et al. Non-insulin dependent diabetes mellitus and fasting glucose and insulin concentrations are associated with arterial stiffness index the ARIC study. Circulation 1995; 91:1432–1443.
73. Suzuki M, Shinozaki K, Kanazawa A, et al. Insulin resistance as an independent risk for carotid wall thickening. Hypetension 1996; 28:593–598.
74. Shinozaki K, Naritomi H, Shimizu T, et al. Role of insulin resistance associated with compensatory hyperinsulinemia in ischemic stroke. Stroke 1996; 27:37–43.
75. Yki-Järvinen H. Thiazolidinediones. N Engl J Med 2004; 351:1106–1118.
76. Promrat K, Lutchman G, Uwaifo GI, et al. A pilot study of pioglitazone treatment for nonalcoholic steatohepatitis. Hepatology 2004; 39:188–196.
77. Assmann G, Schulte H. The Prospective Cardiovascular Munster study: prevalence and hyperlipidaemia in persons with hypertension and/or diabetes mellitus and relationship to coronary heart disease. Am Heart J 1988; 116:1713–1724.
78. Reynisdottir S, Angelin B, Landgin D, et al. Adipose tissue lipoprotiein lipase and hormone-sensitive lipase.Contrasting findgidng in familial combined hyperliipidemia and insulin resistance syndrome. Arterioscler Thromb Vasc Biol 1997; 17:2287–2292.
79. Davy BM, Melby LC. The effect of fiber-rich carbohydrates on features of syndrome, X. J Am Diet Assoc 2003; 103:86–96.
80. Eckel RH. Familial Combined hyperlipidemia and insulin resistance: distant relatives linked by intra-abdominal fat? Arterioscler Thromb Vasc Biol 2001; 21:469–470.
81. Castelli WP. Epidemiology of triglycerides: a view from Framingham. Am J Cardiol 1992; 70:3H–9H.
82. Ballantyne CM, Olsson AG, Cook TJ, et al. Influence of low high-density lipoprotein cholesterol and elevated triglyceride on coronary heart disease events and response ot simvastatin therapy in 4 S. Circulation 2001; 18:3046–3051.
83. Mamo JC, Yu KC, Elsegood CL, et al. Is atherosclerosis exclusively a postprandial phenomenon? Clin Exp Pharmacol Physiol 1997; 24:288–293.
84. Sowers JR. Effects of statins on the vasculature: implications for aggressive lipid management in the cardiovascular metabolics syndrome. Am J Cardiol 2003; 91:14B–22B.
85. Grundy SM, Cleeman JI, Merz CN, et al. Implications of recent clinical trials for the National Cholesterol Education Program Adulat Treatment Panel III guidelines. Circulation 2004; 110:227–239.
86. Knopp RH. Drug treatment of lipid disorders. N Engl J Med 1999; 341:498–511.
87. Deedwania PS, Hunnighake DB, Bays HE, et al. Effects of Rosuvastatin, Atorvastatin, Simvastatin, and Pravastatin on atherogenic dyslipidemia in patient with characteristics of the Metabolic Syndrome. Am J Cardiol 2005; 95:360–366.

88. Cziraky MJ. Mangement of dyslipidemia in patients with metabolic syndrome. J Am Pharm Assoc 2004; 44:478–488.

89. Chapman MJ, Assmann G, Fruchart J-C, et al. Raising high-density lipoprotein cholesterol with reduction of cardiovascular risk: the role of nicotinic acid—a positon paper developed by the European Consensus Panel on HDL-C. Curr Med Res Opin 2004; 20:1253–1268.

90. Dimons L, Tonkon M, Masana L, et al. Effects of ezetimibe added to on-going stain therapy on tlipid profile of hypercholesterolemic patients with diabetes mellitus or metabolic syndrome. Curr Med Res Opin 2004; 20:1437–1445.

91. Ferrannini E, Buzzigoli C, Bonadonna R, et al. Insulin resistance in essential hypertension. N Engl J Med 1987; 317:350–357.

92. Shen DC, Shieh SM, Wu DA, et al. Resistance to insulin stimulated glucose uptake in patients with hypertension. J Clin Endocrinol Meat 1998; 66:580–583.

93. Gress TW, Niet FJ, Shahar E, et al. Hypertesion and atnihypertesiver therapy as risk factors for type 2 diabetes mellitus. Atherosclerosis risk in community study. N Engl J Med 1987; 342:905–912.

94. Sowers JR, Bakris GL. Antihypertensive therapy and the risk of type 2 diabetes mellitus. N Engl J Med 2000; 342:969–970.

95. Sowers JR, Sowers PS, Peuler JD. Role of insulin resistance and hyperinsulinemia in development of hypertension and arherosclrosis. J Lab Clin Med 1994; 123:647–652.

96. Reaven GM, Lithell H, Landsberg L. Hypertension and associated metabolic abnormalities: the role of insulin resistance and sympathetic adrenal system. N Engl J Med 1996; 334:374–381.

97. Nolan JJ, Ludvik B, Baloga J, et al. Mechanisms of the kinetic defect in insulin action in obesity and NIDDDM. Diabetes 1997; 46:494–500.

98. Sowers JR. Insulin and insulin-like growth factor in noral and pathoplogical cardiovascular physiology. Hypertension 1997; 29:691–699.

99. Sowers JR. Effects on insulin and IGF-1 on vscular smooth muscle glucose and cation metabolism. Diabetes 1996; 45:S47–S51.

100. Ren J, Samson WK, Sowers JR. Insulin -like growth gactor 1 as a cardiac hormone: physiological and pahtyophysiological implications inheart disease. J Mol Cell Cardiol 1999; 31:2049–2061.

101. Wang HD, Xu S, Johns DG, et al. Role of NADH oxidase in the vascular hypertrophic and oxidative stress responses to angiotensin II in mice. Circ Res 2001; 88:947–953.

102. Huerta MG, Nadler JL. Role of inflammatory pathways in the development and cardiovascular complications of type 2 diabetes. Curr Diab Rep 2002; 2:396–402.

103. Griendling KK, Sorescu D, Ushio-Fukai M. Nad(P)H oxidase: role in cardiovascular biology and disease. Circ Res 2000; 86:494–501.

104. Sowers JR. Hypertension, angiotensin II, and oxidative stress. N Engl J Med 2002; 20:346–348.

105. Kalinowksi L, Matjie T, Chabelsky E, et al. Angiotensin II AT1 receptor antagonists inhibit platelet adhesion and aggregation by nitci oxide release. Hypertension 2002; 40:521–527.

106. Katovidh MJ, Pachori A. Effects of inhibition of the rennin-angiotensin system of the cardiovascular actions of insulin. Diabet Obes Metab 2002; 2:3–14.

107. Grunfeld B, Balzareti H, Romo H, et al. Hyperinsulinemia in normotensive offspring of hypertensive parents. Hypertension 1994; 23:112–115.
108. Beatty OL, Harper R, Sheridan B. Insuln resistance in offspring of hypertensive parents. BMJ 1993; 3017:92–96.
109. Taittonen L, Uhari M, Nuutinen M, et al. Insulin and blood pressure among healthy children: cardiovasular risk in young Finns. Am J Hypertens 1996; 9:193–199.
110. Hooper L, Barlett C, Davey SG, et al. Advice to reduce dietary salt for prevention of cardiovascular disease. Cochrane Database Syst Rev 2004; CD003656.
111. Vollmer WM, Sacks FM, Ard J, et al. Effects of diet and sodium intake on blood pressure: subfourp analysis of the DASH-sodium trial. Ann Intern Med 2001; 135:1019–1028.
112. Katovidh MJ, Pachori A. Effects of inhibition of the rennin-angiotensin system of the cardiovascular actions of insulin. Diabetes Obes Metab 2002; 2:3–14.
113. Hanson L, Lindholm LH, Niskanen L, et al. Effect of angiotensin-converting-enzyme inhibition compared with conventional therapy on cardiovascular morbidity and mortality in hypertension: The captorpril prevention project randomized trial. Lancet 1999; 353:611–616.
114. Yusuf S, Sleight P, Pgue J, et al. Effects of an angiotensin-converting -enzyme inhibitor, ramipril, on cardiovascular events in high-risk patient's. The Heart Outcomes Prevention Evaluation Study Investigators. N Engl J Med 2000; 342:145–153.
115. Dahlöf B, Devereux RB, Kjeldsen SE, et al. Cardiovasuclar morbidity and mortality in the losartan intervention for endpoint reduction in hypertension study: a randomized trial against atenolol. Lancet 2002; 359:995–1003.
116. Heart Outcomes Prevention Evaluation (HOPE) study Investigators. Effects of ramipril on cardiovascular and mircovascular outcomes in people with diabetes mellitus: results of the HOPE study and MICRO-HOPE substudy. Lancet 2000; 355:253–259.
117. Brenner BM, Cooper ME, De Zeeuw D, et al. Effects of losartan on renal and caridovascular outcomes in patients with type 2 diabetes and nephropathy. N Engl J Med 2001; 345:861–869.
118. Lewis EJ, Hunsicker LG, Clarke WR, et al. Renoprotecive effect of the angiotensin-receptor antagonist irbesartan in patients with nephropathy due to type 2 diabetes. N Engl J Med 2001; 354:851–860.
119. The ALLHAT Officers and Coordinators for the ALLHAT Collaborative Research Group. Major Outcomes in High-Risk Hypertensive Patients Randomized to Angiotensin-Converting Enzyme Inhibitor or Calcium Channel Blocker vs Diuretic The Antihypertensive and Lipid-Lowering Treatment to Prevent Heart Attack Trial (ALLHAT). JAMA 2002; 288:2981–2997.
120. Yudkin JS, Stehouwer CD, Emeis JJ, et al. C-reactive protein in healthy subjects: associations with obesity, insulin resistance, and endothelial dysfunction: a potential role for cytokines originating form adipose tissue? Arterioscler Thromb Vasc Biol 1999; 19:972–978.
121. Pradhan AD, Manson JE, Rifai NC, et al. C-reactive protein, interleukin 6, and risk of developing diabetes mellitud. JAMA 2001; 286:327–334.
122. Ridker PM, Buring JE, Cook NR, et al. C-reactive protein, the metabolic syndrome, and risk of incident cardiovascular events. An 8-year follow up of 14 719 initially healthy American women. Circulation 2003; 107:391–397.

123. Festa A, D'Agostino R, Jr., Howard G, et al. Chronic subclinical inflammation as part of ithe insulin resistance syndrome: the Insulin Resistance Aterhosclerosis Study (IRAS). Circulation 2000; 102:42–47.
124. Chen YQ, Su M, Walia RR, et al. Sp1 sties mediate activation of the plasminogen activator inhibitor-1 promoter by glucose in vascular smooth muscle cells. J Biol Chem 1998; 273:8225–8231.
125. Arand SS, Qilong Y, Gerstein H, et al. Relationship of metabolic syndrome and fibrinolytic dysfunction to cardiovascular disease. Circulation 2003; 108:420–425.
126. Kohler HP, Grant PJ. Mechanisms of disease: plasminogen-activator inhibitor type 1 and coronary artery disease. N Engl J Med 2000; 342:1792–1801.
127. Steinberg HO, Chaker H, Leaming R, et al. Obesity/insulin resistance is associates eith endothelial dysfunction: implications for the syndrome of insulin resistance. J Clin Invest 1996; 97:2601–2610.
128. Higashi Y, Oshima T, Sasaki N, et al. Relationship between isnuin resistance and endothelium-dependent vascular relaxation inpatients with essential hypertension. Hypertension 1997; 29:280–285.
129. Balletshofer BM, Rittig K, Enderle MD, et al. Endothelial dysfunction is detectable in young normotensive first-degree relatives of subjects with type 2 diabetes in association with insulin resistance. Circulation 2000; 101:1780–1784.
130. Chen NG, Holmes M, Reaven GM. Relationship between insulin resistance, soluble adhesion molecules, and mononuclear cell binding in healthy volunteers. J Clin Endocrinol Metab 1999; 84:3485–3489.
131. Enderle MD, Benda N, Schmuelling RM, et al. Preserved endothelial function in IDDM patients, but not in NIDDM patients, compared with healthy subjects. Diabetes Care 1998; 21:271–277.
132. Kawano H, Motoyama T, Hirashima O, et al. Hyperglycemia rapidly suppresses flow-mediated endothelium-dependent vasodilation of brachial artery. its mechanism, measurment, and significance. J Am Coll Cardiol 1999; 34:146–154.
133. Chan NN, Chan CN. Asymmetric dimethylarginine (ADMA): a potent link between endothelial dysfunction and cardiovascular diseases in insulin resistance syndrome? Diabetolgia 2002; 45:1609–1616.
134. Bucala R, Tracey KJ, Cerami A. Advanced glycosylation products quench nitric oxide and mediate defective endothelium-dependent vasodilatation in experimental diabetes. J Clin Invest 1991; 87:432–438.
135. Ridker RM, Hennekens CH, Buring JE, et al. C-reactive protein and other markers of inflammation in the prediction of cardiovascular disease in women. N Engl J Med 2000; 342:836–843.
136. Koenig W, Sund M, Frohlich M, et al. C-reactive protein, a sensitive marker of inflammation, predicts future risk of coronary heart disease in initially healthy middle-aged: results from MONICA (Monitoring trends and determinants in cardiovascular disease) Augsburg cohort study. Circulation 1999; 99:237–242.
137. Forouhi MG, Sattar N, McKeigue PM. Relation of C-reactive protein to body fat distribution and features of the metabolic syndrome in Europeans ans South Asians. Int J Obes Relat Metab Disord 2001; 25:1327–1331.
138. Barzilay JI, Abraham L, Heckbert SR, et al. The relation of markers of inflammation to the development of glucose disorders in the elderly: the Cardiovascular Health Study. Diabetes 2001; 50:2384–2389.

139. Han ATS, Sattar N, Williams K, et al. Prospective study of C-reactive protein in relation ot the development of diabetes and metabolic syndrome in the Mexico City Diabetes Study. Diabetes Care 2002; 25:2016–2020.
140. Sattar N, Gaw A, Scherbakova O, et al. Metabolic syndrome with and without C-reactive protein as a predictor of coronary heart disease and diabetes in the West of Scotland Coronary Prevention Study. Circulation 2003; 108:414–419.
141. Festa A, D'Agostino R, Jr., Tracy RP, et al. Insulin Resistance Atherosclerosis Study. Elevated levels of acute-phase proteins and plasminogen activator inhibitor-1 predict the development of type 2 diabetes: the insulin resistance atherosclerosis study. Diabetes 2002; 51:1131–1137.
142. Pearson TA, Blair SN, Daniels SR, et al. American Heart Association guidelines for primary prevention of cardiovascular disease and stroke: 2002 update: consensus panel guide to comprehensive risk reduction for adult patients without coronary or other atherosclerotic vascular disease. American Hear Association Science Advisory and Coordinating Committee. Circulation 2003; 107:499–511.
143. Ridker PM, Buring JE, Cook NR, et al. C-reactive protein, the metabolic syndrome, and risk of incident cardiovascular events. An 8-year follow up of 14 719 initially healthy American women. Circulation 2003; 107:391–397.
144. Feldman M, Jialal I, Devaraj S, et al. Effects of low-dose aspirin on serum C-reactive protein and throboxane B2 concentrations:A placebo-controlled study using a highly sensitive C-reactive protein assay. J Am Coll Cardiol 2001; 37:2036–2041.
145. Agrawal B, Berger A, Wolf K, et al. Microalbuminuria screening by reagent strip predicts cardiovascular risk in hypertension. J Hypertens 1996; 14:223–228.
146. Dinneen S, Gerstein H. The association of microabuminuria and mortality in non-insulin-dependent diabetes mellitus: A systematic overview of the literature. Arch Intern Med. 1997; 157:1413–1418.
147. Lydakis C, Lip G. Microalbuminuria and cardiovascular risk. QJM 1998; 91:381–391.
148. Miettinen H, Haffner SM, Lehto S, et al. Proteinuria predicts stroke and other atherosclerotic vascular disease events in non-diabetic and non-insulin dependent diabetic subjects. Stroke 1996; 27:2033–2039.
149. Culleton BF, Larson MG, Kannel WB, et al. Serum uric acid and risk for cardiovascular disease and death: the Framingham Heart Study. Ann Intern Med 1999; 131:7–13.
150. Fang J, Alderman MH. Serum uric acid and cardiovascular mortality. JAMA 2000; 283:2404–2410.
151. Verdecchia P, Schillaci G, Reboldi GP, et al. Relation between serum uric acid and cardiovascular disease in essential hypertension. The PIUMA study. Hypertension 2000; 36:1072.
152. Doelle GC. The clinical picture of metabolic syndrome: an update on this complex of conditions and risk factors. Postgrad Med 2004; 116:30–38.
153. Wajchenberg BL. Subcutaneous and visceral adipose tissue: their relation to the metabolic syndrome. Endocr Rev 2000; 21:697–738.
154. Deedwania PC. Metabolic syndrome and vascular disease. Is nature or nurture leading the new epidemic of cardiovascular disease. Circulation 2004; 109:2–4.

2

Lipoprotein Metabolism and Implications for Atherosclerosis Risk Determination and Treatment Decisions

H. Robert Superko, Szilard Voros, and Spencer King III

Fuqua Heart Center/Piedmont Hospital, Cholesterol, Genetics, and Heart Disease Institute, Atlanta, Georgia, U.S.A.

INTRODUCTION

The relationship of lipids and lipoproteins to atherosclerosis is not a recent discovery. Nearly 100 years ago, Ignatowosky noted that wealthy patients who consumed large amounts of meat and dairy products appeared to have more arteriosclerosis on autopsy than poor patients who could not afford this rich type of food (1). Soon after this observation, Anitschkow and Chalatow conducted studies on rabbits that indicated that such high fat diets resulted in hypercholesterolemia and subsequent arteriosclerosis (2). With a tremendous amount of foresight, Aschoff suggested in 1924 that arteriosclerosis might be reversible (3). In the 1950s, Dr. John Gofman and colleagues at the Donner Laboratory (University of California) made another major step forward by investigating the relationship of low-density lipoproteins (LDL) to atherosclerosis in the Framingham and Lawrence Radiation Laboratory at Livermore studies (4). His contributions included the association of multiple lipoprotein subclasses defined by Svedberg floatation (Sf) intervals, assessed in the analytic ultracentrifuge. Gofman and colleagues were also well ahead of their time by reporting that high-density lipoprotein 2 (HDL2) (F3.5–9.0) was reduced 32.1% in patients who developed coronary artery disease (CAD). This raised the possibility of a protective role of HDL and HDL subclasses. An atherogenic index, based on these lipoprotein classes, attempted to quantitate the effect of these lipoproteins on atherosclerosis. With a great degree of prescience, which predated the Adult Treatment Panel guidelines by four decades, it was predicted that if longevity is linked to lipoproteins, then in order to improve longevity, "… a drastic rather than moderate reduction in such parameters is required." Based on the work of Geer and McGill, it was even suggested that alteration in lipoprotein composition might lead to the development of atherosclerosis, even though no alteration in absolute lipoprotein levels occurred. Thus, the field of lipids, lipoproteins, and lipoprotein subclasses within the very-low-density lipoprotein (VLDL), intermediate-density lipoprotein (IDL), LDL, and HDL regions, and their relationship to atherosclerosis, is at least 50 years old.

In the past 20 years investigators have extended the work of Gofman and colleagues to involve a plethora of investigations that assessed the role of lipoprotein subclasses within the entire subclass distribution and their relationship to atherosclerosis (5). These investigations bridged the gap between basic science and clinical research, and most recently have involved genetics and arteriographic trials (6–8).

Topics involving the clinical relevance of lipoprotein disorders are no longer relegated to a small group of "lipidologists." Among interventional cardiologists there is a growing emphasis on the importance of secondary prevention. Words like "secondary" and "prevention" may not engender the aggressive emotions usually associated with interventionalists, but this segment of cardiology must now embrace what happens after the stents are implanted. For more than 20 years the main concern post-intervention has been the prevention of restenosis. Now, with the advent of drug-eluting stents, this complication is becoming rare, although, it is not eliminated. Recent observations show that cardiac events in the five years after percutaneous intervention are much more likely to be due to progression of disease in untreated segments than to restenosis. This was true even before the drug-eluting stents were introduced. With the compelling evidence that effective manipulation of lipoprotein disorders is possible, the interventionalist must now include a post PCI plan that includes aggressive lipoprotein manipulation. As individualized therapies to address multiple inherited disorders are investigated and become available, there is the opportunity for interventionalists to take a central role in their development and clinical application.

BASIC LIPOPROTEIN METABOLISM

Lipoproteins are a diverse group of spherical particles that can be separated into various categories based on their density. The regions include triglyceride-rich, VLDL and IDL, and the relatively cholesterol rich LDL. High-density lipoprotein (HDL) particles may play a role in what has been termed "reverse cholesterol transport" (9). In general, the production and metabolism of lipoproteins follows a path of large particles, rich in triglycerols and relatively poor in cholesterol, that undergoes a series of metabolic interactions, which results in more dense particles that are relatively rich in cholesterol and poor in triglycerols. The large triglyceride-rich transport particles, derived from an intestinal source, are termed chylomicrons. The somewhat smaller, triglyceride-rich particles, derived from a hepatic source, are termed VLDL. After a series of interactions with the enzyme lipoprotein lipase (LPL), the particles become more dense and relatively cholesterol rich. An IDL precedes the appearance of LDL, which is normally the greatest source of cholesterol transport among the lipoproteins. Further metabolism involves the interaction of lecithin-cholesterol acyltransferase (LCAT), apoproteins, and neutral exchange factors (10,11). VLDL particles can be produced in both large and smaller forms and through pathways that involve lipoprotein and hepatic lipase (HL), and cholesteryl ester transfer protein (CETP), develops into either large or small LDL particles (Fig. 1) (12,13).

IDL is a relatively triglyceride-rich particle intermediate between VLDL and LDL. IDL is defined as the lipoprotein mass in the Sf intervals Sf 12–20 and has long been linked to CAD risk and arteriographic progression (14). This is of clinical relevance since the most common laboratory method of determining low-density-lipoprotein cholesterol (LDL-C) involves precipitation of apo B-containing lipoprotein particles, measurement of the cholesterol content of the remaining plasma [high-density-lipoprotein cholesterol (HDL-C)] and then calculation of LDL-C with the Friedawald equation (15). When using this method, intermediate-density-lipoprotein cholesterol (IDL-C) is included in the LDL-C number. When IDL and LDL are individually determined in an ultracentrifuge, it has been shown that the natural history of CAD progression is

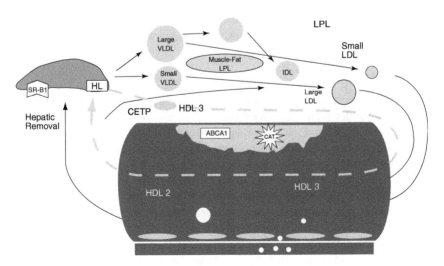

Figure 1 Metabolic pathway of lipoproteins including lipoprotein heterogeneity.

related to IDL and inversely to HDL, but not to LDL (14). It is unclear how much of the atherogeneicity, or treatment benefit, of LDL-C reduction is related to IDL and/or LDL since most clinical research studies employed a calculated LDL-C value that includes IDL. Recently, research using the analytic ultracentrifuge to separate lipoprotein classes has discovered that IDL is significantly associated with atherosclerosis progression as determined by carotid wall intimal media thickness (16).

LDL is not a homogeneous category of lipoproteins but consists of a set of discrete subspecies with distinct molecular properties, including size and density (17,18). In normal subjects, seven major LDL subspecies can be identified. Accurate and reproducible determination of LDL subspecies is made possible by two well-established laboratory methods, gradient gel electrophoresis (GGE), which separates LDL particles on the basis of their differing size, and analytic ultra-centrifugation (ANUC), which separates the particles into 12 regions on the basis of their differing density (19,20). In most healthy people, the major subspecies are large or buoyant, whereas the smaller, denser LDL subspecies are generally present in small amounts (21).

HDL is derived from both intestinal and hepatic sources. Hepatic HDL, in a nascent form, appears as a disk-shaped structure. Intestinally derived HDL is more spherical and varies in its protein composition. Both of these HDL particles are relatively small and cholesterol-poor and can be classified as HDL3. Following interaction with LCAT and LPL in both adipose and muscle tissue, cholesterol ester content is increased and the particle becomes less dense, larger, and classified as HDL2. Based on the relative density obtained in the analytic ultracentrifuge, the more dense, relatively cholesterol-poor form is termed HDL3 (1.125 to 1.21 G per mL) and the less dense, relatively cholesterol-rich form is termed HDL2 (1.062 to 1.125 G per mL) (20,22).

Central to the understanding of lipoprotein metabolism is the action of apoproteins, enzymes, transfer proteins, membrane modulators, and receptors.

Apoproteins

Apoproteins are proteins attached to a lipoprotein particle and are given alphabetical names such as apoprotein A, B, C, D, and E (23). By protruding from the surface of the lipoprotein, they can be recognized by a receptor and assist in uptake or activation of cellular mechanisms. They can also serve as cofactors for specific enzymatic reactions. Each apoprotein probably has more than one function and is in a continuous spectrum of activity. The relative amount of an apoprotein in a lipoprotein particle does not necessarily reflect the biologic importance of the apoprotein. They are identified based on specific antigenic characteristics, and specific apoproteins are associated with various lipoprotein groups. Inherited defects in the amino acid sequence of these proteins can impact normal lipoprotein metabolism by interfering with receptor binding or their actions as cofactors. Some of these apoprotein disorders are relatively common.

The apoprotein content of lipoproteins varies. For example, the relative distribution of apoproteins within a typical HDL particle is: A-I, 46%; A-II, 23%; C-I, 18%; C-II, 2%; C-III, 3%; D, 5%; E, 1% (24). The LDL particle is somewhat unique in that it is in part defined by having only one apoprotein attached, apo B-100.

Apoprotein A can be identified as several forms, including Apo A-I and A-II, and accounts for approximately 70% of the apoproteins on the HDL particle. It is principally associated with the HDL particle. However, A-I is also a constituent of chylomicrons and its synthesis in the intestine is increased after a fatty meal (25). Apo A-I and A-III, along with Apo C-I, are activators of lecithincholesterol acyltransferase (LCAT).

Separation of HDL subclasses can be made on the presence of HDLs with A-I only, or HDL particles with both A-I and A-II attached. Work in France has elucidated HDL subclasses defined as those containing apo A-I only (LpAI) and those containing both apo A-I and A-II (LpAI:II) (26). The LpAI only particle is the HDL subclass most associated with CV protection and is similar to HDL2b. HDL2b, as determined by GGE, is the subclass most associated with cardiovascular protection and has primarily apo A-I as its apoprotein constituent (27).

Apo [a] is an important apoprotein in regard to cardiovascular risk. When attached to apo B and LDL, by a disulfide link, it is termed lipoprotein (a), or Lp(a) for short. The importance of this lipoprotein lies in its very strong association with coronary heart disease and carotid atherosclerosis. Elevated levels may be present in as many as 20–40% of individuals with CAD. The gene is on chromosome 6 and inherited in a dominant fashion, which indicates that approximately 50% of first-degree relatives will express elevated Lp(a) levels (28). This finding may help to explain why some patients with relatively normal blood LDL and HDL cholesterol values still suffer from atherosclerosis (29). This apoprotein is quite large and susceptible to oxidative damage. When oxidized, it is consumed by the scavenger receptor on the macrophage significantly faster than the non-oxidized form (30).

Apo B serves as an identification protein for specific receptors located on hepatic and peripheral cells involved with lipoprotein metabolism (31). Apo B has been identified as primarily two apoproteins that are immunologically distinct. Apo B-100 is produced in the liver and attached to LDL particles. Apo B-48 is derived from the intestines and is approximately half the molecular weight of apo B-100. It is attached to triglyceride-rich particles and not to LDL particles.

Apo C, along with apo A-I, is an activator of LCAT. The hydrolysis of triglycerides by LPL is dependent on apo C-II (32). This is reflected by the substantial elevation in chylomicrons and VLDL seen in persons lacking this apoprotein (33). Apo E plays an important role in hepatic clearance of VLDL remnants and HDL recognition. Apo E can be identified as a number of different

Table 1   Recent Advances in the Understanding of the Role Enzymes, Proteins, Membrane Modulators, and Receptors Play in Atherosclerosis

Name	Function	Recent findings
LPL	TG hydrolysis	Partial defect accounts for substantial amount of plasma TG elevation when exacerbated by lifestyle or diet.
HL	TG and PL hydrolysis	Reconverts HDL2 to HDL3
EL	PL hydrolysis	May be pro or anti atherogenic
LCAT	Esterifies cholesterol	Apo AI is cofactor
ACAT	FC→CE	ACAT1 and ACAT2 discovered
CETP	TG exchange for cholesterol Between VLDL/LDL and HDL	CETP inhibitor in clinical trial
PLTP	Transfers PL from VLDL to HDL	
Paroxonase	Antioxidant	Located to apoAI/HDL2 particles
ABCA1	Transmembrane lipid transport	Genetic disorders discovered
SR-B1	CE uptake from HDL and LDL	May be pro or anti atherogenic

Abbreviations: TG, triglycerides; PL, phospholipids; FC, free cholesterol; CE, cholesterol ester.

isoforms or genotypes that are distinguished on the basis of amino acid or DNA differences (34).

Five major enzymes play a role in basic lipid metabolism: LPL, HL, endothelial lipase (EL), LCAT, and acyl-CoA:cholesterol acyltransferase (ACAT) (Table 1). LPL is a lipolytic enzyme located on the surface of vascular endothelial cells and macrophages (35). It is responsible for Triglycerides hydrolysis. Hepatic lipase (HL) is an enzyme synthesized by hepatocytes and binds to endothelial cells, allowing it to interact with lipoproteins as they traverse the liver (36). Endothelial lipase (EL) is a lipolytic enzyme that uses phospholipids as the substrate (37). LCAT is responsible for the esterification of cholesterol molecules in HDL (38). ACAT serves to convert free cholesterol to esterified cholesterol intracellularly.

Lipoprotein Lipase

LPL is a lipolytic enzyme located on the surface of vascular endothelial cells and on macrophages (39,35). It is responsible for TG hydrolysis and is the rate-limiting step for the uptake of lipoprotein TG and resultant fatty acids into adipose tissue and muscle. Deficiency in LPL activity is often associated with substantial increases in plasma triglycerides and low HDL-C. The relative degree of LPL dysfunction can result in a wide range of triglyceride values that are affected by environmental issues such as diet, body fat, and exercise levels. While mild to moderate elevations in plasma triglycerides is often the result of a polygenic environmental interaction, dramatic elevations in fasting triglycerides, usually greater than 1000 mg/dL, are often associated with inherited defects in triglyceride metabolism. Normal LPL function is essential for normal triglyceride hydrolysis, and apolipoprotein C-II is a cofactor for LPL action. Apo C-II deficiency results in elevated triglycerides due to reduced LPL activity. LPL deficiency is the most common cause of familial chylomcronemia and is an autosomal recessive trait often presenting in childhood with severely elevated plasma triglycerides, pancreatitis, and abdominal pain, along with eruptive xanthomas and lipemia retinales (40). It occurs in approximately 1:5000 individuals, and the heterozygote state is more common than familial heterozygote hypercholesterolemia and in some populations can be found in 1 in 40 individuals (41). Over 26 mutations in the LPL gene have been identified that can result in a spectrum between mild to complete LPL activity deficiency (42). A specific LPL mutation (Asn291Ser) has been identified in 5% of male CAD patients that results in low HDL-C and may contribute to CAD risk (43).

Hepatic Lipase

HL is an enzyme synthesized by hepatocytes and binds to endothelial cells, allowing it to interact with lipoproteins as they traverse the liver (36). Its major function is to hydrolyze triglycerides and phospholipids in lipoprotein particles. In conjunction with CETP activity, HL is believed to reduce the core of large HDL2 particles and play a role in the conversion of HLD2 to HDL3 (44). Apo A-II may assist in HL activation (45). HL may play a pivotal role in the production of small, dense LDL (46).

Endothelial Lipase

EL is a lipolytic enzyme that exclusively uses phospholipids as the substrate (37). The action of EL releases free fatty acids and creates a small HDL particle. The proatherogenic or antiatherogenic role of EL is underinvestigation.

Lecithin-Cholesterol Acyltransferase

LCAT is the enzyme that catalyzes the esterification of free cholesterol in plasma lipoproteins. The HDL3 subfraction appears to be the main substrate for this esterification reaction and the Apo A-I associated with HDL, and possibly apo A-III, act as cofactors for LCAT (47,48). Human apo Al transgenic mice have been shown to increase HDL-C 6.8-fold with larger HDL particles and increased efflux from cholesterol laden cells (49). This illustrates a potential gene transfection approach for treating low HDL-C.

Acyl-CoA:Cholesterol Acyltransferase

ACAT serves to convert free cholesterol to esterified cholesterol intracellularly through an esterification process. Approximately seven years ago, two different forms of ACAT were described: ACAT1 and ACAT2 (50). These two forms differ in regard to cellular location and potential impact on atherosclerosis (51), and ACAT1 appears to be expressed in most tissues in the body. In cholesterol-laden cells it serves to prevent intracellular free cholesterol–induced aptosis. This is particularly important for cell survival in macrophages located in atherosclerotic plaques. ACAT2 is located in small intestine enterocytes and hepatocytes. The role of ACAT2 appears to be to esterify cholesterol that is incorporated in VLDL particles, which eventually transform into LDL particles. It has been suggested that inhibition of ACAT2 may be a therapeutic approach to LDL-C reduction. Conversely, inhibition of ACAT1 may be detrimental due to possible disruption of plaque stability due to toxic macrophage death in existing atherosclerotic lesions. The ACAT inhibitor pactimibe, was recently reported not to have any beneficial effect on intravascular ultrasound–determined coronary atherosclerosis progression in humans (52). Future therapies that target ACAT2 may provide a novel means of reducing LDL-C.

Cholesteryl Ester Transfer Protein

CETP mediates the exchange of triglycerides from VLD/LDL particles for cholesterol ester in HDL particles. This activity may be either proatherogenic if it results in the transferred cholesterol ester being taken up by the arterial wall macrophages, or antiatherogenic if the transferred cholesterol ester is removed through the hepatic apo B receptor. Disorders of CETP function led to the development of medications that inhibit CETP and result in an increase in HDL-C (53).

Phospholipid Transfer Protein

Phospholipid transfer protein (PLTP) mediates transfer of phospholipids from triglyceride-rich lipoproteins to HDL (54). It results in conversion of small HDL3 into larger HDL2 particles.

Paroxonase

Paraoxonase is an enzyme initially of interest in the field of toxicology since it is an "A" esterase and hydrolyses organophosphate compounds used as insecticides and nerve gases (55). Paraoxonase is associated with HDL particles, and in sheep most of the paraoxonase activity is associated with the apoAI only particle (56). Thus, part of the protective effect of some, but perhaps not all, HDL particles may be the association of paraoxonase and its putative role in decreasing lipid peroxide accumulation on LDL particles (57).

Membrane modulators are factors that affect the ability of cholesterol to enter or leave the cell. Lipid-free apo A-I, apo A-II, Apo A-IV, apoC, and apoE can cause an efflux of phospholipids and cholesterol (58). This process can be rapid and result in HDL-like particles. This appears to occur primarily in cholesterol-enriched cells such as aortic smooth muscle cells and macrophages, but not erythrocytes (59). The clinical importance of this knowledge involves the recent reports that the use of apo A products may provide a clinical treatment option in the not-too-distant future (60).

ATP Binding Cassette Transporter 1

ATP binding cassette transporter 1 (ABC1) is a protein that plays an important role in RCT through transmembrane lipid transport via transport channels. This process may serve to "flop" cholesterol and phospholipids from the inner to the outer side of the plasma membrane where it can be picked up by lipid-poor lipoproteins (61).

Scavenger Receptor B1

Scavenger receptor B1 (SR-BI) serves to selectively take up cholesterol esters from HDL and LDL into hepatocytes without taking in the HDL particle itself. Overexpression of SR-BI enhances cholesterol uptake and decreases HDL-C levels (62). Two lipid medications, probucol and atrovastatin, have been reported to increase SR-B1 mRNA and protein expression (63,64). In mice, knockout of the SR-BI gene increased HDL-C two-fold but resulted in increased atherosclerosis (65). This illustrates the complexity of the dynamic RCT process, which is not always reflected by static HDL cholesterol values.

CLASSIC LIPOPROTEIN DISORDERS

Elevated Cholesterol

Elevated total plasma cholesterol was initially identified as a cardiovascular (CV) risk factor through epidemiologic associations that led to the cholesterol hypothesis (66). The cholesterol hypothesis proposed that if total and LDLC were reduced, CV events would be reduced as well. This hypothesis was eventually proven to be correct when the results of the Lipid Research Clinics Coronary Primary Prevention Trial were published in 1984 (67). In this landmark study, a reduction in LDL-C, achieved with cholestyramine, was associated with a statistically significant reduction in clinical events when a 1-tailed t test was used. With the advent of more powerful LDL-C-lowering medications, the cholesterol hypothesis has been verified in both men and women, in subjects with elevated and moderate LDL-C values, and in subjects at risk for CAD and those who have documented CAD. These studies include the Scandinavian Simvastatin Survival Study, the West of Scotland Prevention Study, Cholesterol and Recurrent Events, and the Air Force Coronary Artery Prevention Study (68–71). These studies have consistently shown a 25–35% relative reduction in clinical events. However, review of the actual numbers indicates that a substantial number of subjects who take the active medication continue to have CV events (Fig. 2). This is a reflection of the fact that numerous metabolic issues contribute to CAD events and many are not adequately treated with simple LDL-C reduction alone (72).

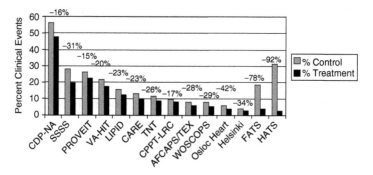

Figure 2 Percent of subjects in the control group (*gray column*) and the treatment group (*black column*) in 14 large clinical trials of cholesterol lowering and coronary events. A consistent approximate 25% reduction in events has been reported in studies using mono-therapy. The difference in the height of the blue and red column represents the approximate 25% reduction in clinical events. The height of the red column represents the percent of patients who took the medication yet still had a Coronary heart disease event. The two studies on the right (FATS, HATS) used combination lipid-altering drug therapy and achieved an 80–90% reduction in clinical events. This percent reduction represents the difference in the number of clinical events in the control versus treatment groups. *Abbreviations*: CDP-NA, nicotinic acid arm of the Coronary Drug Project; SSSS, Scandinavian Simvastatin Survival Study; PROVEIT, Pravastatin or Atorvastatin Evaluation and Infection Therapy; VA-HIT, Veterans Affairs HDL Intervention Trial; LIPID, Long-Term Intervention with Pravastatin in Ischaemic Disease; CARE, Cholesterol and Recurrent Events; TNT, Treating to New Targets; CPPT-LRC, Coronary Primary Prevention Trial-Lipid Research Clinics; AFCAPS/TEX, Air Force/Texas Coronary Atherosclerosis Prevention Study; WOSCOPS, West of Scotland Coronary Prevention Study; Oslo Heart, Oslo Heart Study; Helsinki, Helsinki Heart Study; FATS, Familial Atherosclerosis Treatment Study; HATS, HDL Atherosclerosis Treatment Study. *Source:* Modified from Ref. 107.

Recently, the studies PROVE-IT and TNT suggest that LDL-C goals of <70 mg/dL should be considered as new LDL-C goals (73,74). However, close examination of the results of these trials reveals that a large number of patients continue to experience cardiovascular events. The Incremental Decrease in clinical Endpoints through Aggressive Lipid lowering (IDEAL) trial reported a greater reduction in coronary events (-11%) in a group of 4439 subjects treated with 80 mg/day atorvastatin compared to a group of 4449 subjects treated with 20–40 mg/day simvastatin (p=0.07) (75). However, this was the difference between 463 (10.4%) events in the simvastatin group compared to 411 (9.3%) in the atorvastatin group. Although these results are statistically (mathematically) significant, the clinical relevance may be viewed as less than significant. A successful approach to cardiovascular event reduction should achieve clinical event reductions of approximately 90%. National Institutes of Health funded studies that employed coronary arteriographic endpoints and used combination drug therapy have reported clinical cardiovascular event reduction in the 90% range (76,77).

Familial Defective Apo B

A disorder that presents with elevations in LDL-C similar to familial heterozygous (FH) hypercholesterolemia is familial defective apo B (FDB). FDB is a genetic disorder resulting from a single nucleotide mutation at codon 3500 (78). It occurs in approximately one in 500 people in the general population and is associated with LDL-C values between 270–370 mg/dL (79). Unlike FH, LDL receptor function is normal; however, due to the abnormal apo B, only 32% of receptor-binding activity is found. One major difference between FDB and FH is that only one genetic defect has been found for FDB, while approximately 30 mutations have been found for the LDL receptor that results in FH.

Fish Eye Disease

LCAT deficiency, or fish eye disease (FED), is caused by respective mutations of the LCAT gene and associated with low HDL-C (80). FED was initially described in a Swedish family with corneal opacifications that resembled boiled fish; excess amounts of VLDL, IDL, and LDL; and low levels of HDL-C. The functional abnormalities of LCAT are known to cause two diseases characterized by severe corneal opacity: familial LCAT deficiency, which is accompanied with anemia and often renal failure, and FED with few other symptoms (81).

Low HDL-C

Low HDL-C has been identified as a cardiovascular risk factor for many years (82). One problem with attributing independent risk to low HDL-C is the powerful inverse correlation HDL-C has with other risk factors such as triglycerides and small LDL (12). This correlation issue compounds the ability to attribute CV benefit to HDL-C change since most lifestyle and pharmacologic therapies that increase HDL-C also reduce body fat, triglycerides, small LDL, and IDL, each of which is associated with CV risk. Thus, it is often unclear if it is the HDL-C increase that causes the benefit or the triglyceride and small LDL reduction, or a combination of the two. Evidence that HDL-C raising is of CV benefit was presented with the results of the VA-HIT results (83). In this investigation, men with relatively low HDL-C were randomized to gemfibrozil or a placebo and the resulting reduction in CV events was statistically attributed to an increase in HDL-C, which was attributed to gemfibrozil therapy. However, the issue of which parameter was responsible for the cardiovascular benefit remains unclear since gemfibrozil treatment reduces triglycerides and small LDL as well as increases HDL-C (84). From a clinician's standpoint, the argument of statistical independence is less important since clinical trials using combination drug therapy, which both lowers LDL-C, small LDL, and IDL and increases

HDL-C and HDL2, have demonstrated both clinical event and arteriographic benefit (76,77).

Low HDL-C is not rare in the CAD population and as many as 36% of men with premature CAD have been reported to express this trait, which is a broad spectrum of overlapping disorders (85–87). Primary hypoalphalipoproteinemia (HALP) is seen in approximately 4% of CAD patients and, equally important, approximately 50% of the offspring appear to be affected since it is inherited in an autosomal co-dominant pattern (88). In these cases, the HDL particles are particularly small (HDL3), suggesting impaired reverse cholesterol transport and impaired antioxidation capabilities. Low HDL2 has been observed in post–myocardial infarction (MI) patients, even in the setting of "normal" risk factors (89). Low HDL2b has been associated with arteriographic severity and arteriographic progression, particularly in normotriglyceridemic patients (90). In HATS, treatment with nicotinic acid and a statin resulted in a significant increase in LpAI, which was associated with significant arteriographic benefit and reduced clinical events (91).

One inherited example of low HDL-C is a specific LPL mutation (Asn291Ser), which has been identified in 5% of male CAD patients and results in low HDL-C and may contribute to CAD risk (92). Another genetic cause is a polymorphism in the region between the apolipoprotein A-I and apolipoprotein C-III genes that results in abnormally low HDL values (93). In these cases, elevated triglycerides or elevated LDL-C are not common and isolated low HDL is the main contributor to premature CAD. The role of impaired reverse cholesterol transport may be emphasized in different ethnic populations. Males of Asian Indian descent have been found to have abnormally low HDL2b compared to matched Caucasian subjects (94).

Elevated HDL-C generally reflects reduced cardiovascular risk with rare but notable exceptions. Other metabolic disorders such as hyperhomocysteinemia have been associated with CAD even in the presence of elevated HDL-C (95). CETP deficiency results in markedly increased HDL-C values. While elevated HDL-C most often reflects reduced CAD risk, it should be noted that a genetic CETP mutation, resulting in CETP deficiency and associated with HDL-C equal to 205 mg/dL has been reported in a patient with arteriographically documented CAD with angina (96). Sixty percent of the Japanese cases of HALP are associated with CETP deficiency (97). It has been suggested that the HDL observed in CETP deficiency is an atherogenic lipoprotein, as it contains a large amount of CE (98).

Elevated Triglycerides

Elevations in plasma triglyceride levels (hypertriglyceridemia) may be the result of multiple genetic and metabolic issues that can often be exacerbated by environmental issues such as diets rich in simple carbohydrates, excess body fat, and lack of physical activity. Some of the genetic causes that contribute to elevated triglycerides include the apo E 2/2 genotype and partial LPL deficiency

(34,35). Values in excess of 200 mg/dL have been defined as elevated and values > 150 mg/dL as grounds for concern (99). Although elevated triglycerides are associated with a predominance of small LDL particles, it is important to appreciate that populations with elevated triglyceride values are a mix of individuals with the small LDL pattern B trait, and those in which the mild to moderately elevated triglycerides (150–250 mg/dL) are not associated with the small LDL trait. In healthy family members, the mean fasting triglycerides in small LDL pattern B subjects is 140 mg/dL while in large LDL pattern A subjects it is 70 mg/dL (100). It may be more physiologically appropriate to define a "normal" triglyceride as less than 100 mg/dL and values in excess of 150 mg/dL as suspicious for the presence of the small LDL trait.

Combined Hyperlipidemia

The combination of elevated triglycerides and elevated LDL-C is termed combined hyperlipidemia, and when a family history of hyperlipidemia or atherosclerosis is present, it is termed familial combined hyperlipidemia (FCH). FCH is associated with a four-fold increased CAD risk (101,102). The variability in phenotypic expression has involved a number of related disorders, including LDL subclass pattern B, hyperapobetalipoproteinemia, familial dyslipidemic hypertension, and syndrome X (103–106). One attribute of FCH involves LDL particles more susceptible to oxidative damage than LDLs from non-FCH individuals (107,108).

ADVANCED LIPOPROTEIN DISORDERS

Many nontraditional lipoprotein disorders are more common than classic elevations in LDL-C, or low HDL-C, and knowledge of these disorders is useful in diagnosing individual patient disorders, estimating risk, and developing individualized treatment plans that are matched to the patient's individual disorder(s) (109). These issues include disorders of IDL and remnant particles and postprandial lipemia, disorders of LDL subclass distribution, disorders of HDL subclass distribution, and apoprotein abnormalities.

IDL and Remnant Particles

Clinical trial evidence for the relevance of IDL dates back to the 1960s. The Framingham and Lawrence Livermore trials revealed a significant relation of triglyceride-rich lipoproteins to atherosclerosis risk (4). Recently, it has been reported that IDL is significantly associated with atherosclerosis progression as determined by carotid wall intima medial thickness (IMT) (16). In a revealing study of the natural progression of CAD assessed with coronary arteriography, it was reported that IDL-C correlated with disease progression while LDL-C did not (14). The standard "indirect" laboratory method of calculating LDL-C results in an LDL-C value that includes IDL-C in the LDL-C number. In this investigation, the patients were typical CAD patients and not selected for elevated blood cholesterol levels. The somewhat surprising results are clarified when it is understood that the IDL-C and LDL-C were directly determined with ultracentrifugation and thus, the LDL-C number did not include IDL-C as does the standard calculated LDL-C value.

Remnant lipoprotein particles (RLP) are another type of triglyceride-rich lipoprotein that are the result of triglyceride-rich particle metabolism (110). An association of elevated remnant particles to CAD risk has been established and laboratory assays are currently available (111,112). Elevated remnant-lipoprotein-partide cholesterol (RLP-C) levels have been reported to be a significant and independent risk factor for impaired flow-mediated endothelium-dependent dilatation and angiographically proven CAD in patients with the metabolic syndrome (113). Large studies designed to specifically reduce IDL or RLP and investigate the effect on clinical endpoints or arteriographic change, have not been reported. The issue of the independent role RLP may play in CAD risk is complicated by the association of other triglyceride-rich particles, small LDL, and low HDL2 in the setting of elevated RLP.

LDL Subclass Distribution

The small LDL pattern B trait is linked to several metabolic issues that help explain its atherogenicity and has been termed the Atherogenic Lipoprotein Profile (ALP). Pattern B is a term used to describe individuals with a predominance of small LDL particles compared to pattern A, which describes individuals with predominately large LDL particles. Small LDL particles are able to infiltrate the arterial wall approximately 40% to 50% faster than large LDL particles. These particles are more susceptible to oxidative damage, and the HDL subclass that is associated with low CV risk (FIDL2) is reduced in LDL pattern B subjects. Further, this trait is associated with significantly increased blood fats following a meal, increased plasminogen activator inhibitor 1 (PAI-I), low antioxidant lipoprotein content, increased susceptibility to oxidative damage, increased IDL, and increased insulin resistance and risk for the development of Type 2 diabetes (114–117). Elevated plasma triglycerides are often, but not always, associated with LDL pattern B, and epidemiological analysis has now identified elevated triglycerides as an independent coronary heart disease risk factor (118). Thus, the LDL pattern B trait is associated with a plethora of metabolic disorders, each contributing to increased CAD risk.

The dense LDL subclass pattern (ALP or LDL pattern B) is a heritable trait determined by a single major dominant gene (the alp locus) (119,120). The gene for this trait has been localized to chromosome #19 near the LDL receptor, and expression is affected by at least three other loci, the apo AI/CIII/AIV gene cluster on chromosome #11, the manganese super oxide dismutase gene on chromosome #6, and the CETP gene on chromosome #16 (121–123). There is no linkage with the LDL receptor gene. The full expression of this trait occurs following puberty in men and after menopause in women. Based on Hardy–Weinberg equilibrium, 30% to 35% of the Caucasian population is heterozygous for ALP, and another 5% are homozygous. The dense LDL subspecies is a marker for a common genetic trait that affects lipoprotein metabolism and increases CAD risk.

Low-density lipoprotein subclass distribution determination contributes information to CAD risk determination that is independent of TC and LDL-C. The Boston Area Health Study, the Physicians Health Survey, the Stanford Five City Project, and the Quebec Cardiovascular Study all confirmed that the presence of an abundance of small, dense LDL particles signifies an approximate three-fold increased risk for cardiovascular events (118,124–127). This is clinically important because this common genetically determined CAD risk factor is not reflected by measurement of LDL-C. It helps explain the incidence of CAD in patients who do not have classic hypercholesterolemia.

Seemingly contrary to the abundant evidence that small LDL is a significant risk factor is a report that larger LDL particles are associated with increased CHD risk and not small LDL. This report assessed baseline values only (as a percent distribution) and statistical adjustments for triglycerides and other variables associated with the small LDL trait were required to expose the relationship of CHD risk to larger LDL size (128). Contradicting this report are numerous studies supporting the independent role small, dense LDL plays in CV risk and the recent quantitation of small LDL-C further strengthens the role of small versus large LDL in CHD risk (129). Taken as a whole, the body of evidence supports the conclusion that an abundance of small LDL is a significant risk factor for CHD events. However, this does not exclude the role of larger LDL particles in CHD risk.

Carotid artery wall IMT has been reported to be a useful tool in predicting the risk for MI and stroke in older adults (130). Change in carotid artery IMT is correlated with change in the severity of CAD as assessed by coronary arteriography (131). Evidence that small LDL III plays a role in peripheral vascular disease is present using ultrasonography measure of carotid artery IMT. Investigators in Stockholm reported the relationship of small LDL-III to IMT progression in a group of healthy middle-aged mate subjects (132). Importantly, small LDL III had a significant relationship to IMT thickness ($r = 0.44$, $p < 0.001$) while LDL-C did not. Nicotinic acid is reported to preferentially reduce small LDLs compared to large LDLs (133). In another study utilizing IMT as an outcome variable, the addition of 1000 mg/day nicotinic acid to patients treated with an HMGCoA reductase inhibitor resulted in a significant reduction in carotid IMT-determined atherosclerosis progression (134).

Evidence that LDL heterogeneity is clinically important in determining arteriographic change over time is derived from several investigations. The NHLBI-II was the first investigation to report significantly less arteriographic progression in subjects with reduction in IDL and dense LDL (135). The Stanford Coronary Risk Intervention Project has revealed that individuals with predominantly dense LDLs in the control group had an approximate two-fold greater rate of arteriographic progression compared to patients with predominantly buoyant LDL, but with multi-factorial risk intervention. The patients with predominantly dense LDL did significantly better than patients with predominantly buoyant LDL in regard to arteriographic benefit (136). The risk of arteriographic progression is independently linked to the smallest of the LDL particles, LDL IVb (137). The St. Thomas Atheroma Regression Study (STARS) investigated the effect of a low fat diet and cholestyramine on arteriographic rates of progression in men with CAD and reported that a reduction in dense LDL was one of the best predictors of arteriographic benefit (138). The Familial Atherosclerosis Treatment Study reported that change in LDL buoyancy was the best predictor of arteriographic outcome in this investigation, which used colestipol + niacin, or colestipol + statin as treatment modalities (139).

The gold-standard laboratory method of determining lipoprotein subclass distribution is based on density as determined in the ANUC (4). This method employs a highly accurate and reproducible ultracentrifugation method that characterizes lipoprotein subclasses by floatation intervals. It is time consuming, expensive, and available only in a limited number of research laboratories. Non-denaturing GGE was developed as a less expensive method of determining lipoprotein subclass distribution (19). A rapid ultracentrifugation method, termed vertical auto profile (VAP), has been used to determine relative floatation index as a determination of change in LDL buoyancy (140). This method determines the cholesterol concentration of multiple lipoprotein fractions based on density. During profile decomposition, peak heights for predefined sub-curves for all classes are simultaneously varied until the sum of the squared deviations between the sum of the sub-curves and the parent profile is minimized using linear regression. A relatively new method used to estimate lipoprotein subclass distribution is nuclear magnetic resonance (NMR) (141). Signals are derived from methyl groups on phospholipids, cholesterol, cholesterol ester, and triglycerides. NMR assumes a constancy of lipid mass contained within a particle of given diameter and phospholipid composition and thus methyl lipid NMR signal. This system uses a library of reference spectra of lipoprotein subclasses incorporated into a linear least-square fitting computer program which works backward from the shape of the composite plasma methyl signal to compute the subclass signal intensities.

National standardization programs do not monitor the accuracy of lipoprotein subclass determination by any of these methods. A split sample assessment of the traditional enzymatic methods of determining lipoprotein cholesterol and the established GGE method of determining LDL subclass distribution, compared to VAP and NMR, revealed significant differences ($p < 0.001$) between methods for total cholesterol, triglycerides, LDL-C, HDL-C, Lp(a), and LDL and HDL subclass distribution (142). Other laboratory methods designed to accurately determine LDL and HDL subclass distribution are under development (143–145). These new methods may provide an accurate, rapid, and cost-effective means to determine subclass distribution in the hospital and clinical setting.

Individual Versus Group Determination of LDL Subclass Distribution

The presence of predominantly small LDL in large populations is often, but not always, associated with other physiologic parameters and laboratory measurements. Chief among these are fasting triglycerides, HDL-C (inversely), insulin, and body mass index. Use of these surrogate markers provides researchers an inexpensive method of assessing relative differences in large groups who are most likely to have a predominance of small or large LDL. However, within any of these surrogate marker groups, subgroups exist that have a greater or lesser probability of an individual having a predominance of small LDL. In general, the higher the triglyceride value the smaller the LDL size, and the lower the HDL-C the smaller the LDL size (Fig. 3). However, this relationship is most useful clinically when triglycerides are in excess of 250 mg/dL or less than 70 mg/dL and HDL-C is less than 40 mg/dL or greater than 70 mg/dL. The significant relationship between HDL-C and LDL size follows a similar but inverse relationship (Fig. 4). Higher HDL-C values are associated with larger LDL particles and lower HDL-C values with smaller LDL particles. The scatter plots in Figures 4 and 5 are based on 5366 patients with CAD examined at the

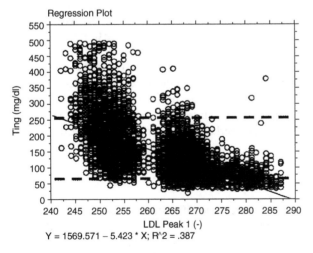

Figure 3 Scatter-plot of fasting triglycerides and LDL peak particle diameter in angstroms ($r = 0.62$, $p < 0.0001$) in 5366 CAD patients seen at the Fuqua Heart Center in Atlanta, Georgia. Large LDL particles have a diameter ≥ 263 angstroms and small LDL particles a diameter ≤ 257 angstroms.

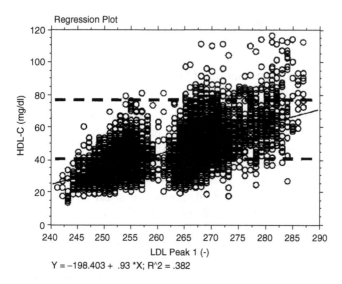

Figure 4   Scatter-plot of fasting HDL-C and LDL peak particle diameter in angstroms ($r = 0.62$, $p < 0.0001$) in 5366 CAD patients seen at the Fuqua Heart Center in Atlanta, Georgia. Large LDL particles have a diameter ≥ 263 angstroms and small LDL particles a diameter ≤ 257 angstroms.

Fuqua Heart Center in Atlanta, Georgia. In the case of fasting triglycerides, the significant correlation of fasting triglycerides to LDL peak particle diameter ($r = 0.62$, $p < 0.0001$) reveals a group with fasting triglycerides greater than 250 mg/dL that predominantly express small LDL (< 257 angstroms). Likewise, patients with fasting triglycerides less than 75 mg/dL predominantly express large LDL (> 262 angstroms). However, when fasting triglycerides are less than 250 mg/dL and greater than 75 mg/dL, a significant overlap exists between individual patients with predominantly large or small LDL particles, which makes fasting triglycerides, in this range, unreliable for clinical decision making in an individual patient. A similar overlap occurs for HDL-C and LDL size as illustrated in Figure 4.

HDL Subclass Distribution

There are three basic methods to determine HDL subclass distribution: density, size, and apolipoprotein content. Based on the relative density obtained in the analytic ultracentrifuge, the more dense, relatively cholesterol-poor form is termed HDL3 (1.125 to 1.21 G per mL) and the less dense, relatively cholesterol-rich form is termed HDL2 (1.062 to 1.125 G per mL) (20). GGE can be used to characterize the distribution of HDL particles based on size (146). Sequential immunoaffinity chromatography can isolate two HDL subclasses defined by their apo A-I and A-II content as those with A-I only and those with AI and AII (AI:AII) (147). A relationship exists between HDL subclasses as determined by all three methods. HDL2a and HDL3b as determined by GGE contain both apo A-I and A-II, while HDL2b and HDL3c contain apo A-I only (147). The cardiovascular benefit of these particles may also be related to the ability of apo A-I to reduce VCAM-1 expression and damage that results in neointimal proliferation (148). In patients with low HDL-C and documented CAD the Lp(A-I) particle has been correlated with phospholipid transfer protein, which may also play a role in determining Lp(A-I) levels (149).

While low total HDL-C is an established CAD risk factor in epidemiological investigations, differences in HDL subclass distribution (proportion of HDL2 versus HDL3) exist within the "normal" HDL-C range and may contribute to CAD risk in individuals with "normal" HDL-C values. Low HDL2b has been linked to both arteriographically determined CAD severity and arteriographic progression of CAD (150,151). While focus has been mainly placed on low HDL-C and low HDL2b as a risk factor for CAD, it is of interest to note that the cardio protection in high HDL-C patients appears to also be related to differences in HDL subclass. HALP (very elevated HDL-C values) that is primarily HDL2 or HDL A-I only is also associated with decreased HL activity and cardio protection, while those that have high HDL-C values but are primarily composed of A-I:A-II exhibit less protection (152). In the FATS and HATS investigations, increases in HDL2-C, and/or the HDL A-I only particle were one of the best predictors of improvement in coronary stenosis and in HATS were associated with a reduction in clinical events (46). Finally, the inheritance of HDL subclasses has revealed correlations among family members for specific HDL subclasses, which are independent of HDL cholesterol and apo A-I (153).

Lipoprotein a

When apo [a] is attached to apo B and LDL, the particle is termed lipoprotein (a), or Lp(a) for short. Apo [a] is a protein with structural similarities to plasminogen (154). The importance of this lipoprotein lies in its strong independent association with coronary heart disease and carotid atherosclerosis. Elevated levels may be present in as many as 20–40% of individuals with CAD. This finding may help to explain why some patients with relatively normal blood LDL-C and HDL-C values still suffer from atherosclerosis.

Rapid progression of arteriographically quantitated CAD has been reported to be significantly more common in subjects with Lp(a) > 25 mg/dL (155). Lp(a) has been reported to be an independent risk factor for myocardial infarction in young men, is independently associated with arteriographically defined coronary disease, and has been reported to be more closely linked to the extent of coronary atherosclerosis than other lipid parameters (156–158). This inherited disorder appears to increase CAD risk, particularly in the presence of more traditional risk factors such as elevated LDL-C and low HDL-C (159). The presence of elevated

Lp(a) (> fifth quintile) has been reported to significantly increase the future risk of angina approximately three-fold and the combination of elevated LDL-C and elevated Lp(a) increases the risk 12-fold (160). The contribution of elevated LDL-C to increased CHD risk associated with elevated Lp(a) has been observed in several investigations (161–163). The contribution of low HDL-C and elevated Lp(a) to atherogenic risk has also been reported (164).

Most studies investigating the atherogenic potential of elevated Lp(a) have been conducted in large population samples of middle age. Recently the role of elevated Lp(a) in men and women > 65 years of age was reported from the Cardiovascular Health Study (165). Those with Lp(a) in the highest quintile had three times the risk of stroke and death associated with vascular events.

Lp(a) isoforms exist that represent a range of different [a] sizes (166). The smaller the [a] isoform, the greater the associated atherogenecity. Lp(a) size has an inverse relationship with Lp(a) concentration so that higher Lp(a) values are associated with small Lp(a) isoforms. The Physician's Health Study has reported that in apo(a) size is an independent predictor of angina regardless of Lp(a) concentration (160). In the Stanford Five City Project, Lp(a) size was found to be predictive of CAD risk in men but not women (167). Lp(a) size difference may help explain why elevated Lp(a) values reflect greater CAD risk in caucasian men compared to African American men. Gender differences may also exist since it has been reported that Lp(a) size is associated with CAD in African American men but not women (168).

Laboratory methods to determine Lp(a) are varied and clinical use hindered by the lack of standardization and accuracy (169). Commercially available methods use antibodies that recognize kringle 4 type 2 repeated epitopes, which are not specific for apo(a) size. A reference ELISA method has been developed that utilizes apo(a) kringle 4 type 9 that is unaffected by apo(a) size (170).

One emerging aspect of Lp(a) atherogenecity involves the potential to adversely interfere with natural thrombolysis (171). Elevated Lp(a) in combination with resistance to activated protein C attributed to the factor V Leiden mutation, and is associated with an odds ratio of 30 for stroke in children. The combination of elevated Lp(a) with any thrombophilic risk factor appears to increase the risk of a thromboembolic event by 2.6 and increases to 6.2 when the Leiden V mutation is present (172).

While the evidence that Lp(a) has a strong link to CAD and PVD is abundant, the clinical evidence that reducing Lp(a) is beneficial is sparse, due to a lack of clinical trials designed to test the hypothesis that reduction of Lp(a) results in a reduction in clinical events. However, some evidence derived from retrospective analysis exists. Reduction of Lp(a) following apheresis has been associated with a significant reduction in restenosis following PTCA (173). Most recently, reduction of Lp(a) in postmenopausal women with elevated Lp(a) has been associated with a significant 17% reduction in CV events and the authors reported Lp(a) to be an independent and modifiable risk factor for CAD events in postmenopausal women with known CAD (174). The treatment in this investigation was hormone replacement therapy (HRT). Of particular interest in regard to the atherogenecity of elevated Lp(a) associated with elevated LDL-C is the retrospective evidence from FATS suggesting that significant reduction of LDL-C in patients with elevated Lp(a) may retard the rate of arteriographic progression and blunt the adverse affect of elevated Lp(a) (175).

Apolipoprotein B and Hyperapobetalipoproteinemia

LDL cholesterol values are commonly determined by a precipitation method, which results in an LDL cholesterol concentration value but no information in regard to the absolute number of LDL particles. Each LDL particle contains one apoprotein B, and determination of plasma LDL apoprotein B values allows the determination of LDL particle number. It has been suggested that measurement of apo B may be a more reliable indicator of LDL particle number and of more clinical utility than the standard calculated LDL-C value (176). In the setting of normolipemia, plasma apo B values are consistently lower than the LDL-C value. However, the condition described as hyperapobetalipoproteinemia exists in which the apo B value is higher than predicted based on the LDL-C value (177). A remarkable high incidence of hyperapobetalipoproteinemia (81%) has been reported in the post-MI population that exhibits relatively "normal" LDL-C values yet have disproportionately elevated LDL apo B (178). Individuals with this condition have an overabundance of small, dense LDL particles that are similar to those noted in patients with FCH and patients shown to have more progression of CAD demonstrated on arteriography (179). This condition appears to be due to increased apoprotein B-100 synthesis and transmitted as a dominant trait. Incorporation of fatty acids into lipid esters appears to be decreased, which results in abnormal processing of dietary fat and postprandial increases in free fatty acids. Thus, in this relatively common disorder, several abnormalities in lipoprotein metabolism that are not reflected in the LDL-C measurement could contribute to CAD risk.

The clinical importance of determining apo B values lies not only in the identification of hyperapobetalipoproteinemia, but in the association of elevated apo B with other cardiovascular risk predictors that result in identification of a group of patients at extremely high risk for cardiovascular events. The Quebec Cardiovascular Study investigated the relationship of small LDL, elevated fasting insulin values, and apo B in relation to CAD risk. Each abnormality individually contributed to CAD risk as demonstrated in previous investigations. However, in the Quebec Cardiovascular Study, the combination of all three abnormalities (an abundance of small LDL, elevated fasting insulin, and elevated apo B) identified a group of individuals who were at a 20-fold increased risk for cardiovascular events (179). In the new millennium of cardiovascular risk prediction, it is important to assess multiple risk determinants, since interaction between various metabolic abnormalities has important implications for accurate risk prediction and treatment that are not apparent from standard blood cholesterol measurements.

Apo E Polymorphism

The most common gene affecting LDL cholesterol levels is apo E, which has three major genotypes, or isoforms, designated as E2, E3, and E4 (180). The most common allele, E3, has a frequency of approximately 0.78, while E4 has a frequency of 0.15, and E2 a frequency of 0.07 (181). While these are the most common genotypes, analysis of amino acid substitution has revealed at least 25 mutations in apolipoprotein E. The plasma lipoprotein profile that results from genotype differences relates to the greater fractional catabolic rate of LDL in individuals with the apo E2 genotype compared to those with the common apo E3 (182). This is consistent with the suggestion that hepatic LDL receptor activity is relatively higher in individuals with apo E2 because of decreased uptake of apo E2 containing triglyceride-rich lipoproteins, which results in less suppression of LDL receptors (183). Conversely, fractional catabolic rate of LDL is reduced in individuals with the apo E4 genotype, and this appears to be related to enhanced clearance of apo E4–containing remnants and suppression of LDL receptors. The disease, type III hyperlipoproteinemia, is an example of an interaction of the apo E2 homozygous state with another genetic or environmental factor leading to marked accumulation of triglyceride-rich lipoprotein remnants and accelerated atherosclerosis. Over 90% of individuals with type III hyperlipoproteinemia are apo E2 homozygotes. However, the disease is caused by interaction of the apo E2/E2 state with another genetic or environmental factor because while about 1% of the population expresses the E2/E2 isoform, only 2% of these develop type III hyperlipidemia and most individuals with E2/E2 do not exhibit the abnormal lipid profile.

Apo E isoforms explain part of individual differences in LDL-C response to a reduced fat diet. Men with the apo E3/E4 pattern respond to a reduced fat diet with significantly greater LDL-C reduction compared to men with the apo E3/E3 pattern (184). A differential effect of reduced fat diet–induced reduction in LDL appears to affect large LDL particles greater in individuals with the apo E4 allele and least in E3/E2 subjects, indicating the reduction in large LDL is mediated by an apo E–dependent mechanism. Because of this, diet-induced LDL-C reduction may have a variable benefit in individuals with different E genotypes and LDL subclass patterns (185). Postprandial lipid metabolism differences also exist between E3/E4 and E3/E3 subjects. Subjects with the E4 allele have enhanced postprandial lipemia, which may contribute to increased CAD risk (186).

Apo E isoforms can be of use in CAD risk prediction. The Etude Cas-Temoins sur l'Infarctus du Myocarde (ECTIM) study reported a relative risk for MI of 1.33 ($p=0.02$) for subjects carrying the E4 allele, which explained approximately 12% of MI cases in the populations studied (187). This finding is consistent with the European Atherosclerosis Research Study in which the population adjusted odds ratios for the phenotype E4/E3 and E4/E4 were 1.16 and 1.33, respectively, and it was concluded that the apo E polymorphism is one major factor responsible for the familial predisposition to CAD (188). However, the E4 genotype has recently been associated with Alzheimer's disease risk. In families with a history of Alzheimer's disease, the presence of the E4 allele increases the risk for developing Alzheimer's disease, but the interaction is probably complex and may involve interaction with the amyloid B protein precursor gene on chromosome 21q (189). It has been recommended that the Apo E4 test not be used for the prediction of Alzheimer's disease risk (190).

Cholesteryl Ester Transfer Protein Dysfunction

CETP mediates the exchange of triglycerides from VLD/LDL particles for cholesterol ester in HDL particles. This activity may be either proatherogenic, if it results in the transferred cholesterol ester being taken up by the arterial wall macrophages, or antiatherogenic, if the transferred cholesterol ester is removed through the hepatic apo B receptor. Disorders of CETP function led to the development of medications that inhibit CETP and result in an increase in HDL-C (191). In the rabbit model, inhibition of CETP activity with a vaccine or a pharmacologic approach has been shown to reduce atherosclerotic lesions (192,193). Total inhibition of CETP activity in families appears to be associated with increased CVD risk compared to partial inhibition that may reduce CVD risk (194). This may be due to the production of large, cholesterol-rich dysfunctional HDL particles when CETP activity is completely inhibited.

ATP Binding Cassette Transporter 1

Cholesterol efflux from cells is regulated in part by the ABC1 transporter (195). It serves to efflux cholesterol from an intracellular location to lipid-poor apo A-I and forms nascent HDL particles, which can then be converted into mature HDL particles by the action of LCAT. The important role of ABC1 in lipoprotein metabolism and atherosclerosis was discovered through the investigation of the low HDL-C disorder described as Tangier disease and now known to be the result of ABC1 mutations. In order to efflux cholesterol from cells, specific amphipathic helical structures of apoproteins must interact with ABC1. This knowledge has resulted in the production of amphipathic apo A-I mimetic peptides of 18–36 amino acids long that stimulate cholesterol efflux via the ABC1 pathway (196). ABC1 activity can be regulated by several environmental issues including sterols, retinoids, thiazolidinediones, and unsaturated fatty acids (197).

The end result of manipulating ABC1 activity on the atherosclerositic process in humans remains to be elucidated. Overexpression of hepatic ABC1 transporter could increase atherosclerosis by increasing flux into apo B–containing atherogenic particles, or assist in the removal of cholesterol from lipid laden plaques. Overexpression of the ABC1 transporter in mice has been reported to result in decreased diet-induced atherosclerosis (198).

Metabolic Syndrome

The metabolic syndrome combines aspects of lipid disorders, insulin resistance, hypertension, and thrombosis (199). Disorders of lipid metabolism are found in a majority of these patients. Forty-eight percent of metabolic syndrome patients exhibit elevations in plasma triglycerides (>150 mg/dL) compared to 10% of individuals without the metabolic syndrome, and 85% exhibit low HDL-C (<40 mg/dL in men and <50 mg/dL in women) (200). The metabolic disorders associated with the small LDL trait outlined above match many of the characteristics of the "metabolic syndrome." This cardiovascular health threat is rapidly enlarging the population at risk for CAD as can be seen from the startling increase in individuals defined as obese (200). In 1980 14.5% of the U.S. population was determined to be obese and in 2002 this had increased to 31% (201).

ADVANCES IN TREATMENT

Diet

Low fat diets have been recommended as the foundation for treating lipid disorders that involve elevations in LDL-C (99). However, when diets are reduced in fat content, the eliminated fat calories are frequently replaced by calories derived from simple carbohydrates and elevations in plasma triglycerides are often observed. Low fat, high carbohydrate diets have been investigated in regard to LDL and HDL subclass distribution. Dreon and colleagues initially reported that an isocaloric reduction in the percent of fat calories from 46% to 20% resulted in a significant reduction in LDL-C and apo B in subjects with predominantly small LDL, but unexpectedly, 40% of the subjects who exhibited a predominance of large LDL on the 46% fat diet converted to predominantly small LDL on the 20% fat diet (202). This was attributed to the increase of simple carbohydrates in the isocaloric lower fat diet. Further studies by Dreon and colleagues revealed that reduction of total calories from 20% to 10% has no effect on standard lipid measurements or LDL and HDL subclass distribution in individuals classified as very unlikely to carry the small LDL trait based on family history. However, patients who were predominantly large LDL but had the potential to express small LDL revealed no change in LDL-C or total LDL mass, but a significant increase in small, dense LDL balanced by a significant reduction in large, buoyant LDL accompanied by a dramatic reduction in HDL2 (203). This suggests that dietary advice to reduce calories from fat, without attention to the source of replacement calories, may be detrimental to individuals who carry the ALP trait. One popular new diet that reflects a Mediterranean diet influence has been shown to shift LDL subclass distribution towards the less atherogenic large LDL region (204).

Exercise/Weight Loss

Exercise and associated fat weight loss can have a significant effect on reducing small, dense LDL and increasing HDL2 (205). These investigations have indicated that reductions in small LDL, induced by loss of excess body fat, are accompanied by increases in large LDL for no net change in total LDL mass or LDL-C. This effect on LDL and HDL subclass distribution appears to be linked to loss of excess body fat, which can be induced by either dietary caloric restriction or increased exercise caloric expenditure (206).

Nicotinic Acid

Nicotinic acid has been reported to have a differential effect on LDL subclass distribution in subjects classified as having predominantly large or small LDL (207). In response to nicotinic acid, the reduction in small, dense LDL is counterbalanced by less of an increase in large, buoyant LDL, which results in an LDL-C reduction that does not reflect the greater reduction in small LDL (208). Similarly, nicotinic acid has a significant effect on increasing HDL2 that is greater than appreciated from the change in HDL-C. The nicotinic acid–induced increase in HDL2 is due to a reduction in the removal rate of HDL2 particles (209). Niacin selectively and directly inhibits hepatic diacylglycerol acyltransferase 2, but not diacylglycerol acyltransferase 1, thus inhibiting hepatic triglyceride synthesis and VLDL secretion. The recent discovery and characterization of a membrane-bound nicotinic acid receptor (HM74) explains niacin's acute inhibition of adipocyte lipolysis, but the role of HM74 in lowering triglycerides is unclear. Niacin possesses antioxidant, anti-inflammatory, and other beneficial effects on atherosclerosis unrelated to lipid lowering.

Fibric Acid Derivatives (Gemibrozil and Fenoibrate)

In general, fibrates reduce small LDL, particularly when elevated triglycerides are reduced, and they may increase HDL2. However, different fibrates can have different effects on HDL subclass distribution. Gemfibrozil has been shown to reduce small, dense LDL significantly in subjects with predominantly small LDL but has little to no effect on small LDL in subjects who have predominantly large LDL (84,210). A similar effect of fenofibrate on increasing LDL peak particle diameter has been reported (211). This effect of fibrates on LDL and HDL subclass distribution may have implications for the interpretation of the VA-HIT study that associated an increase in HDL-C, attributed to gemfibrozil treatment, with fewer cardiovascular events (83). The Diabetes Atherosclerosis Intervention Study (DAIS) showed that treatment with fenofibrate decreases progression of coronary atherosclerosis in subjects with type 2 diabetes (212). LDL size increased significantly more in the fenofibrate group than in the placebo group ($p < 0.001$) and small LDL was significantly associated with progression of CAD.

HMGCoA Reductase Inhibitors

The effect of HMGCoA reductase inhibitors including pravastatin, lovastatin, simvastatin, and fluvastatin has been investigated using GGE and no significant differential effect on LDL subclass distribution has been reported (213–217). A pilot study of atorvastatin has reported that in patients with elevated fasting triglycerides, atorvastatin has a statistically significant effect on reducing the small LDL subtraction IIIa (218). In a small study of patients with chronic renal failure, atorvastatin significantly increased LDL size (219).

CETP Inibition

Inhibition of CETP activity can result in increased HDL-C and may improve reverse cholesterol transport. Partial CETP inhibition appears to provide some CVD protection in animals. Anti-CETP antibodies increase HDL-C and reduce aortic atherosclerosis in rabbits, and the use of the CETP inhibitor JTT-705 increased HDL-C two-fold, which was associated with reduced atherosclerosis in rabbits (220,221). However, the use of JTT-705 in rabbits fed a high cholesterol diet resulted in no atherosclerosis benefit (222).

Two CETP inhibitor agents have been tried in human subjects: JTT-705, and torce trapib. Initial small human trials with torcetrapib have revealed a 16% to 91% increase in HDL-C when doses of 10 mg to 240 mg/day are utilized (223). In patients with low HDL-C (< 40 mg/dL) 120 mg–240 mg/day resulted in a 46% to 106% increase in HDL-C with an associated increase in mean HDL particle size (224).

Lipid Drug Combinations

Combination lipid drug therapy can produce dramatic improvement in the lipoprotein abnormalities associated with combined hyperlipidemia (225). In regard to LDL subclass distribution, combinations of lipid lowering medications that have been reported to have a beneficial effect on LDL subclass distribution include pravastatin + niacin, niacin + resin, and niacin + gemfibrozil (226–228). Combination drug therapy has been used in numerous successful clinical trials including CLAS, SCRIP, SCOR, FATS, and HATS.

Alpha- and Beta-Blockers

Selective and nonselective beta-blocker medications are known to be associated with an increase in triglycerides and a reduction in HDL-C (229). The effect on triglycerides and HDL-C is accompanied by an increase in small, dense LDL counterbalanced by a reduction in large, buoyant LDL particles (230). The reduction in HDL-C induced by nonselective beta blockade is also associated with reductions in the HDL2 distribution (231). The alpha-blocker prazosin is associated with mild reductions in triglycerides and increases in HDL-C, which are further associated with reductions in small, dense LDL counterbalanced by increases in large, buoyant LDL particles.

Hormone Replacement Therapy

The hormonal components of oral contraceptives exert major effects on plasma lipoprotein metabolism that suggests that hormone replacement therapy in postmenopausal women may impact lipoprotein subclass distribution (232). HRT may be beneficial in postmenopausal women for a variety of reasons and have a differential effect in different subsets of postmenopausal women (233). Treatment with 0.625 mg/day conjugated equine estrogen and 2.5 mg/day medroxyprogesterone in postmenopausal women has been reported to have a significantly greater effect on reducing LDL-C and apo B in postmenopausal women with a predominance of small LDL compared to women with a predominance of large LDL (234). This reduction in LDL-C was accompanied by a significant reduction in small dense LDL, increase in HDL2, and increase in LPL. Postmenopausal women in the highest quartile for Lp(a) have been reported to have a significant reduction in cardiovascular events associated with a reduction in Lp(a) attributed to the HRT (174).

Novel Treatments

Novel therapeutic approaches to optimizing lipoprotein metabolism in order to treat atherosclerosis involve immunization, recombinant HDL, peptide infusion, and gene transfection. In mice, a recombinant adenovirus was constructed in which the human LCAT cDNA was expressed under the control of the human cytomegalovirus immediate/early promoter followed by a chimeric intron (AdCMV human LCAT), which resulted in overexpression of LCAT and a 580% increase in HDL-C and a 149% increase in human apo A-I (235). A CETP vaccine has been used in phase I human trials and reported to develop anti-CETP antibodies in 58% of the human subjects (236). In a rabbit model of atherosclerosis, production of anti-CETP antibodies reduced atherosclerosis by 48% (237).

Human apo A-I transgenic mice have shown a significant inhibition of early atherosclerosis (238). This may be related to alterations in the efficiency of reverse cholesterol transport. Infusion of recombinant apo A-I Milano has been shown in apo E deficient mice to increase cholesterol efflux capacity 60% in one hour and reduce plaque lipid content 50% in 48 hours (239). A small investigation in humans that employed intravascular ultrasound as an outcome variable, reported that infusion of a recombinant apo A-I Milano phospholipids complex significantly reduced atheroma thickness following five weekly injections (240). These novel approaches to therapy illustrate the future role of lipoprotein metabolism manipulation as possible treatment modalities for atherosclerosis.

ROLE OF NONINVASIVE TESTS

While the presence of circulating atherogenic lipoproteins is an expression of a disorder phenotype, it is the development of atherosclerosis disease in the vessel wall that leads to clinical cardiovascular syndromes. Thus, the detection of subclinical atherosclerosis and the noninvasive visualization of plaque composition in the vessel wall are critical in the prevention of cardiovascular disease.

Traditional models of assessing atherosclerosis have grown out of large longitudinal databases and rely on calculating the likelihood of atherosclerosis based on the presence or absence of known atherosclerotic risk factors. Thus, when faced with a given patient, one can calculate the probability of disease by using phenotypic blood markers. However, whether or not atherosclerosis is truly present in an individual cannot be determined from these models. Noninvasive imaging methodologies of atherosclerosis directly visualize disease, thus moving the assessment of atherosclerosis from the paradigm of probability to the paradigm of certainty.

The presence or absence of atherosclerosis can assist with treatment decisions when faced with an asymptomatic individual with a risk factor profile that reflects increased CHD probability. Furthermore, the same noninvasive imaging approaches can be used in individuals to follow the effectiveness of treatment over time. Finally, these imaging endpoints can be used in clinical trials investigating novel therapeutic approaches to modulate atherosclerosis.

Non-Coronary Arterial Beds

Several imaging modalities can be used to visualize atherosclerosis in non-coronary beds. Carotid intima-media thickness (CIMT) is a simple, easy-to-perform method that can be implemented in the outpatient setting and measures the thickness of the posterior wall of the common carotid artery or the internal carotid artery in a standardized fashion. Although not imaging lipoproteins directly, CIMT can visualize atherosclerotic plaques. Both absolute CIMT and change in CIMT over time have been validated in predicting major cardiovascular endpoints (241,242). One of the challenges of CIMT is its dependence on the operator and its relatively low reproducibility, making CIMT an excellent research tool in large populations, but rendering it less reliable in individual patients. Another limitation of CIMT is that it is a one-dimensional evaluation of the three-dimensional process of atherosclerosis.

More recently, cardiovascular magnetic resonance (CMR) has been introduced as a noninvasive modality to image atherosclerosis, since it has many theoretical advantages. First, it is a three-dimensional technique and can therefore more accurately assess atherosclerotic plaque volume. Furthermore, CMR is capable of tissue characterization based on intrinsic signal property differences using different imaging pulse sequences. The most common approach is referred to as a "multi-spectral" approach, where an atherosclerotic plaque is imaged with a combination of T1-weighted, T2-weighted, and other pulse sequences and different plaque components are evaluated based on the different signal characteristics with different pulse sequences. For example, intra-plaque lipids are characteristically bright on T1-weighted images and dark on T2-weighted images. Moreover, the signal characteristics of lipoproteins are determined by the oxidative state and the surrounding molecular milieu. Such approaches can be used to quantify the relative content of different tissue components in plaques.

This multi-spectral approach has been validated in humans in vivo and has been shown to be quite accurate in classifying human carotid atherosclerotic plaques based on a modified AHA-classification using histology of surgically removed carotid endarterectomy specimens as reference standards (243). The thickness of the fibrous cap in carotid plaques can also be evaluated and has been shown to predict symptomatic patients (244). Injection of gadolinium-based contrast agents can further enhance plaque characterization by highlighting neo-vascularization and inflammation in plaques (245,246).

More novel plaque imaging approaches rely on molecular or cellular targeting approaches. Fibrin-specific gadolinium-based contrast agents are being developed for thrombus imaging and activated macrophages can be detected by their selective uptake of iron oxide–based MR contrast agents (247,248). While these CMR-based approaches are very promising in non-coronary vascular beds, their implementation is much more challenging in the coronary arteries, although some groups have reported some success (249).

Coronary Arterial Beds

Although intra-vascular ultrasound (IVUS) has made significant contributions to the understanding of plaque remodeling in atherosclerosis, it is invasive and is beyond the scope of this review. Of the noninvasive modalities, cardiovascular computed tomography (CCT) has emerged as a major tool in atherosclerosis imaging in the coronary arteries.

Coronary Artery Calcium

The evaluation of coronary artery calcium (CAC) has been validated in large patient populations, primarily utilizing electron-beam computed tomography (EBCT) approaches. More recently, multi-slice CT, which is much more widely available, has been shown to be equally accurate and reproducible in the assessment of CAC. The predictive value of CAC has been validated in large patient populations and has been shown to have independent and incremental predictive value over the traditional cardiovascular risk factors (250,251). CAC distribution tables have been created and each patient's percentile can be determined based on age and gender. CAC establishes the diagnosis of CAD and moves patients into a secondary prevention category.

Coronary Artery Computed Tomography Angiography

The introduction of the 64-detector CT technology and fast gantry rotation speeds have allowed for greatly improved spatial resolution ($400\mu \times 400\mu$ isotopic resolution) and temporal resolution (~ 160 ms), putting coronary artery computed tomography angiography (CCTA) in competitive range with invasive X-ray angiography. The accuracy of this technology has been recently validated using quantitative X-ray angiography as a reference standard, revealing a sensitivity of 99%, specificity of 95%, positive predictive value of 76%, and negative predictive value of 99% on a per-segment basis (252). The superior sensitivity and negative predictive value make this technique very attractive as an initial imaging tool in the evaluation of patients for obstructive CAD.

A very exciting aspect of CCTA is its ability to detect even non-obstructive, non-calcified atherosclerotic plaques in the coronary arteries. There is tremendous interest in developing strategies directed toward the treatment of these plaques to prevent plaque rupture and subsequent acute coronary syndromes. The 64-detector CCT technology was recently validated against IVUS and was shown to be very accurate in the noninvasive assessment of basic atherosclerotic plaque composition (253). Studies are ongoing at our institution to evaluate the role of CCTA in the assessment of non-obstructive coronary atherosclerotic plaques.

Evaluation of Treatment Effects Using Noninvasive Imaging

CIMT imaging has been used to study the effect of statin treatment on carotid plaque remodeling and showed that more aggressive LDL lowering with a potent statin was more effective in slowing atherosclerosis progression, compared to a less potent statin (254). Furthermore, it has been shown using CIMT that HDL reduction with nicotinic acid resulted in plaque regression, while LDL lowering with a potent statin only induced slowing or halting of progression (255) (Table 2).

CAC evaluation by EBCT has been used to follow treatment with different lipid-modifying medications that have shown minimal or no effect on coronary artery calcification. This suggests that calcification is a late and irreversible process in atherosclerosis. Coronary artery CTA is very promising in the evaluation of changes in plaque characteristics over time. These studies are currently under way.

CMR has been used to study changes in atherosclerotic plaque volume over time in patients treated with simvastatin for two years (256–258). In this study, statin therapy reduced vessel wall area by 15% at 12 months and by 18% at 24 months. Furthermore, there was a significant 5% increase in luminal area at 24 months. Importantly, these changes in vessel wall area were caused by a reduction in maximal wall thickness rather than in minimal wall thickness, indicating a negative (beneficial) remodeling of the atherosclerotic plaque. CMR

Table 2 Recent Advances in the Understanding of the Role of Apoproteins in Lipid Metabolism and Atherosclerosis

Name	Chylomicron	VLDL	IDL	LDL	HDL	Primary function
AI	X				X	Activates LCAT
AII	X				X	Influences HDL functional states
AIV	X				X	Satiety signal
B100		X	X	X		Hepatic receptor uptake
B48	X					Dietary fat adsorption
CII	X	X	X		X	Activates LPL
CIII	X	X	X		X	Inhibits LPL
D					X	Transporter of small, hydrophobic ligands
E	X	X	X		X	Ligand for LDL receptors

The primary particle associated with each apoprotein and its primary metabolic function is listed.

is not only able to follow atherosclerotic plaque volume, but also plaque composition over time. In a case–control study from the FATS database it was demonstrated that aggressive triple lipid lowering therapy was associated with significantly fewer plaque lipid components (1% vs. 17%) and significantly more fibrous tissue (84% vs. 77%), compared to placebo (259).

Noninvasive imaging of atherosclerosis is starting to play an important role in the comprehensive evaluation of patients at risk for cardiovascular disease. It complements the evaluation of lipoprotein disorders by providing a phenotypical evaluation of disease expression in the arterial wall. At our institution, we routinely use coronary artery plaque characterization by coronary CTA and carotid arterial plaque characterization by CMR in asymptomatic patients with atherogenic lipoprotein phenotypes.

CONCLUSION

The dawn of the 21st century has witnessed a profound revolution in our understanding of atherosclerosis and the role of metabolic disorders other than the traditional hyperlipidemias. This revolution includes new understanding of the role of apoproteins, metabolic fat processing, and a dramatic expansion of clinical aspects of multiple lipoprotein subclasses that until recently were lumped under one name. This is most clinically applicable in the role small, dense LDL particles and HDL2 play in atherosclerosis progression, stability, and regression. It can no longer be assumed that a "normal" LDL-C reflects a normal CAD risk

Table 3 Prevalence of Metabolic Disorders Contributing to CAD in 1489 Subjects with Established CAD Seen by Invasive Cardiologists

	All	NCEP-NL	NCEP-HR	p
N	1489	874 (59%)	615 (41%)	
LDL IIIa + b > 20%	50.1%	44.3%	54.1%	0.005
LDL PPD (A) < 257 A	32.2%	20.4%	43.3%	0.0001
HDL2b < 20%	55.2%	42.1%	73.0%	0.0001
Insulin > 12 uU/ml	23.2%	17.0%	26.4%	0.008
Lp(a) > 25 mg/dl	25.0%	25.1%	22.0%	0.29
Hcy > 14 (umol/l)	10.0%	11.3%	9.2%	0.32
Fibrinogen > 350 mg/dl	37.9%	36.7%	41.5%	0.25
hs-CRP > 0.40 mg/dl	29.5%	27.8%	31.8%	0.42

The prevalence is presented for the entire group and for the group who were at high CAD risk (NCEP-HR) according to ATP-III LDL-C (LDL-C < 100 mg/dL) and HDL-C (HDL-C > 40 mg/dL), and those who were normal risk (NCEP-NL).

status. Disorders other than LDL-C concentrations are common in the CAD population. One thousand four hundred eighty nine patients seen by invasive cardiologists associated with the Fuqua Heart Center in Atlanta, Georgia, were examined in regard to the prevalence of these disorders in patients who met ATP-III LDL-C and HDL-C goals (n = 874) and those who did not (n = 615) (Table 3). An abundance of small LDL was found in 50.1% of the entire population with 44.3% of the patients who met ATP-III goals expressing an abundance of small LDL compared to 54.1% of those who did not. Seventeen percent of the patients who met ATP-III goals exhibited elevated insulin levels compared to 26.4% of those who did not. This higher incidence of small LDL and insulin levels in patients who do not meet ATP-III goals is expected due to the association of the small LDL trait with low HDL-C. However, metabolic disorders not linked to the small LDL trait, nor to plasma cholesterol values, show no difference in incidence in groups who did and did not meet ATP-III LDL-C and HDL-C goals. These issues include elevated Lp(a), elevated homocysteine, elevated fibrinogen, and elevated hs-CRP. In the group that met ATP LDL-C and HDL-C goals, 83.2% had one or more of the metabolic disorders listed above. This has clinical relevance since it has been reported that 45% of patients with CAD, as defined by the presence of coronary calcification, met ATP-III lipid goals (243).

This level of sophistication in the understanding of lipoproteins and CAD is important to clinicians for several reasons. The knowledge allows significantly more accuracy in predicting both primary and secondary risk for clinical events and disease progression or regression. It allows an explanation for the presence of CAD in patients with few to no traditional CAD risk factors. With this knowledge, individual patient treatment goals can be established that create the optimal milieu in which to achieve improved outcomes similar to those reported in multiple National Institute of Health (NIH)-funded arteriographic investigations. Since many of these disorders are inherited in a dominant fashion, family members can be identified who carry the trait(s) and appropriate noninvasive testing can be recommended. Most importantly, this knowledge allows selection of the most appropriate medication for the individual patient and avoids the issue of treating all patients as if they were in a large clinical trial, an approach that ignores individual variability. Once therapy is initiated, this knowledge allows patient monitoring as lifestyle and pharmacologic treatments take effect and are modified. Intelligent application of detailed knowledge of lipoprotein metabolism and noninvasive test results will contribute to improved patient care now and in the future.

REFERENCES

1. Ignatowsky IA. Influence de la nourriture animale sur l'organisme des lapins. Arch Med Exp Anat Pathol 1908; 20:1–20.
2. Anitschkow N, Chalatow S. Uber experimentelle cholesterinteatose and ihre beduting fur die entstehung einiger pathologische prozesse. Zentralbl Allg Pathol 1913; 24:1.
3. Aschoff L. Lectures in Pathology. New York: Hueber, 1924.
4. Gofman JW, Young W, Tandy R. Ischemic heart disease, atherosclerosis and longevity. Circulation 1966; 34:679–697.
5. Krauss RM. Atherogenicity of triglyceride-rich lipoproteins. Am J Cardiol 1998; 81:13B–17B.
6. Superko HR. What can we learn about dense LDL and lipoprotein particles from clinical trials? Current opinion in lipidology 1996; 7:363–368.
7. Nishina PM, Johnson JP, Naggert JK, Krauss RM. Linkage of atherogenic lipoprotein phenotype to the low-density lipoprotein receptor locus on the short arm of chromosome 19. Proc Natl Acad Sci USA 1992; 89:708–712.
8. Zhao XQ, Kosinski AJS, Barnhart HX, Superko HR, King SB. Prediction of native coronary artery disease progression following PTCA or CABG in the emory angioplasty verus surgery trial. Med Sci Monit 2003; 9:48–54.
9. Chapman MJ. The potential role of HDL- and LDL-cholesterol modulation in atheromatous plaque development. Curr Med Res Opin 2005; 21:S17–S22.
10. Deckelaum RJ, Olivecrona T, Eisenberg S. Plasma lipoproteins in hyperlipidemia: roles of neutral lipid exchange and lipase. In: Carlson LA, Olsson AG, eds. Treatment of Hyperlipoproteinemia. New York: Raven Press, 1984:85–93.
11. Glomset JA, Janssen ET, Kennedy R, et al. Role of plasma lecithin: cholesterol acyltransferase in the metabolism of high density lipoproteins. J Lipid Res 1966; 7:638–648.
12. Krauss RM. Atherogenicity of triglyceride- rich lipoproteins. Am J Cardiol 1998; 81:13B–17B.
13. Ruggeri RB. Cholesteryl ester transfer protein: pharmacological inhibition for the modulation of plasma cholesterol levels and promising target for the prevention of atherosclerosis. Curr Top Med Chem 2005; 5:257–264.

14. Phillips NR, Waters D, Havel RJ. Plasma lipoproteins and progression of coronary artery disease evaluated by angiography and clinical events. Circulation 1993; 88:2762–2770.

15. Friedewald WT, Levy RI, Fredrickson DS. Estimation of the concentration of low-density lipoprotein cholesterol in plasma, without use of the preparative ultracentrifuge. Clin Chem 1972; 18:499–502.

16. Hodis HN, Mack WJ, Dunn M, Liu C, Selzer RH, Krauss RM. Intermediate density lipoproteins and progression of carotid arterial wall intima-media thickness. Circulation 1997; 95:2022–2026.

17. Shen MMS, Krauss RM, Lindgren FT, et al. Heterogeneity of serum low density lipoproteins in normal human subjects. J Lipid Res 1981; 22:236–244.

18. Krauss RM, Burke DJ. Identification of multiple subclasses of plasma low density lipoproteins in normal humans. J Lipid Res 1982; 23:97–104.

19. Krauss RM, Blanche PJ. Detection and quantitation of LDL subfractions. Curr Opin Lipidol 1992; 3:377–383.

20. Lindgren FT, Jensen LC, Hatach FT. The isolation and quantitative analysis of serum lipoproteins. In: Nelson GJ, ed. Blood Lipids and Lipoproteins: Quantitation, Composition and Metabolism. New York: John Wiley, 1972:181–274.

21. Krauss RM, Burke DJ. Identifcation of multiple subclasses of plasma low density lipoproteins in normal humans. J Lipid Res 1982; 23:97–104.

22. Blanche PJ, Gong EL, Forte TM. Characterization of human high-density lipoproteins by gradient gel electrophoresis. Biochim Biophys Acta 1981; 665:408–419.

23. Alaupovic P. Apolipoproteins and lipoproteins. Atherosclerosis 1971; 13:141–145.

24. Gotto MA. High-density lipoproteins: biochemical and metabolic factors. Am J Cardiol 1983; 52:2B–4B.

25. Green PH, Glickman RM. Intestinal lipoprotein metabolism. J Lipid Res 1981; 22:1153–1173.

26. Fruchart JC, Ailhaud G. Recent progress in the study of ApoA-containing lipoprotein particles. Pro Lipid Res 1991; 30:145–150.

27. Cheung MC, Brown BG, Wolf AC, Albers JJ. Altered particle size distribution of apolipoprotein A-I containing lipoproteins in subjects with coronary artery disease. J Lipid Res 1991; 32:383–394.

28. Mihalich A, Magnaghi P, Sessa L, Trubia M, Acquati F, Taramelli R. Genomic structure and organization of kringles type 3 to 10 of the apolipoprotein (a) gene in 6q26-27. Gene 1997; 196:1–8.

29. Scanu AM, Gless GM. Lipoprotein (a). Heterogeneity and biological relevance. J Clin Invest 1990; 85:1709–1715.

30. Naruszewicze M, Giroux LM, Davignon J. Oxidative modifcation of Lp(a) causes changes in the structure and biological properties of apo (a). Chem Phys Lipids 1994; 68:167–174.

31. Goldstein JL, Brown MS. Atherosclerosis—the low density lipoprotein receptor hypothesis. Metabolism 1977; 26:1257–1275.

32. Tan MH, Sata T, Havel RJ. The significance of lipoprotein lipase in rat skeletal muscles. J Lipid Res 1977; 18:363–370.

33. Breckenridge WC, Alaupovic P, Cox DW, et al. Apoprotein and lipoprotein concentrations in familial apolipoprotein C-II defciency. Atherosclerosis 1982; 44:223–235.

34. Weisgraber KH, Rall SC, Mahley RW. Human E apoprotein heterogeneity. J Biol Chem 1981; 256:9077–9081.

35. Kinnunen PK, Virtanen JA, Vainio P. Lipoprotein lipase and hepatic endothelial lipase: their roles in plasma lipoprotein metabolism. Atheroscler Rev 1983; 11:65–105.

36. Jensen GL, Baly DL, Brannon PM, et al. Synthesis and secretion of lipolytic enzymes by cultured chicken hepatocytes. J Biol Chem 1980; 25:11141–11148.

37. Von Eckardstein A, Nofer JR, Assmann G. High density lipoproteins and arteriosclerosis. Arterioscler Thromb Vasc Biol 2001; 21:13–27.

38. Glomset JA, Janssen ET, Kennedy R, et al. Role of plasma lecithin: cholesterol acyltransferase in the metabolism of high density lipoproteins. J Lipid Res 1966; 7:638–648.

39. Khoo JC, Mahoney EM, Witxtum JL. Secretion of lipoprotein lipase by macrophages in culture. J Biol Chem 1981; 256:7105–7108.

40. Santamarina-Fojo S, Brewer HB, Jr. The familial hyperchylomicronemia syndrome. New insights into underlying genetic defects. JAMA 1991; 265:904–908.

41. Gagne C, Brum LD, Julien P, Moorjani S, Lupien PJ. Primary lipoprotein lipase activity deficiency. Clinical investigation of a French Canadian population. Can Med Assoc J 1989; 140:405–411.

42. Santamarina-Fojo S. Genetic dyslipoproetinemias: rote of lipoprotein lipase and apolipoprotein C-II. Curr Opin Lipidol 1992; 3:186–195.

43. Reymer PW, Gagne E, Groenemeyer BE, et al. A lipoprotein lipase mutation (Asn291 Ser) is associated with reduced HDL cholesterol levels in premature atherosclerosis. Nat Genet 1995; 10:28–34.

44. Collet X, Tall AR, Serajuddin H, et al. Remodeling of HDL by CETP and hepatic lipase in vitro results in enhanced uptake of HDL CE by cells expressing scavenger receptor B-1. J Lipid Res 1999; 40:1185–1193.

45. Jahn C, Osborne JC, Schaefer EJ, et al. In vitro activation of the enzyme activity of hepatic lipase by A-II. FEBS Lett 1981; 131:366–368.

46. Zambon A, Brown G, Deeb S, Brunzell J. Hepatic pilase as a focal point for the development and treatment of coronary artery disease. J Invest Med 2001; 49:112–118.

47. Fielding CJ, Shore VG, Fielding PE. A protein cofactor of lecithin: cholesterol acyltransferase. Biochem Biophys Res Commun 1972; 46:1493–1498.

48. Kastner G. Studies on the cofactor requirements for lecithin-cholesterol acyltransferase. Scand J Lab Invest 1974; 33:19–21.

49. Seguret-Mace S, Latta-Mahieu M, Castro G, et al. Potential gene therapy for lecithin-cholesterol acyltransferase (LCAT)-deficient and hypo alpha lipoproteinemic patients with adenovirus-mediated transfer of human LCAT gene. Circulation 1996; 94:2177–2184.

50. Meiner VL, Cases S, Myers HM, et al. Diruption of the acyl-CoA:cholesterol acyltransferase gene in mice: evidence suggesting multiple cholesterol esterifcation enzymes in mammals. Proc Natl Acad Sci USA 1996; 93:14041–14046.

51. Rudel LL, Lee RG, Parini P. ACAT2 os a target fpr treat,emt pf cprpmaru jeart dosease asspcoated wotj ju[ercjp;esterp;e,ia. Arterioscler Thromb Vasc Biol 2005; 25:1112–1118.

52. Nissen S. Efect of ACAT inhibition on the progression of coronary atherosclerosis: a randomized controlled trial. Am Heart Assoc Late Breaking Clin Trials 2005;15.

53. Barter PJ, Brewer HB, Jr., Chapman JM, Hennekens CH, Rader DJ, Tall AR. Cholesterol ester transfer protein: a novel target for raising HDL and inhibiting atherosclerosis. ATVB 2003; 23:160–167.

54. Navab M, Berliner JA, Watson AD, et al. The Yin and Yang of oxidation in the development of the fatty streak. Arteriocler Thromb Vasc Biol 1996; 16:831–842.

55. Mackness MI, Mackness B, Durrington PN, Connelly PW, Hegele RA. Paroxonase: biochemistry, genetics and relationship to plasma lipoproteins. Curr Opin Lipidol 1996; 7:69–76.

56. Mackness MI, Walker CH. Multiple forms of sheep serum A-esterase activity associated with the high-density lipoprotein. Biochem J 1988; 250:539–545.

57. Mackness MI, Arrol S, Abbott CA, Durrington PN. Protection of low-density lipoprotein against oxidative modifcation by high-density lipoprotein associated paraoxonase. Atherosclerosis 1993; 104:129–135.

58. Oram JF, Yokoyama S. Apolipoprotein-mediated removal of cellular cholesterol and phospholipids. J Lipid Res 1997; 37:2473–2491.

59. Mendez AJ. Cholesterol efflux mediated by apolipoproteirts is an active cellular process distinct from efflux mediated by passive diffusion. J Lipid Res 1997; 38:1807–1821.

60. Domingo N, Mastellone I, Gres S, et al. The endothelial cholesterol efflux is promoted by the high-density lipoprotein anionic peptide factor. Metabolism 2005; 54:1087–1094.

61. Hamon Y, Broccardo C, Chambenoit O, et al. ABC1 promotes engulfment of apoptotic cells and transbilayer redistribution of phosphatidylerine. Nat Cell Biol 2000; 2:399–406.

62. Kozarsky KF, Donahee MH, Rigotti A, lqbal SN, Edelman ER, Krieger M. Overexpression of the HDL receptor SR-BI alters plasma HDL and bile cholesterol levels. Nature 1997; 387:414–417.

63. Zhao SP, Wu ZH, Hong SC, Ye HJ, Wu J. Effect of atorvastatin on SR81 expression and HDL-induced cholesterol efflux in adipocytes of hypercholesterolemic rabbits. Clin Chim Acta 2005; Sep (Epub).

64. Hirano KI, legami C, Tsujii HL, et al. Probucol enhances the expression of human hepatic scavenger receptor class B tye I, possibly through a species specific mechanism. Arterioscler Thromb vasc Biol 2005; Sep:8 (Epub).

65. Trigatti B, Rayburn H, Vinals M, et al. Influence of the high density lipoprotein receptor SR-BI on reproductive and cardiovascular pathophysiology. Proc Natl Acad Sci USA 1999; 96:9322–9327.

66. Levy RI, Brensike JF, Epstein SE, et al. The influence of changes in lipid values induced by cholestyramine and diet on progression of coronary artery disease: results of the NHLBI type II coronary intervention study. Circulation 1984; 69:325–337.

67. Lipid Research Clinics Program. The lipid research clinics coronary primary prevention trial results: I. Reduction of incidence of coronary heart disease, and II. The relationship of reduction in incidence of coronary heart disease to cholesterol lowering. JAMA 1984; 251:351–374.

68. Scandinavian Simvastatin Survival Study Group. Randomised trial of cholesterol lowering in 4,444 patients with coronary heart disease: the Scandinavian Simvastatin Survival Stduy (4S). Lancet 1994; 349:1383–1389.

69. Shepherd J, Cobbe SM, Isles CG, et al. Prevention of coronary heart disease with pravastatin in men with hypercholesterolemia. NEJM 1995; 333:1301–1307.

70. Sacks FM, Pfeffer MA, Moye LA, et al. The effect of pravastatin on coronary events after myocardial infarction in patients with average cholesterol levels. NEJM 1996; 335:1001–1009.

71. Downs JR, Clearfeld M, Weis S, et al. Primary prevention of acute coronary events with lovastatin in men and women with average cholesterol levels. JAMA 1998; 279:1615–1622.

72. Superko HR. Did Grandma give you heart disease ? The new battle against coronary artery disease Am J Card 1998; 82:34–46.

73. Cannon CP, Braunwald E, McCabe CH, et al. Pravastatin or Atorvastatin evaluation and infection therapy-thrombolysis in myocardial infarction, 22 investigators. Intensive versus moderate lipid lowering with statins afer acute coronary syndromes. N Engl J Med 2004; 350:1495–1504.

74. LaRosa JC, Grundy SM, Waters DD, et al. Treating to New Targets (TNT) investigators. Intensive lipid lowering with atorvastatin in patients with stable coronary disease. N Engl J Med 2005; 352:1425–1435.

75. Pedersen Terje R, Faergeman Ole, Kastelein John JP, et al. The Incremental Decrease in End Points Through Aggressive Lipid Lowering (IDEAL) study group. High-Dose atorvastatin vs usual-dose simvastatin for secondary prevention after myocardial infarction. JAMA 2005; 294:2437–2445.

76. Brown BG, Hillger L, Zhao XQ, Poulin D, Albers JJ. Types of change in coronary stenosis severity and their relative importance in overall progression and regression of coronary disease. Observations from the FATS trial. Familial Atherosclerosis Treatment Study. Ann N Y Acad Sci 1995; 748:407–417.

77. Brown GB, Zhao XQ, Chait A, et al. Simvastatin and niacin, antioxidant vitamins, or the combination for the prevention of coronary disease. NEJM 2001; 345:1583–1592.

78. Soria LF, Ludwig EH, Clarke HRG, Vega GL, Grundy SM, McCarthy BJ. Association between a specifc apolipprotein B mutation and familial defective apolipoprotein B-100. Proc Natl Acad Sci USA 1989; 86:587–591.

79. Innerarity TL. Familial hypobetalipoproteinemia and familial defective apolipo-protein B100: genetic disorders associated with apolipoprotein B. Curr Opin Lipidol 1990; 1:104–109.

80. Winder AF, Owen JS, Pritchard PH, et al. A first British case of fish-eye disease presenting at age 75 years: a double heterozygote for defined and new mutations affecting LCAT structure and expression. J Clin Pathol 1999; 52:228–230.

81. Hirano K, Kachi S, Ushida C, Naito M. Corneal and macular manifestations in a case of deficient lecithin: cholesterol acyltransferase. Jpn J Ophthalmol 2004; 48:82–84.

82. Gordon T, Castelli WP, Hjortland MC, et al. High density lipoprotein as a protective factor against coronary heart disease: the Framingham study. Am J Med 1977; 62:707–714.

83. Rubins HB, Robins SJ, Collins D, et al. Gemfibrozil for the secondary prevention of coronary heart disease in men with low levels of high-density lipoprotein cholesterol. Veterans affairs high-density lipoprotein cholesterol intervention trial study group. NEJM 1999; 341:410–418.

84. Superko HR, Berneis KK, Williams PT, Rizzo M, Wood PD. Differential effect of Gemfibrozil in Normolipemic subjects with predominantly dense or buoyant low density lipoprotein particles and the effect on postprandial lipemia and Lp(a). Am J Card 2005; November.

85. Frohlich J, Pritchard PH. Analysius of familial hypoalphalipoproteinemia syn. Mol Cell Biochem 1992; 18:141–149.

86. Genest J, Bard JM, Fruchart JC, Ordovas JM, Schaefer EJ. Familial hypoalpha-lipoproteinemia in premature CAD. Arterioscler Thromb 1993; 13:1728–1737.

87. Vega GL, Grundy SM. Two patterns of LDL metabolism in normotriglyceridemic patients with hypoalphalipoproteinemia. Arterioscler Thromb 1993; 13:579–589.

88. Marcil M, Boucher B, Krimbou L, et al. Severe familial HDL deficiency in French-Canadian kindreds. Arterioscler Thromb Vasc Biol 1995; 15:1015–1024.

89. Franceschini G, Bondioli A, Granata D, et al. Reduced HDL2 levels in myocardial infarction patients without risk factors for atherosclerosis. Atherosclerosis 1987; 68:213–219.

90. Johansson J, Carlson LA, Landow C, Hamsten A. High density lipoproteins and coronary atherosclerosis. A strong inverse relation with the largest particles is confined to normotriglyceridemic patients. Arterioscler Thromb 1991; 11:174–182.

91. Zambon A, Deeb SS, Brown BG, Hokanson JE, Brunzell JD. Common hepatic lipase gene promoter variant determines clinical response to intensive lipid lowering treatment. Circulation 2001; 103:792–798.

92. Reymer PW, Gagne E, Groenemeyer BE, et al. A lipoprotein lipase mutation (Asn291Ser) is associated with reduced HDL cholesterol levels in premature atherosclerosis. Nat Genet 1995; 10:28–34.

93. Ordovas JM, Schaefer EJ, Salem D, et al. Apolipoprotein A-I gene polymorphism associated with premature coronary artery disease and familial hypoalphalipopro-teinemia. NEJM 1986; 314:671–677.

94. Superko HR, Enas EA, Kotha P, Bhat NK, Garrett B. HDL subclass distribution in individuals of Asian Indian descent. The national Asian Indian heart disease project. Prev Cardiol 2004; 8:81–86.

95. Superko HR, High HDLC. Not protective in the presence of homocysteinemia. Am J Card 1997; 79:705–706.

96. Nagano M, Nakamura M, Kobayashi N, Kamata J, Hiramori K. Effort angina in a middle-aged woman with abnormally high levels of serum high-density lipoprotein cholesterol: a case of cholesteryl-ester transfer protein deficiency. Circ J 2005; 69:609–612.

97. Maruyama T, Sakai N, Ishigami M, et al. Prevalence and phenotypic spectrum of cholesteryl ester transfer protein gene mutations in Japanese hyperalphalipoptoei-nemia. Atherosclerosis 2003; 166:177–185.

98. Kinoshita M, Fujita M, Usui S, et al. Scavenger receptor type BI potentiates reverse cholesterol transport system by removing cholesterol ester from HDL. Athero-sclerosis 2004; 173:197–202.

99. NCEP ATP-III. Expert Panel on Detection, Evaluation, and Treatment of High Blood Cholesterol in Adults. Executive Summary of The Third Report of The National Cholesterol Education Program (NCEP) Expert Panel on Detection, Evaluation, And Treatment of High Blood Cholesterol In Adults (Adult Treatment Panel III). JAMA 2001; 285:2486–2497.

100. Austin MA, King MC, Vranizan KM, Krauss RM. Atherogenic lipoprotein phenotype. A proposed genetic marker for coronary heart disease risk. Circulation 1990; 82:495–506.

101. Goldstein JL, Schrott HG, Hazzard WR, Bierman EL, Motulsky AG. Hyperlipidemia in coronary heart disease II. Genetic analysis of lipid levels in 176 families and delineation of a new inherited disorder, combined hyperlipidemia. J Clin Invest 1973; 52:1544–1568.

102. Kwiterovich PO. Genetics and molecular biology of familial combined hyperlipidemia. Curr Opin Lipidol 1993; 4:133–143.

103. Sniderman A, Shapiro S, Marpole D, Malcolm I, Skinner B, Kwiterovich PO, Jr. The association of coronary Atherosclerosis and Hyperapobetalipoproteinemia (increased protein but normal cholesterol content in human plasma low density lipoprotein). Proc Natl Acad Sci USA 1980; 97:604–608.

104. Williams RR, Hunt SC, Hopkins PN, et al. Familial dyslipidemic hypertension: evidence from 58 utah families for a syndrome present in approximately 15% of patients with essential hypertension. JAMA 1988; 259:3579–3586.

105. Hunt SC, Wu LL, Hopkins PN, et al. Apolipoprotein, low density lipoprotein subfraction, and insulin associations with familial combined hyperlipidemia (Study of utah patients with familial dyslipidemic hypertension). Arteriosclerosis 1989; 9:335–344.

106. Reaven GM. Banting lecture1988. Role of insulin resistance in human disease. Diabetes 1988; 37:1595–1607.

107. Dejager S, Bruckert E, Chapman MJ. Dense low density lipoprotein subspecies with diminished oxidative resistance predominate in combined hyperlipidemia. J Lipid Res 1993; 34:295–308.

108. Chait A, Brazg RL, Tribble DL, Krauss RM. Susceptibility of small, dense, low-density lipoproteins to oxidative modification in subjects with the atherogenic lipoprotein phenotype, pattern B. Am J Med 1993; 94:350–356.

109. Superko HR. Beyond LDL-C reduction. Circulation 1996; 94:2351–2354.

110. Nakamura T, Takano H, Umetani K, et al. Remnant lipoproteinemia is a risk factor for endothelial vasomotor dysfunction and coronary artery disease in metabolic syndrome. Atherosclerosis 2005; 181:321–327.

111. Kishi K, Ochiai K, Ohta Y, et al. Highly sensitive cholesterol assay with enzymatic cycling applied to measurement of remnant lipoprotein-cholesterol in serum. Clin Chem 2002; 48:737–741.

112. Hulley SB, Rosenman RH, Bawol RD, et al. Epidemiology as a guide to clinical decisions: the association between triglyceride and coronary heart disease. N Engl J Med 1980; 302:1383–1389.

113. Nakamura T, Takano H, Umetani K, et al. Remnant lipoproteinemia is a risk factor for endothelial vasomotor dysfunction and coronary artery disease in metabolic syndrome. Atherosclerosis 2005; 181:321–327.

114. Austin MA. Review: plasma triglyceride and coronary heart disease. Arterioscler Thromb 1991; 1:11–14.

115. Superko HR, Wood PD, Laughton C, Krauss RM. Low density lipoprotein (LDL) subclass patterns and postprandial lipemia. Arteriosclerosis 1990; 10:826a.

116. Tribble DL, Holl LG, Wood PD, Krauss RM. Variations in oxidative susceptibility among six low density lipoprotein subfractions of differing density and particle size. Atherosclerosis 1992; 3:189–199.

117. Reaven GM. Why Syndrome X? From Harold Himsworth to the insulin resistance syndrome. Cell Metab 2005; 1:9–14.

118. Austin MA, Kamigaki A, Hokanson JE. Low-density lipoprotein particle size is a risk factor for coronary heart disease independent of triglyceride and HDL cholesterol: a meta-analysis of three prospective studies in men. Circulation 1999; 99:1124.

119. Austin MA, King MC, Vranizan KM, et al. Atherogenic lipoprotein phenotype. A proposed genetic marker for coronary heart disease risk. Circulation 1990; 82:495–506.

120. Austin MA, Breslow JL, Hennekens CH, et al. Low density lipoprotein subclass patterns and risk of myocardial infarction. JAMA 1988; 260:1917–1921.

121. Nishina PM, Johnson JP, Naggert JK, et al. Linkage of atherogenic lipoprotein phenotype to the low-density lipoprotein receptor locus on the short arm of chromosome 19. Proc Natl Acad Sci USA 1992; 89:708–712.

122. Rotter JI, Bu X, Cantor R, et al. Multilocus genetic determination of LDL particle size in coronary artery disease families (abstr). Clin Res 1994; 42:16A.

123. Hogue JC, Lamarche B, Gaudet D, et al. Relationship between cholesteryl ester transfer protein and LDL heterogeneity in familial hypercholesterolemia. J Lipid Res 2004; 45:1077–1083.

124. Stampfer MJ, Krauss RM, Blanche PJ, Noll LG, Sacks FM, Hennekens CH. A prospective study of triglyceride level, low density lipoprotein particle diameter, and risk of myocardial infarction. JAMA 1996; 276:882–888.

125. Gardner CD, Fortmann SP, Krauss RM. Small low density lipoprotein particles are associated with the incidence of coronary artery disease in men and women. JAMA 1996; 276:875–881.

126. Lamarche B, Tchernof A, Moorjani S, et al. Small, dense low-density lipoprotein particles as a predictor of the risk of ischemic heart disease in men. Prespective results from the Quebec cardiovascular study. Circulation 1997; 95:69–75.

127. St. Pierre AC, Cantin B, Dagenais GR, et al. Los-density lipoprotein subfractions and the long-term risk of ischemic heart disease in men. Arterioscler Thromb Vasc Biol 2005; 25:553–559.

128. Campos H, Moye LA, Glasser SP, Stampfer MJ, Sacks FM. Low-density lipoprotein size, pravastatin treatment, and coronary events. JAMA 2001; 286:1468–1474.

129. Krauss R. Is the size of low-density lipoprotein particles related to the risk of coronary heart disease? JAMA 2002; 287:712–713.

130. O'Leary DH, Polak JF, Kronmal RA, Manolio TA, Burke GL, Wolfson SK. Carotid-artery intima and media thickness as a risk factor for myocardial infarction and stroke in older adulats. NEJM 1999; 340:14–22.

131. Mack WJ, LaBree L, Liu C, Selzer RH, Hodis HN. Correlations between measures of atherosclerosis change using carotid ultrasonography and coronary angiography. Atherosclerosis 2000; 150:371–379.

132. Skoglund-Anderson C, Tang R, Bond MG, de Faire U, Hamsten A, Karpe F. LDL particle size distribution is associated with carotid intima-media thickness in healthy 50-year-old men. Arterioscler Thromb Vasc Biol 1999; 19:2422–2430.
133. Robert Superko H, McGovern Mark E, Brenda Garrett Elaine Raul. Nicotinic acid has a differential effect on low density lipoprotein subclass distribution in patients classified as LDL pattern A, B, or I. Am J Cardiol 2004; 94:588–594.
134. Taylor AJ, Sullenberger LE, Lee HJ, Lee JK, Grace KA. Arterial biology for the investigation of the treatment effects of reducing cholesterol (ARBITER) 2: a double-blind, placebo-controlled study of extended-release niacin on athero-sclerosis progression in secondary prevention patients treated with statins. Circulation 2004; 110:3512–3517.
135. Krauss RM, Lindgren FT, Wlliams PT, et al. Intermedicate-density lipoproteins and progression of coronary artery disease in hypercholesterolaemic men. Lancet 1987; 2:62–65.
136. Miller BD, Alderman EL, Haskell WL, Fair JM, Krauss RM. Predominance of dense low-density lipoprotein particles predicts angiographic beneft or therapy in the Stanford Coronary Risk Intervention project. Circulation 1996; 94:2146–2153.
137. Williams PT, Superko HR, Haskell WL, et al. Smallest LDL particles are most strongly related to coronary disease progression in men. Arterioscler Thromb Vasc Biol 2003; 23:314–321.
138. Watts GF, Lewis B, Brunt JNH, et al. Efects on coronary artery disease of lipid-lowering diet, or diet plus cholestyramine, in the St Thomas' Atherosclerosis Regression Study (STARS). Lancet 1992; 339:563–569.
139. Zambon A, Hokanson JE, Brown BG, Brunzell JD. Evidence for a new pathophysiological mechanism for coronary artery disease regression. Circulation 1999; 99:1959–1964.
140. Kulkarni KR, Garber DW, Marcovina SM, Segrest JP. Quantification of cholesterol in all lipoprotein classes by VAP-II method. J Lipid Res 1994; 35:159–168.
141. Otvas JD, Jeyarajah EJ, Bennett DW, Krauss RM. Development of a proton nuclear magnetic resonance spectroscopic method for determining plasma lipoprotein concentrations and subspecies distributions from a single, rapid measurement. Clin Chem 1992; 38:1632–1638.
142. Superko HR, Schott RJ, Barr C, Raul E. Comparison of traditional and alternative laboratory methods for the determination of lipid measurements, Lp(a) and LDL phenotype. Circulation 2002; 105:14.
143. Cheung MC, Albers JJ. Characterization of lipoprotein particles isolated by immunoaffinity chromatography: particles containing A-I and A-II and particles containing A-I but no A-II. J Biol Chem 1984; 259:12201–12209.
144. Mao H, Yang T, Gremon PS. A micro fluids device with linear temperature gradient for parallel and combinatorial measurements. J Am Chem Soc 2002; 124:4432–4435.
145. Okazaki M, Usui S, Ishigami M, et al. Identifcation of unique lipoprotein subclasses for visceral obesit by component analysis of cholesterol profile in high-performance liquid chromatography. Arterioscler Thromb Vasc Biol 2005; 25:578–584.

146. Blanche PJ, Gong EL, Forte TM, Nichols AV. Characterization of human high-density lipoproteins by gradient gel electrophoresis. Biochim Biophys Acta 1981; 665:408–419.

147. Cheung MC, Albers JJ. Distribution of high density lipoprotein particles with diferent apoprotein composition; particles with A-I and A-II and particles with A-I but not A-II. J Lipid Res 1982; 23:747–753.

148. Dimayuga P, Zhu J, Oguchi S, et al. Reconstituted HDL containing human apolipoprotein A-1 reduces CAM-1 expression and neointima formation following periadventitial cuff-indced carotid injury in apoE null mice. Biochem Biophys Res Commun 1999; 22:465–468.

149. Cheung MC, Wolfbauer G, Brown BG, Albers JJ. Relationship between plasma phospholipid transfer protein activity and HDL subclasses among patients with low HDL and cardiovascular disease. Atherosclerosis 1999; 142:201–205.

150. Johansson J, Carlson LA, Landow C, Hamsten A. High density lipoproteins and coronary atherosclerosis. A strong inverse relation wit the largest particles is confined to normotriglyceridemic patients. Arterioscler Thromb 1991; 11:174–182.

151. Miller NE. Associations of high-density lipoprotein subclasses and apolipoproteins with ischemic heart disease and coronary atherosclerosis. Am Heart J 1987; 113:589–597.

152. Sich D, Saidi Y, Giral P, et al. Hyperalphalipoproteinemia:characterization of a cardioprotective profile associating increased high-density lipoprotein 2 levels and decreased hepatic lipase activity. Metabolism 1998; 47:965–973.

153. Williams PT, Vranizan KM, Austin MA, Krauss RM. Familial correlations wof HDL subclasses based on gradient gel electrophoresis. Arterioscler Thromb 1992; 12:1467–1474.

154. Scanu AM, Gless GM. Lipoprotein(a). Heterogeneity and biological relevance. J Clin Invest 1990; 85:1709–1715.

155. Terres W, Tatsis E, Pfalzer B, Beil U, Beisiegel U, Hamm CW. Rapid angiographic progression of coronary artery disease in patients with elevated lipoprotein(a). Circulation 1995; 91:948–950.

156. Sandkamp M, Funke H, Schelte H, Kohler E, Assmann G. Lipoprotein(a) is an independent risk factor for myocardial infarction at a young age. Clin Chern 1990; 36:20–23.

157. Dahlen GH, Guyton JR, Attar M, et al. Association of levels of lipoprotein Lp(a), plasma lipids, and other lipoproteins with coronary artery disease documented by angiography. Circulation 1986; 74:758–765.

158. Budde T, Fechtrup C, Bosenberg E, et al. Plasma lp(a) levels correlate with number, severity, and length-extension of coronary lesions in male patients undergoing coronary arteriography for clinically suspected coronary atherosclerosis. Arterioscler Thromb 1994; 14:1730–1736.

159. Schaefer EJ, Lamon-Fava S, Jenner JL, et al. Lipoprotein(a) levels and risk of coronary heart disease in men. JAMA 1994; 271:999–1003.

160. Rifai N, Ma J, Sacks FM, et al. Apolipoprotein(a) size and lipoprotein(a) concentration and future risk of angina pectoris with evidence of severe coronary atherosclerosis in men: the physicians' health study. Clin Chem 2004; 50:1364–1371.

161. Luc G, Bard JM, Arveiler D, et al. Lipoprotein(a) as a predictor of coronary heart disease: the PRIME study. Atherosclerosis 2002; 163:377–384.

162. Cantin B, Gagnon F, Moorjani S, et al. Is Lipoprotein(a) an independent risk factor for ischemic heart disease in men? The Quebec cardiovascular study JACC 1998; 31:519–525.

163. Luc G, Bard JM, Arveiler D, et al. Lipoprotein(a) as a predictor of coronary heart disease: the PRIME study. Atherosclerosis 2002; 163:377–384.

164. von Eckardstein A, Schulte H, Cullen P, Assmann G. Lipoprotein(a) further increases the risk of coronary events in men with high global cardiovascular risk. J Am Coll Cardiol 2001; 37:434–439.

165. Ariyo AA, Thach C, Tracy R. Cardiovascular health study investigators. Lp(a) lipoprotein, vascular disease, and mortality in the elderly. N Engl J Med 2003; 349:2108–2115.

166. Koschirisky ML, Beislegel U, Henne-Bruns D, Eaton DL, lawn RM. Apolipoprotein(a) size heterogeneity is related to variable number of repeat sequences in its mRNA. Biochemistry 1990; 29:640–644.

167. Wild SH, Fortmann SP, Marcovina SM. A prospective case-control study of lipoprotein(a) levels and apo(a) size and risk of coronary heart disease in Stanford Five-City Project participants. Arterioscler Thromb Vasc Biol 1997; 17:239–245.

168. Paultre F, Pearson TA, Weil HF, et al. High levels of Lp(a) with a small apo(a) isoform are associated with coronary artery disease in African American and white men. Arterioscler Thromb Vasc Biol 2000; 20:2619–2624.

169. Marcovina SM, Albers JJ, Scanu AM, et al. Use of a reference material proposed by the international federation of clinical chemistry and laboratory medicine to evaluate analytical methods for the determination of plasma lipoprotein(a). Clin Chem 2000; 46:1956–1967.

170. Tate JR, Berg K, Couderc R, et al. International Federation of Clinical Chemistry and Laboratory Medicine (IFCC) standardization project for the measurement of lipoprotein(a). Clin Chem Lab Med 1999; 37:949–958.

171. Marcovina SM, Koschinsky ML. Evaluation of lipoprotein(a) as a prothrombotic factor: progress from bench to bedside. Curr Opin Lipidol 2003; 14:361–366.

172. Strater R, Becker S, von Eckardstein A, et al. Prospective assessment of risk factors for recurrent stroke during childhood—a 5-year follow-up study. Lancet 2002; 360:1540–1545.

173. Daida H, Lee YJ, Yokoi H, et al. Prevention of restenos after percutaneous transluminal coronary angioplasty by reducing lipoprotein(a) levels with low-density lipoprotein apheresis. Am J Card 1994; 73:1037–1040.

174. Shlipak MG, Simon JA, Vittinghof E, et al. Estrogen and Progestin, Lipoprotein(a), and the risk of recurrent coronary heart disease events after menopause. JAMA 2000; 283:1845–1852.

175. Maher VMG, Brown BG, Marcovina S, Hilger LA, Zhao XQ, Albers JJ. Effects of lowering elevated LDL cholesterol on the cardiovascular risk of lipoprotein(a). JAMA 1995; 274:1771–1774.

176. Genest J, Sniderman A, Cianflone K, Teng B, et al. Hyperapobetalipoproteinemia. Plasma lipoprotein responses to oral fat load. Arteriosclerosis 1986; 6:297–304.

177. Kwiterovich PO. HyperapoB: a pleiotropic phenotype characterized by dense low-density lipoprotein and associated with coronary artery disease. Clin Chem 1988; 34:B71–B77.

178. Sniderman AD, Wolfson C, Teng B, Franklin FA, Bachorik PS, Kwiterovich PO. Association of hyperapobetalipoproteinemia with endogenous hypertriglyceridemia and atherosclerosis. Ann Internal Med 1982; 97:833–839.

179. Lamarche B, Tchernof A, Mauriege P, et al. Fasting insulin and apolipoprotein B levels and low-density lipoprotein particle size as risk factors for ischemic heart disease. JAMA 1998; 279:1955–1961.

180. Utermann G. Apolipoprotein E polmorphism in health and disease. Am Heart J 1987; 113:433–440.

181. Gregg RE, Zech LA, Schaefer EJ, Brewer HB. Type III hyperlipoproteineima: defective metabolism of an abnormal apolipoprotein E. Science 1981; 211:584–586.

182. Gregg RE, Zech LA, Schaefer EJ, Stark D, Wilson O, Brewer HB, Jr. Abnormal in vivo metabolism of apolipoprotein E4 in humans. J Clin Invest 1986; 78:815–821.

183. Mahley RW. Atherogenic hyperlipoproteinemia. The cellular and molecular biology of plasma lipoproteins altered by dietary fat and cholesterol. Med Clin N Am 1982; 66:375–400.

184. Lopez-Miranda J, Ordovas JM, Mata P, et al. Effect of apolipoprotein E phenotype on diet-induced lowering of plasma low density lipoprotein cholesterol. J Lipid Res 1994; 35:1965–1975.

185. Dreon DM, Fernstrom HA, Miller B, Krauss RM. Apolipoprotein E isoform phenotype and LDL subclass response to a reduced-fat diet. Arterioscler Thromb Vasc Biol 1995; 15:105–111.

186. Superko HR. The effect of apolipoprotein E isoform difference on postprandial lipoprotein composition in patients matched for triglycerides, LDL-cholesterol and HDL cholesterol. Artery 1991; 18:315–325.

187. Luc G, Bard JM, Arveiler D, et al. Impact of apolipoprotein E polymorphism on lipoproteins and risk of myocardial infarction. The ECTIM study. Arterioscler Thromb 1994; 14:1412–1419.

188. Tirot L, Knijff P, Menzel H, Ehnholm C, Nicaud V, Havekes LM. ApoE polymorphism and predisposition to coronary heart disease in youths of diferent european populations. Arterioscler Thromb 1994; 14:1617–1624.

189. Corder EH, Saunders AM, Strittmatter WJ, et al. Gene dose of apolipoprotein E type 4 allele and the risk of Alzheimer's disease in late onset families. Science 1993; 261:921–923.

190. American College of Medical Genetics/American Society of Human Genetics Working Group on ApoE and Alzheimer Disease. Statement on use of apolipoprotein E testing for alzheimer disease. JAMA 1995; 274:1627–1629.

191. Barter PJ, Brewer HB, Jr., Chapman MJ, Hennekens CH, Rader DJ, Tall AR. Cholesteryl ester transfer protein: a novel target for raising HDL and inhibiting atherosclerosis. Arterioscler Thromb Vasc Biol 2003; 23:160–167.

192. Rittershaus CW, Miller DP, Thomas LJ, et al. Vaccine-induced antibodies inhibit CETP activity in vivo and reduce aortic lesions in a rabbit model of atherosclerosis. Arterioscler Thromb Vasc Biol 2000; 20:2106–2112.

193. Okamoto H, Yonemori F, Wakitani K, Minowa T, Maeda K, Shinkai H. A cholesteryl ester transfer protein inhibitor attenuates atherosclerosis in rabbits. Nature 2000; 406:203–207.

194. Hirano K, Yamashita S, Matsuzawa Y. Pros and cons of inhibitint cholesteryl ester transfer protein. Curr Opin Lipidol 2000; 11:589–596.

195. Brewer HB, Jr., Remaley AT, Neufeld EB, Basso F, Jayce C. Regulation of plasma high-density lipoprotein levels by the ABCA1 transporter and the emerging role of high-density lipoprotein in the treatment of cardiovascular disease. ATVB 2004; 24:1755–1760.

196. Naveb M, Anantharamaiah GM, Reddy ST, et al. Human apolipoprotein AI mimetic peptides for the treatment of atherosclerosis. Curr opin Investig Drugs 2003; 4:1100–1104.

197. Oram JF. HDL apolipoproteins and ABCA1: partners in the removal of excess cellular cholesterol. Arterioscler Thromb Vasc Biol 2003; 23:720–727.

198. Joyce C, Amar MJA, Lambert G, et al. The ATP binding cassette transporter Al (ABCA1) modulates the development of aortic atherosclerosis in C57BL/6 and apoE-knockout mice. Proc Nat Acad Sci 2002; 99:407–412.

199. Robert Superko H. The metabolic syndrome and coronary artery disease. In: Fuster V, et al. ed. Hurst's the Heart. New York: McGraw-Hill, 2004:2127–2141.

200. Malik S, Wong ND, Franklin SS, et al. Impact of the metabolic syndrome on mortality from coronary heart disease, cardiovascular disease, and all causes in United States adults. Circulation 2004; 110:1245–1250.

201. Flegal KM, Carroll MD, Ogden CL, Johnson CL. Prevalence and trends in obesity among U.S. adults, 1999-2000. JAMA 2002; 288:1723–1727.

202. Dreon DM, Fernstrom H, Miller B, Krauss RM. Low density lipoprotein subclass patterns and lipoprotein response to a reduced-fat diet in men. FASEB J 1994; 8:121–126.

203. Dreon DM, Fernstrom HA, Williams PT, Krauss RM. LDL subclass pattern sand lipoprotein response to a low-fat, high-carbohydrate diet in women. Arterioscler Thromb Vasc Biol 1997; 17:7007–7714.

204. Aude YW, Lamas GA, Lopez-Jimenez F, et al. Results of a randomized trial comparing a high fat low carbohydrate diet to the NCEP step 2 diet; effect on LDL cholesterol subclasses. JACC 2001; 37:280A.

205. Williams PT, Krauss RM, Vranizan KM, Albers JJ, Terry RB, Wood PD. Effects of exercise induced weight loss on low density lipoprotein subfractions in healthy men. Arteriosclerosis 1989; 9:623–632.

206. Williams PT, Krauss RM, Vranizan KM, Wood PD. Changes in lipoprotein subfractions during diet-induced and exercise-induced weight loss in moderately overweight men. Circulation 1990; 81:1293–1304.

207. Superko HR, Krauss RM. Differential effects of nicotinic acid in subjects with diferent LDL subclass patterns. Atherosclerosis 1992; 95:69–76.

208. Robert Superko H, McGovern Mark E, Brenda Garrett Elaine Raul RN. Nicotinic acid has a differential effect on low density lipoprotein subclass distribution in patients classified as LDL pattern, A., B, or I. Am J Card 2004; 94:588–594.

209. Meyers CD, Kamanna VS, Kashyap ML. Niacin therapy in atherosclerosis. Curr Opin Lipidol 2004; 15:659–665.

210. Franceschini G, Lovati MR, Manzoni C, et al. Effect of gemfibrozil treatment in hypercholesterolemia on low density lipoprotein (LDL) subclass distribution and LDL-cell interaction. Atherosclerosis 1995; 114:61–71.

211. Guerin M, Bruckert E, Dolphin PJ, Turpin G, Chapman MJ. Fenofibrate reduces plasma cholesteryl ester transfer from HDL to VLDL and normalizes the athergenic, dense LDL profile in combined hyperlipidemia. Arterioscler Thromb Vasc Biol 1996; 16:763–772.

212. Vakkilainen J, Steiner G, Ansquer JC, et al. DAIS Group. Relationships between low-density lipoprotein particle size, plasma lipoproteins, and progression of coronary artery disease: the Diabetes Atherosclerosis Intervention Study (DAIS). Circulation 2003; 107:1733–1741.

213. Cheung MC, Austin MA, Moulin P, Wolf AC, Cryer D, Knopp RH. Effects of pravastatin on apolipoprotein-specifc high density lipoprotein subpopulations and low density lipoprotein subclass phenotypes in patients with primary hypercholesterolemia. Atherosclerosis 1993; 102:107–119.

214. Vega GL, Krauss RM, Grundy SM. Pravastatin therapy in primary moderate hypercholesterolaemia: changes in metabolism of apolipoprotein B-containing lipoproteins. J Intern Med 1990; 227:81–94.

215. Franceschini G, Sirtori M, Vaccarino V, Gianfranceschi G, Chiesa G, Sirtori CR. Plasma lipoprotein changes after treatment with pravastatin and gemfibrozil in patients with familial hypercholesterolemia. J Lab Clin Med Sep 1989; 114:250–259.

216. Krauss RM, Isaacsohn J, Hunninghake D, et al. Changes in atherogenic lipoprotein fractions with simvastatin in patients with hypertriglyceridemia. Circulation 1999; 100:1–470.

217. Superko HR, Krauss RM, DiRicco C. Effect of HMGCoA reductase inhibitor (fluvastatin) on LDL peak particle diameter. Am J Cardiol 1997; 80:78–81.

218. Superko HR, Raul E, Davis V, Aron C. Atorvastatin and LDL subclass distribution. JACC 2001; 37:248A.

219. Ikejiri A, Hirano T, Murayama S, et al. Effects of atorvastatin on triglyceride-rich lipoproteins, low-density lipoprotein subclass, and C-reactive protein in hemodialysis patients. Metabolism 2004; 53:1113–1117.

220. Rittershaus CW, Miller DP, Thomas LJ, et al. Vaccine-Induced antibodies inhibit CETP activity in vivo and reduce aortic lesions in a rabbit model of atherosclerosis. ATVB 2000;2106–2112.

221. Okamoto H, Yonemori F, Wakitani K, Minowa T, Maeda K, Shinkai H. A cholesteryl ester transfer protein inhibitor attenuates atherosclerosis in rabbits. Nature 2000; 406:203–207.

222. Huang Z, Inazu A, Nohara A, Higashikata T, Mabuchi H. Cholesteryl ester transfer protein inhibitor (JTT-705) and the development of atherosclerosis in rabbits with severe hypercholesterolaemia. Clin Sci (Lond) 2002; 103:587–594.

223. Clark RW, Sutfin TA, Ruggeri RB, et al. Raising high-density lipoprotein in humans through inhibition of cholesterylester transfer protein: an initial multidose study of torcetrapib. Arterioscler Thromb Vase Biol 2004; 24:490–497.

224. Brousseau ME, Schaefer EJ, Wolfe ML, et al. Effects of an inhibitor of cholesteryl ester transfer protein on HDL cholesterol. N Engl J Med 2004; 350:1505–1515.

225. Brown BG, Zambon A, Poulin D, et al. Use of niacin, statins, and resins in patients with combined hyperlipidemia. Am J Cardiol 1998; 81:52B–59B.

226. O'Keefe JH, Jr., Harris WS, Nelson J, Windsor SL. Effects of pravastatin with niacin or magnesium on lipid levels and postprandial lipemia. Am J Cardiol 1995; 76:480–484.
227. Superko HR, Krauss RM. Differential effect on HDL of niacin and resin in LDL subclass pattern A and B subjects. Circulation 1993; 88:1–386.
228. Superko HR, Krauss RM. LDL subclass distribution change in familial combined hyperlipidemia patients following Gemfibrozil and Niacin treatment. JACC 1997; 29:46A.
229. Miller NE. Effects of adrenoceptor-blocking drugs on plasma lipoprotein concentrations. Am J Card 1987; 60:17–23.
230. Superko HR, Wood PD, Krauss RM. Effect of alpha-and selective beta blockade for hypertension control on plasma lipoproteins, apoproteins, lipoprotein subclasses, and postprandial lipemia. Am J Med 1989; 1:26–31.
231. Superko HR, Krauss RM, Haskell WL. Stanford coronary risk intervention project investigators. Association of lipoprotein subclass distribution with use of selective and non-selective beta-blocker medications in patients with coronary heart disease. Atherosclerosis 1993; 101:1–8.
232. Krauss RM, Burkman RT, Jr. The metabolic impact of oral contraceptives. Am J Obstet Gynecol 1992; 167:1177–1184.
233. Grodstein F, Stampfer MJ, Colditz GA, et al. Postmenopausal hormone therapy and mortality. NEJM 1997; 336:1769–1775.
234. Superko HR, Blanche P, Holl L, Orr J, Shoenfeld MJ, Krauss RM. Reduction of plasma LDL and apo B levels with combined estrogen + progestin therapy in post-menopausal women is greater in women with dense rather than buoyant LDL. Circulation 1998; 98:1–7.
235. Seguret-Mace S, Latta-Mahieu M, Castro G, et al. Potential gene therapy for lecithin-cholesterol acyltransferase (LCAT)-deficient and hypoalphalipoproteine-mic patients with adenovirus-mediated transfer of human LCAT gene. Circulation 1996; 94:2177–2184.
236. Davidson MH, Maki K, Umporowicz D, Wheeler A, Rittershaus C, Ryan U. The safety and immunogenicity of a CETP vaccine in healthy adults. Atherosclerosis 2003; 169:113–120.
237. Gaofu Q, Jun L, Xiuyun Z, Wentao L, Jie W, Jingjing L. Antibody against cholesteryl ester transfer protein (CETP) elicited by a recombinant chimeric enzyme vaccine attenuated atherosclerosis in a rabbit model. Life Sci 2005; 77:2690–2702.
238. Rubin EM, Krauss RM, Spangler EA, Verstuyft JG, Clift SM. Inhibition of early atherogenesis in transgenic mice by human apolipoprotein Al. Nature 1991; 353:265–267.
239. Shah PK, Yano J, Reyes O, et al. High-dose recombinant apolipoprotein A-I(milano) mobilizes tissue cholesterol and rapidly reduces plaque lipid and macrophage content in apolipoprotein e-deficient mice. Potential implications for acute plaque stabilization. Circulation 2001; 103:3047–3050.
240. Nissen SE, Tsunoda T, Tuzcu EM, et al. Effect of recombinant ApoA-I Milano on coronary atherosclerosis in patients with acute coronary syndromes: a randomized controlled trial. JAMA 2003; 290:2292–2300.
241. Chambless LE, Heiss G, Folsom AR, et al. Association of coronary heart disease incidence with carotid arterial wall thickness and major risk factors: the Atherosclerosis Risk in Communities (ARIC) study, 1987–1993. Am J Epidemiol 1997; 146:483–494.

242. Hodis HN, Mack WJ, LaBree L, et al. The role of carotid arterial intima-media thickness in predicting clinical coronary events. Ann Intern Med 1998; 128:262–269.
243. Cai JM, Hatsukami TS, Ferguson MS, Small R, Polissar NL, Yuan C. Classifcation of human carotid atherosclerotic lesions with in vivo multicontrast magnetic resonance imaging. Circulation 2002; 106:1368–1373.
244. Chun Yuan, Shao-xiong Zhang, Nayak L, et al. Identification of fibrous cap rupture with magnetic resonance imaging is highly associated with recent transient ischemic attack or stroke. Circulation 2002; 105:181–185.
245. Yuan C, Kerwin WS, Ferguson MS, et al. Contrast-enhanced high resolution MRI for atherosclerotic carotid artery tissue characterization. J Magn Reson Imaging 2002; 15:62–67.
246. Brent A, French Zequan Yang, Berr Stuart S, Kramer CM. Of mice and men…and broken hearts. Circulation 2001; 104:110.
247. Sirol M, Fuster V, Badimon JJ, et al. Chronic thrombus detection with in vivo magnetic resonance imaging and a fibrin-targeted contrast agent. Circulation 2005; 112:1594–1600.
248. Ruehm SG, Corot C, Vogt P, Kolb S, Debatin JF. Magnetic resonance imaging of atherosclerotic plaque with ultrasmall superparamagnetic particles of iron oxide in hyperlipidemic rabbits. Circulation 2001; 103:415–422.
249. Yong Kim W, Stuber Matthias, Börnert Peter, Kissinger Kraig V, Manning Warren J, Botnar René M. Three-dmensional black-blood cardiac magnetic resonance coronary vessel wall imaging detects positive arterial remodeling in patients with nonsignificant coronary artery disease. Circulation 2002; 106:296–299.
250. Arad Y, Spadaro LA, Roth M, Newstein D, Guerci AD. Treatment of asymptomatic adults with elevated coronary calcium scores with atorvastatin, vitamin, C and vitamin E: the St. Francis Heart Study randomized clinical trial. J Am Coll Cardiol 2005; 46:166–172.
251. LaMonte MJ, FitzGerald SJ, Church TS, et al. Coronary artery calcium score and coronary heart disease events in a large cohort of asymptomatic men and women. Am J Epidemiol 2005; 162:421–429.
252. MoJlet NR, Cademartiri F, van Mieghem CA, et al. High-resolution spiral computed tomography coronary angiography in patients referred for diagnostic conventional coronary angiography. Circulation 2005; 112:2318–2323.
253. Leber AW, Knez A, von Ziegler F, et al. Quantification of obstructive and nonobstructive coronary lesions by 64-slice computed tomography: a comparative study with quantitative coronary angiography and intravascular ultrasound. J Am Coll Cardiol 2005; 46:147–154.
254. Taylor AJ, Kent SM, Flaherty PJ, Coyle LC, Markwood TT, Vernalis MN. ARBITER: arterial biology for the investigation of the treatment effects of reducing cholesterol: a randomized trial comparing the effects of atorvastatin and pravastatin on carotid intima medial thickness. Circulation 2002; 106:2055–2060.
255. Taylor AJ, Sullenberger LE, Lee HJ, Lee JK, Grace KA. Arterial Biology for the Investigation of the Treatment Effects of Reducing Cholesterol (ARBITER) 2: a double-blind, placebo-controlled study of extended-release niacin on athero-sclerosis progression in secondary prevention patients treated with statins. Circulation 2004; 110:3512–3517.

256. Corti R, Fayad ZA, Fuster V, et al. Effects of lipid-lowering by simvastatin on human atherosclerotic lesions: a longitudinal study by high-resolution, noninvasive magnetic resonance imaging. Circulation 2001; 104:249–252.

257. Corti R, Fuster V, Fayad ZA, et al. Lipid lowering by simvastatin induces regression of human atherosclerotic lesions: two years' follow-up by high-resolution noninvasive magnetic resonance imaging. Circulation 2002; 106:2884–2887.

258. Corti R, Fuster V, Fayad ZA, et al. Effects of aggressive versus conventional lipid-lowering therapy by simvastatin on human atherosclerotic lesions: a prospective, randomized, double-blind trial with high-resolution magnetic resonance imaging. J Am Coll Cardiol 2005; 46:106–112.

259. Zhao XQ, Yuan C, Hatsukami TS, et al. Effects of prolonged intensive lipid-lowering therapy on the characteristics of carotid atherosclerotic plaques in vivo by MRI: a case-control study. Arterioscler Thromb Vasc Biol 2001; 21:1623–1629.

260. Superko HR, Hecht H. Metabolic disorders contributing to subclinical coronary atherosclerosis in patients with coronary calcification. Am J Card 2001; 88:260–264.

3

Hemostatic Risk Factors for Atherothrombosis

P. K. Shah

Atherosclerosis Research Center, Division of Cardiology and Department of Medicine, Cedars-Sinai Medical Center and David Geffen School of Medicine, University of California, Los Angeles, California, U.S.A.

Atherosclerosis predisposes to arterial thrombosis and thrombosis superimposed on a disrupted (ruptured or eroded) plaque is the proximate event that triggers acute ischemic syndromes and sudden death (1,2). Although a number of risk factors for atherothrombosis have been defined through observational and epidemiologic studies, a significant number of atherothrombotic events occur in individuals without traditional atherosclerosis related risk factors (3). A number of studies have also focused on novel risk factors, predominantly related to hemostasis and coagulation, to identify a potential role for primary hemostatic abnormalities and cardiovascular risk (4–7). Normal hemostasis is orchestrated through a closely regulated interaction between prothrombotic and antithrombotic/thrombolytic processes mediated by cellular components, soluble plasma proteins, and endothelium-derived mediators. Genetic or acquired abnormalities that alter the production, activity, bioavailability, or metabolism of specific factors can alter this intricate balance resulting in predisposition thrombotic events.

COAGULATION FACTORS AND ATHEROTHROMBOTIC DISEASE

Fibrinogen

Fibrinogen, precursor of fibrin, is an important coagulation protein that also plays an important role in plasma viscosity and platelet aggregation. Fibrinogen levels are strongly correlated with traditional vascular risk factors such as age, physical inactivity, hypertension, smoking, and features of the insulin resistance syndrome. Furthermore, fibrinogen is an acute-phase reactant, and the acute-phase response arising from viral infection, inflammatory stimuli, and smoking has been implicated in the development of atherothrombosis. Several prospective studies—Northwick Park Heart study, the Prospective Cardiovascular Munster (PROCAM) study, and the Prospective Epidemiological Study of Myocardial Infarction (PRIME)—of both healthy subjects and those with established vascular disease have identified an association between fibrinogen levels and myocardial infarction, stroke, and peripheral vascular disease (8–10) with an independent relative risk of arterial disease around 2–2.5% in the highest fibrinogen quartile compared with the lowest fibrinogen quartile. Several genetic polymorphisms of the fibrinogen gene have been identified that influence fibrinogen levels as well as other functional aspects of clot formation, but the relationship of these polymorphisms to atherothrombotic vascular disease has in general yielded weak or inconsistent results (4). Recently, results were reported from a detailed individual participant meta-analysis of a large data set with 6944 first nonfatal acute myocardial infarction or stroke events, and 13,210 deaths with cause-specific mortality data, among 154,211 participants from 31 studies (10). The age and sex adjusted hazard ratio per 1 gram increase in usual level of fibrinogen was 2.42 (95% CI: 2.24–2.60) for coronary heart disease, 2.06 (95% CI: 1.83–2.33) for stroke, 2.76 (95% CI: 2.28–3.35) for vascular mortality, and 2.03 (95% CI: 1.90–2.18) for nonvascular mortality (11). The hazard ratios, after adjustment for established risk factors, were reduced to 1.8 for coronary heart disease and stroke. Thus, overwhelming evidence suggests a moderately strong relationship between fibrinogen levels and cardiovascular risk. Although biologically plausible explanations could account for a causal relationship between fibrinogen levels and atherothrombosis, it is also possible that elevated fibrinogen levels reflect the inflammation associated with atherosclerosis rather than reflecting a cause and effect relationship (12).

Factor VII

Factor VII (FVII) is a vitamin K dependent coagulation factor, and its levels are influenced by age, body mass index, and plasma triglyceride levels (4). Several prospective studies have examined the relationship between FVII mediated pro-coagulant activity (FVIIc) and atherothrombosis, but the results have been inconsistent. The Northwick Park heart study found a significant association between FVIIc and coronary heart disease that was stronger than that with cholesterol levels (8); however, subsequent reports, taking into account confounding variables, failed to confirm this finding (13). Similarly, several genetic polymorphisms of FVII gene that influence its levels have been described, but the relationship of these polymorphisms with coronary heart disease have again been weak, negative, or inconsistent (4,14–21).

Factor XIII

This coagulation factor is involved in stabilizing a fibrin clot. Several genetic polymorphisms have been identified in the Factor XIII gene, but once again no consistent relationship of these polymorphisms to atherothrombotic vascular disease has been confirmed; in fact, some of the polymorphisms have actually shown an inverse relationship (22–28).

Factor V/Prothrombin

Several studies have evaluated the relationship between genetic abnormalities in the Factor V and Prothrombin genes and risk of arterial thrombosis. In general, the studies examining the association of Factor V Leiden (1691 G/A) mutation and prothrombin 20210G/A to arterial thrombotic disease have been negative even among young subjects (4). Positive associations have, in general, been observed in studies involving highly selected populations or among children or have considered interactions with environmental risk factors (29,30). Thus, Factor V Leiden mutation was shown to be associated with a 2.5-fold increased risk of nonfatal myocardial infarction among young women predominantly among smokers (31). Similar findings were noted among carriers of the prothrombin 20210A allele who had a 4-fold increase in the risk of myocardial infarction that was again increased more than 40-fold among smokers (32). A combined analysis of Factor V Leiden and the prothrombin 20210A allele in this population showed that the effect of major coronary risk factors was increased 4- to 6-fold by the presence of one of these inherited, prothrombotic risk factors. Subsequently, two case-control studies of men showed an increased risk of myocardial infarction associated with Factor V Leiden and the prothrombin 20210G/A mutations predominantly in the presence of other cardiovascular risk factors (33,34).

Thrombomodulin

Thrombomodulin is an endothelial cell surface receptor for thrombin that accelerates thrombin-induced activation of the natural anticoagulant protein C. Reduced plasma thrombomodulin levels were associated with an increased risk of myocardial infarction in a prospective case-control study (35). The association of certain genetic polymorphisms in the thrombomodulin gene with atherothrombotic disease have been inconsistent (36,37).

Platelets and Atherothrombotic Vascular Disease

Platelet adhesion and aggregation at the site of vascular injury plays an important role in clot formation. Platelet surface receptors such as the glycoprotein IIb/IIIa bind fibrinogen and von Willebrand factor are essential final common steps in platelet aggregation. Genetic polymorphisms of this receptor complex, in particular the presence of glycoprotein IIIa isoforms known as the PL A2, have been linked to a markedly increased risk for coronary heart disease among young subjects, especially smokers, in some studies, but these findings have not been substantiated in larger studies after accounting for confounding variables (38–48). Similarly, other platelet glycoprotein receptor gene polymorphisms have also yielded inconsistent results (4).

Role of Endothelium-Derived Hemostatic Mediators in Atherothrombosis

Endogenous fibrinolysis is dominantly mediated by endothelium-derived tissue-type plasminogen activator (t-PA) whose action, in turn, is opposed by its inhibitor known as the plasminogen activator inhibitor-1 (PAI-1). Circulating t-PA is mostly complexed with PAI-1, and thus circulating levels of t-PA do not necessarily reflect functionally active t-PA. Elevated levels of both t-PA and PAI-1 have been associated with an increased risk of arterial thrombotic disease in some but not in other studies (13). An imbalance of this fibrinolytic equilibrium is encountered primarily in the insulin resistance syndrome and hypertriglyceridemia (elevated triglycerides are associated with increased PAI-1 levels), which leads to increased plasma PAI-1 and t-PA antigen levels (reflecting inactive t-PA/PAI-1 complexes) with a consequent decrease in fibrinolytic activity (49). Genetic polymorphisms of t-PA and PAI-1 genes have not shown uniform relationship to atherothrombotic vascular disease (4).

A recently identified inhibitor of fibrinolysis is a plasma carboxypeptidase called Thrombin-activatable fibrinolysis inhibitor (TAFI) (50). Plasma TAFI concentrations demonstrate high interindividual variability that is poorly explained by environmental factors (51). Activation of TAFI occurs by the thrombin–thrombomodulin complex and results in prolongation of clot lysis time. Increased plasma TAFI levels have been associated with an increased risk of both deep-vein thrombosis and symptomatic or angiographic coronary artery disease in some studies, whereas others have shown an inverse relationship to risk of myocardial infarction (52–54). In the past few years, several polymorphisms that have been described in the TAFI gene have been identified without a consistent relationship to atherothrombotic risk (4).

Endothelium-derived nitric oxide, produced by the action of endothelial nitric oxide synthase (eNOS) from Arginine, exerts antithrombotic actions in addition to its anti-inflammatory, anti-oxidant, vasodilator, and anti-proliferative effects (55). Several genetic polymorphisms of the eNOS gene have been identified, but their relationship to atherothrombosis has been inconsistent at best (4).

White Blood Cell Count and Atherothrombosis

Inflammation is critically linked to various pathophysiologic events leading to initiation, progression, and destabilization of atherosclerosis (2). A number of epidemiologic studies have shown an association between elevated white blood cell (WBC) count and coronary heart disease (56–64). Similarly, in acute coronary syndromes, elevated WBC count has been linked to increased risk for fatal and nonfatal cardiovascular events (65–68). A recent study suggested that the cardiovascular risk of elevated WBC counts is carried by increased circulating neutrophil counts and decreased total mononuclear cell counts (lymphocytes plus monocytes) (69). However, some studies have failed to confirm these relationships after correction for confounding risk factors such as smoking (15,70).

CONCLUSION

The relationship between hemostatic factors and risk for arterial atherothrombosis, after correction for all known risk factors and confounding variables, is at best weak and at worst unconvincing. In contrast to venous thromboembolic disease, wherein the role of certain thrombophilia markers is well established, there is little clarity in relation to arterial thrombotic disease except possibly in the case of fibrinogen levels. Although early reports in the literature revealed positive associations, numerous negative studies have followed, and the initial hope that inherited risk factors might contribute significantly to the development of atherothrombotic disease remains largely unconfirmed.

REFERENCES

1. Ross R. Atherosclerosis: an inflammatory disease. N Engl J Med 1999; 340:115–126.
2. Shah PK. Mechanisms of plaque vulnerability and rupture. J Am Coll Cardiol 2003; 41:15S–22S.
3. Kullo IJ, Gau GT, Tajik AJ. Novel risk factors for atherosclerosis. Mayo Clin Proc 2000; 75:369–380.
4. Voetsch B, Loscelzo J. Genetic determinants of arterial thrombosis. ATVB 2005; 24:216–229.
5. Andreotic F, Becker RC. Atherothrombolic disorders: new insights from hematology. Circulation 2005; 3:1855–1863.
6. Rosenberg RD, Aird WC. Vascular-bed-specific hemostasis and hypercoagulable states. N Engl J Med 1999; 340:1555–1564.
7. Folsom AR. Hemostatic risk factors for atherothrombotic disease: an epidemiologic view. Thromb Haemost 2001; 86:366–373.
8. Meade TW, Mellows S, Brozovic M, et al. Haemostatic function and ischaemic heart disease: principal results of the Northwick Park heart study. Lancet 1986; 2:533–537.
9. Heinrich J, Balleisen L, Schulte H, Assmann G, van de Loo J. Fibrinogen and factor VII in the prediction of coronary risk: results from the PROCAM study in healthy men. Arterioscler Thromb 1994; 14:54–59.
10. Scarabin PY, Arveiler D, Amouyel P, et al. Plasma fibrinogen explains much of the difference in risk of coronary heart disease between France and Northern Ireland. The PRIME study. Atherosclerosis 2003; 166:103–109.

11. Fibrinogen Studies Collaboration. Plasma fibrinogen level and the risk of major cardiovascular diseases and non-vascular mortality: an individual participant meta-analysis. JAMA 2005; 294:1799–1809.

12. Sakkinen PA, Wahl P, Cushman M, Lewis MR, Tracy RP. Clustering of procoagulation, inflammation, and fibrinolysis variables with metabolic factors in insulin resistance syndrome. Am J Epidemiol 2000; 152:897–907.

13. Lane DA, Grant PJ. Role of hemostatic gene polymorphisms in venous and arterial thrombotic disease. Blood 2000; 95:1517–1532.

14. Hunault M, Arbini AA, Lopaciuk S, Carew JA, Bauer KA. The Arg353Gln polymorphism reduces the level of coagulation factor VII: in vivo and in vitro studies. Arterioscler Thromb Vasc Biol 1997; 17:2825–2829.

15. Pinotti M, Toso R, Girelli D, et al. Modulation of factor VII levels by intron 7 polymorphisms: population and in vitro studies. Blood 2000; 95:3423–3428.

16. van 't Hooft FM, Silveira A, Tornvall P, et al. Two common functional polymorphisms in the promoter region of the coagulation factor VII gene determining plasma factor VII activity and mass concentration. Blood 1999; 93:3432–3441.

17. Kavlie A, Hiltunen L, Rasi V, Prydz H. Two novel mutations in the human coagulation factor VII promoter. Thromb Haemost 2003; 90:194–205.

18. Iacoviello L, Di Castelnuovo A, De Knijff P. Polymorphisms in the coagulation factor VII gene and the risk of myocardial infarction. N Engl J Med 1998; 338:79–85.

19. Folsom AR, Wu KK, Rosamond WD, Sharrett AR, Chambless LE. Prospective study of hemostatic factors and incidence of coronary heart disease: the atherosclerosis risk in communities (ARIC) study. Circulation 1997; 96:1102–1108.

20. Smith FB, Lee AJ, Fowkes FG, Price JF, Rumley A, Lowe GD. Hemostatic factors as predictors of ischemic heart disease and stroke in the edinburgh artery study. Arterioscler Thromb Vasc Biol 1997; 17:3321–3325.

21. Doggen CJ, Manger Cats V, Bertina RM, Reitsma PH, Vandenbroucke JP, Rosendaal FR. A genetic propensity to high factor VII is not associated with the risk of myocardial infarction in men. Thromb Haemost 1998; 80:281–285.

22. Ariens RA, Lai TS, Weisel JW, Greenberg CS, Grant PJ. Role of factor XIII in fibrin clot formation and effects of genetic polymorphisms. Blood 2002; 100:743–754.

23. Kohler HP, Ariens RA, Whitaker P, Grant PJ. A common coding polymorphism in the FXIII A-subunit gene (FXIIIVal34Leu) affects cross-linking activity. Thromb Haemost 1998; 80:704.

24. Ariens RA, Philippou H, Nagaswami C, Weisel JW, Lane DA, Grant PJ. The factor XIII V34L polymorphism accelerates thrombin activation of factor XIII and affects cross-linked fibrin structure. Blood 2000; 96:988–995.

25. Lim BC, Ariens RA, Carter AM, Weisel JW, Grant PJ. Genetic regulation of fibrin structure and function: complex gene-environment interactions may modulate vascular risk. Lancet 2003; 361:1424–1431.

26. Elbaz A, Poirier O, Canaple S, Chedru F, Cambien F, Amarenco P. The association between the Val34Leu polymorphism in the factor XIII gene and brain infarction. Blood 2000; 95:586–591.

27. Franco RF, Pazin-Filho A, Tavella MH, Simoes MV, Marin-Neto JA, Zago MA. Factor XIII Val34Leu and the risk of myocardial infarction. Haematologica 2000; 85:67–71.

28. Dardik R, Solomon A, Loscalzo J, et al. Novel proangiogenic effect of factor XIII associated with suppression of thrombospondin 1 expression. Arterioscler Thromb Vasc Biol 2003; 23:1472–1477.
29. Margaglione M, D'Andrea G, Giuliani N, et al. Inherited prothrombotic conditions and premature ischemic stroke: sex difference in the association with factor V Leiden. Arterioscler Thromb Vasc Biol 1999; 19:1751–1756.
30. Nowak-Gottl U, Strater R, Heinecke A, et al. Lipoprotein(a) and genetic polymorphisms of clotting factor V, prothrombin, and methylenetetrahydrofolate reductase are risk factors of spontaneous ischemic stroke in childhood. Blood 1999; 94:3678–3682.
31. Rosendaal FR, Siscovick DS, Schwartz SM, et al. Factor V Leiden (resistance to activated protein C) increases the risk of myocardial infarction in young women. Blood 1997; 89:2817–2821.
32. Rosendaal FR, Siscovick DS, Schwartz SM, Psaty BM, Raghunathan TE, Vos HL. A common prothrombin variant (20210 G to A) increases the risk of myocardial infarction in young women. Blood 1997; 90:1747–1750.
33. Doggen CJ, Cats VM, Bertina RM, Rosendaal FR. Interaction of coagulation defects and cardiovascular risk factors: increased risk of myocardial infarction associated with factor V Leiden or prothrombin 20210A. Circulation 1998; 97:1037–1041.
34. Inbal A, Freimark D, Modan B, et al. Synergistic effects of prothrombotic polymorphisms and atherogenic factors on the risk of myocardial infarction in young males. Blood 1999; 93:2186–2190.
35. Salomaa V, Matei C, Aleksic N, et al. Soluble thrombomodulin as a predictor of incident coronary heart disease and symptomless carotid artery atherosclerosis in the atherosclerosis risk in communities (ARIC) study: a case-cohort study. Lancet 1999; 353:1729–1734 [CrossRef][Medline] [Order article via Infotrieve].
36. Norlund L, Holm J, Zoller B, Ohlin AK. A common thrombomodulin amino acid dimorphism is associated with myocardial infarction. Thromb Haemost 1997; 77:248–251.
37. Doggen CJ, Kunz G, Rosendaal FR, et al. A mutation in the thrombomodulin gene, 127G to A coding for Ala25Thr, and the risk of myocardial infarction in men. Thromb Haemost 1998; 80:743–748.
38. Honda S, Honda Y, Bauer B, Ruan C, Kunicki TJ. The impact of three-dimensional structure on the expression of PlA alloantigens on human integrin â3. Blood 1995; 86:234–242.
39. Newman PJ. Platelet alloantigens: cardiovascular as well as immunological risk factors? Lancet 1997; 349:370–371.
40. Weiss EJ, Bray PF, Tayback M, et al. A polymorphism of a platelet glycoprotein receptor as an inherited risk factor for coronary thrombosis. N Engl J Med 1996; 334:1090–1094.
41. Carter AM, Ossei-Gerning N, Wilson IJ, Grant PJ. Association of the platelet Pl(A) polymorphism of glycoprotein IIb/IIIa and the fibrinogen B â 448 polymorphism with myocardial infarction and extent of coronary artery disease. Circulation 1997; 96:1424–1431.
42. Wagner KR, Giles WH, Johnson CJ, et al. Platelet glycoprotein receptor IIIa polymorphism P1A2 and ischemic stroke risk: the stroke prevention in young women study. Stroke 1998; 29:581–585.

43. Ridker PM, Hennekens CH, Schmitz C, Stampfer MJ, Lindpaintner K. PIA1/A2 polymorphism of platelet glycoprotein IIIa and risks of myocardial infarction, stroke, and venous thrombosis. Lancet 1997; 349:385–388.
44. Herrmann SM, Poirier O, Marques-Vidal P, et al. The Leu33/Pro polymorphism (PlA1/PlA2) of the glycoprotein IIIa (GPIIIa) receptor is not related to myocardial infarction in the ECTIM Study. Etude Cas-Temoins de l'infarctus du myocarde. Thromb Haemost 1997; 77:1179–1181.
45. Ardissino D, Mannucci PM, Merlini PA, et al. Prothrombotic genetic risk factors in young survivors of myocardial infarction. Blood 1999; 94:46–51.
46. Bray PF. Integrin polymorphisms as risk factors for thrombosis. Thromb Haemost 1999; 82:337–344.
47. Gonzalez-Conejero R, Lozano ML, Rivera J, et al. Polymorphisms of platelet membrane glycoprotein Ib associated with arterial thrombotic disease. Blood 1998; 92:2771–2776.
48. Santoso S, Kunicki TJ, Kroll H, Haberbosch W, Gardemann A. Association of the platelet glycoprotein Ia C807T gene polymorphism with nonfatal myocardial infarction in younger patients. Blood 1999; 93:2449–2453.
49. Juhan-Vague I, Morange P, Alessi MC. Fibrinolytic function and coronary risk. Curr Cardiol Rep 1999; 1:119–124.
50. Sakharov DV, Plow EF, Rijken DC. On the mechanism of the antifibrinolytic activity of plasma carboxypeptidase B. J Biol Chem 1997; 272:14477–14482.
51. Juhan-Vague I, Renucci JF, Grimaux M, et al. Thrombin-activatable fibrinolysis inhibitor antigen levels and cardiovascular risk factors. Arterioscler Thromb Vasc Biol 2000; 20:2156–2161.
52. van Tilburg NH, Rosendaal FR, Bertina RM. Thrombin activatable fibrinolysis inhibitor and the risk for deep vein thrombosis. Blood 2000; 95:2855–2859.
53. Silveira A, Schatteman K, Goossens F, et al. Plasma procarboxypeptidase U in men with symptomatic coronary artery disease. Thromb Haemost 2000; 84:364–368.
54. Morange PE, Juhan-Vague I, Scarabin PY, et al. Association between TAFI antigen and Ala147Thr polymorphism of the TAFI gene and the angina pectoris incidence. Thromb Haemost 2003; 89:554–560.
55. Loscalzo J, Welch G. Nitric oxide and its role in the cardiovascular system. Prog Cardiovasc Dis 1995; 38:87–104.
56. Ensrud K, Grimm RJ. The white blood cell count and risk for coronary heart disease. Am Heart J 1992; 124:207–213.
57. Kannel, Anderson K, Wilson P. White blood cell count and cardiovascular disease. insights from the framingham study. JAMA 1992; 267:1253–1256.
58. Phillips A, Neaton J, Cook D, Grimm RJ, Shaper A. Leukocyte count and risk of major coronary heart disease event. Am J Epidemiol 1992; 136:59–70.
59. Gillum, Ingram D, Makuc D. White blood cell count, coronary hear disease, and death the NHANES I epidemiologic follow-up study. Am Heart J 1993; 125:855–863.
60. Sweetnam P, Thomas H, Yarnell J, Baker I, Elwood P. Total and differential leukocyte counts as predictors of ischemic heart disease the caerphilly and speedwell studies. Am J Epidemiol 1997; 145:416–421.
61. Danesh J, Collins R, Appleby P, Peto R. Association of fibrinogen, C-reactive protein, albumin, or leukocyte count with coronary heart disease meta-analyses of prospective studies. JAMA 1998; 279:1477–1482.

62. Brown E, Giles W, Croft J. White blood cell count an independent predictor of coronary heart disease mortality among a national cohort. J Clin Epidemiol 2001; 54:316–322.
63. Lee C, Folsom A, Nieto F, Chambless L, Shahar E, Wolfe D. White blood cell count and incidence of coronary heart disease and ischemic stroke and mortality from cardiovascular disease in African–American and white men and women atherosclerosis risk in communities study. Am J Epidemiol 2001; 154:758–764.
64. Haim M, Boyko V, Goldbourt U, Battler A, Behar S. Predictive value of elevated white blood cell count in patients with preexisting coronary heart disease the bezafibrate infarction prevention study. Arch Intern Med 2004; 164:433–439.
65. Barron H, Cannon C, Murphy S, Braunwald E, Gibson C. Association between white blood cell count, epicardial blood flow, myocardial perfusion, and clinical outcomes in the setting of acute myocardial infarction a thrombolysis in myocardial infarction 10 substudy. Circulation 2000; 102:2329–2334.
66. Barron H, Harr S, Radford M, Wang Y, Krumholz H. The association between white blood cell count and acute myocardial infarction mortality in patients >or =65 years of age findings from the cooperative cardiovascular project. J Am Coll Cardiol 2001; 38:1654–1661.
67. Cannon C, McCabe C, Wilcox R, Bentley J, Braunwald E. Association of white blood cell count with increased mortality in acute myocardial infarction and unstable angina pectoris. OPUS TIMI 16 investigators. Am J Cardiol 2001; 87:636–639.
68. Pelizzon G, Dixon S, Stone G, et al. Relation of admission white blood cell count to long-term outcomes after primary coronary angioplasty for acute myocardial infarction (The stent PAMI trial). Am J Cardiol 2003; 91:729–731.
69. Horne BD, Anderson JL, John JM, et al. Intermountain heart collaborative study group. J Am Coll Cardiol 2005; 45:1638–1643.
70. Huang Z-C, Chien K, Yang C, Wang C-H, Chang T, Chen C. Peripheral differential leukocyte counts and subsequent mortality form all diseases, cancers, and cardiovascular diseases in Taiwanese. J Formos Med Assoc 2003; 102:775–781.

4

Homocysteine: A Risk Factor for Atherothrombotic Cardiovascular Disease

Mathew J. Price

*Division of Cardiovascular Diseases, Scripps Clinic,
La Jolla, California, U.S.A.*

Andrew A. Zadeh

*Department of Medicine, Cedars-Sinai Medical Center and the David
Geffen School of Medicine, University of California,
Los Angeles, California, U.S.A.*

Sanjay Kaul

*Division of Cardiology, Cedars-Sinai Medical Center and the David Geffen
School of Medicine, University of California,
Los Angeles, California, U.S.A.*

The recognition of hypercholesterolemia, tobacco use, hypertension, family history, and diabetes mellitus as risk factors for cardiovascular disease has contributed to the significant decline in cardiovascular morbidity and mortality over the last 50 years. However, we are still far from defining the physiological milieu necessary for the development of cardiovascular disease. The traditional risk factors only explain 50% or less of the variation in atherosclerotic cardiovascular disease. As such, other variables besides the traditional risk factors might offer some insights. Chief among them include homocysteine, a sulfur amino acid formed during the metabolism of methionine. In homocystinuria, an inborn error of this metabolism, homocysteine levels are severely elevated, often to more than 50 times that of normal. The cardiovascular hallmark of this disease is premature atherothrombosis of the peripheral, coronary, and cerebral vasculature. From this observation, three hypotheses can be proposed: first, that homocysteine directly promotes atherothrombosis; second, that in doing so, the homocysteine concentration in otherwise normal individuals is a measure of cardiovascular risk; and third, that by reducing the homocysteine level, one can diminish this risk. A similar line of reasoning links familial hypercholesterolemia and the established risk factor, low-density lipoprotein, in the general population. Different types of data are needed to prove each of the three hypotheses listed above. First, basic science investigation must establish a coherent mechanism for how homocysteine may cause atherothrombosis in vivo. Second, epidemiological studies must show a strong, consistent, independent association between elevated homocysteine levels and cardiovascular morbidity and mortality. Third, prospective, randomized trials must establish that decreasing the level of homocysteine modifies this risk. Only by fulfilling these criteria can homocysteine join the canon of the classical cardiovascular risk factors of hypertension, diabetes mellitus, hypercholesterolemia, and tobacco use. If it does not fulfill these criteria completely, or does so only partially, homocysteine measurement may still provide prognostic information for patients with unstable angina, acute myocardial infarction, deep venous thrombosis, or stroke.

HOMOCYSTEINE METABOLISM

Homocysteine is a sulfur amino acid formed during the metabolism of methionine, an essential amino acid that is found in dietary protein. Homocysteine is metabolized by remethylation or transsulfuration (Fig. 1) (1). Remethylation is a salvage pathway; homocysteine acquires a methyl group from 5-methyl-tetrahydrofolate to form methionine in a reaction catalyzed by the vitamin B12-dependent enzyme, methionine synthase. 5-methyl-tetrahydrofolate is derived from folate in a cycle catalyzed by methylene tetrahydrofolate reductase (MTHFR). An alternative pathway for remethylation occurs in the liver, where betaine acts as the methyl donor. Transsulfuration occurs during times of methionine excess or cysteine depletion. Homocysteine combines with serine to form cystathionine via a rate-limiting reaction catalyzed by the B6-dependent enzyme, cystathionine-beta-synthase. Cystathionine-gamma-lyase, another B6-dependent enzyme, then catalyzes the hydrolysis of cystathionine to cysteine, which is then further metabolized to glutathione or sulfate (2).

HOMOCYSTEINE: CIRCULATING FORMS

Homocysteine is a four-carbon thiol amino acid that exists in various forms within human plasma depending on the redox status of its sulfhydryl group (Fig. 2). Approximately 1% of circulating homocysteine circulates in the reduced form of the free thiol itself. When this is bound to another molecule of homocysteine, it forms the symmetrical disulfide, homocystine. When bound to

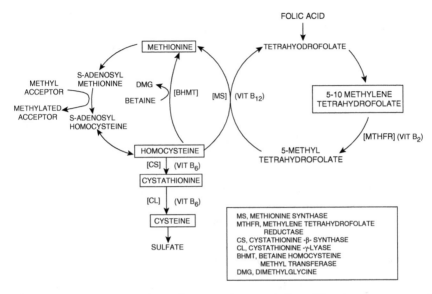

Figure 1 Outline of methionine/homocysteine metabolism. Vitamin coenzymes and substrates: THF, tetrahydrofolate; B_2, riboflavin; B_6, vitamin B_6 as its biological active form, i.e., pyridoxal 5'-phosphate; and B_{12}, methyl cobalamin. Intermediate metabolite: DMG, dimethylglycine. *Source*: From Ref. 1.

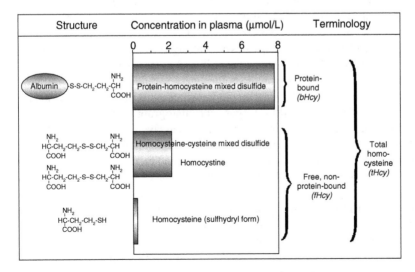

Figure 2 Homocysteine and the major related disulfides in normal human plasma. *Source*: From Ref. 3.

other types of thiols, it forms mixed disulfides, predominantly homocysteine-cysteine disulfide. Roughly 75% of circulating homocysteine is protein-bound, mostly to albumin, by disulfide linkage to protein-cysteine. The term "free" homocysteine refers to those forms of homocysteine that are not protein bound (including disulfides), while "total" homocysteine (tHcy) refers to both protein-bound and free states (3).

The saturation of plasma protein-binding sites only occurs at very high levels of total homocysteine (homocystinuric range > 100 micromol) (4). Thus, the relatively large differences in measured total homocysteine between individuals in the general population (on the order of 5 μmol/L) represent very small changes in circulating reduced homocysteine. Serum plasma protein concentration also significantly affects measured total homocysteine given that a large proportion of total homocysteine is protein bound; a positive correlation between tHcy and serum albumin level has been observed (5).

HOMOCYSTEINE: LABORATORY MEASUREMENTS

The clinician must confront three factors when interpreting a laboratory value for homocysteine concentration: the methodologic variability of homocysteine concentration analysis, the biological variability of homocysteine concentration in the subject, and, given these variations, the estimation of patient risk.

Methodologic variability is introduced during sample collection, storage, and laboratory analysis. Food ingestion may change the circulating homocysteine concentration (6,7). Thus, it is recommended that the representative sample be gathered while the subject is fasting. Homocysteine is an unstable compound ex vivo; total homocysteine in whole blood increases at room temperature because of its synthesis and release from erythrocytes. After phlebotomy, levels rise at a rate of 10% per hour in stored blood even with additives such as ethylenediamine tetra-acetic acid (EDTA). Thus, to avoid falsely elevated results, the sample should be promptly placed on ice and centrifuged or stored at 0° C (8).

There are three primary methods for measuring the plasma concentration of homocysteine: electrochemical or fluorescence-detection high-performance liquid chromatography (HPLC), gas chromatography-mass spectrometry (GC-MS), and fluorescence or enzyme immunoassay. In general, HPLC and GC-MS are expensive, cumbersome, and require highly skilled technicians. The immunoassays offer the hope of improved speed and ease.

Analytical quality specifications analysis of these methods by the Centers for Disease Control (CDC), revealed significant inter-laboratory and intra-laboratory variations with none of the laboratories showing optimum performance (9). This variation was less than 10% of the sample measurement; however, this may still present a difficulty for the interpreting physician, because the relationship between homocysteine level and cardiovascular risk may be a graded phenomenon and small differences in levels may have substantial clinical implications.

Even with the accurate measurement of homocysteine concentration, reference ranges must be established so that the clinician can differentiate between normal and pathological levels. Because some studies show that the relationship between total homocysteine and cardiovascular risk is a graded phenomenon, the precise definition of the "upper limit of normal" is unclear. Moreover, many studies that show a strong correlation between total homocysteine levels and risk derive this association not by comparing absolute levels, but by comparing a given cohort's highest and lowest inter-quartile levels. Mean levels of homocysteine differ according to gender and increase with age (10), so that proper reference values must incorporate both of these patient variables.

The patient's clinical situation also affects the measured homocysteine concentration. An acute atherothrombotic event may transiently alter total homocysteine levels because a large proportion of total homocysteine is bound to albumin, which decreases during the acute inflammatory response. In patients presenting with acute coronary syndrome, homocysteine levels do not change, or slightly decrease, between the day of admission and hospital day 2 (11), and then rise significantly thereafter; this rise persists as long as 6 months (12,13). Similar findings have been observed in homocysteine levels measured during the acute and convalescent phases of stroke (14). It is unclear whether homocysteine levels drop initially and then recover, or alternatively, rise from baseline for an undetermined amount of time. This could have a significant clinical impact because the hospital admission for an acute atherothrombotic event is likely to be when the physician assesses a patient's risk factors and the homocysteine level is first measured. It is uncertain how accurately such an admission level reflects future risk given the flux in homocysteine concentrations around this time. Conversely, because of the persistent rise in levels after events, retrospective studies that measure the homocysteine levels of index cases in the initial months after an acute event may overestimate the association between elevated homocysteine and risk.

THE ORAL METHIONINE LOAD

Similar in approach to the oral glucose tolerance test, the oral methionine load is a provocative test to uncover patients who may be at atherothrombotic risk but have a fasting total homocysteine in the normal range. By expanding the definition of hyperhomocysteinemia to include those individuals with a high post-methionine load and normal fasting total homocysteine, it has been stated that as many as 40% of at risk patients are not identified by screening with fasting total homocysteine alone (15). The standard procedure is to administer 0.1 gm/kg of L-methionine orally, usually in fruit juice to mask this amino acid's unpleasant taste. Total homocysteine is measured 4 hours later. An abnormal post-methionine load homocysteine level is generally defined as higher than two standard deviations above the mean, although some cohort studies also define it based on inter-quartile comparison.

Homocysteine metabolism is dependent on two pathways: remethylation to methionine, which is thought to be primary during basal metabolism and periods of methionine scarcity, and transsulfuration to cysteine, a process active during periods of methionine excess. An abnormally elevated response to a methionine load primarily reflects a defect in the transsulfuration pathway. However, the remethylation and transsulfuration pathways may be inter-regulated, so that aberrations of one pathway influence the other (16).

The response to a methionine load depends on age and sex, as well as vitamin status. Women and younger individuals have a statistically significant higher than average post-load homocysteine concentration compared to older males, so any set of standardized reference ranges must take this into account (17).

An important question is whether the hyperhomocysteinemia induced by a methionine load has clinical significance. The magnitude of homocysteine elevation that is induced physiologically by routine dietary stress on the transsulfuration pathway is likely quite small. However, epidemiological data show that patients with an abnormal response to a methionine load despite a normal fasting homocysteine level have an increase in cardiovascular risk (18).

DETERMINANTS OF ELEVATED HOMOCYSTEINE

Plasma homocysteine concentration is dependent on the interplay between genetics, nutritional intake, disease states, and environmental factors.

Genetic causes of hyperhomocysteinemia involve mutations in the enzymes that regulate the metabolic pathways of methionine synthesis. Homozygous cystathionine-beta-synthase (CBS) deficiency is responsible for homocystinuria, in which fasting total homocysteine can reach levels as high as 400 μmol/L. In the United States this disease occurs at a frequency of about 1 in 400,000 births. Approximately 1% of patients with coronary artery disease and hyperhomocysteinemia are heterozygous for the mutation; thus, it is not a major contributor to atherosclerosis in the general population (19). Deficiency of the MTHFR gene also leads to homocystinuria, but this entity is exceedingly rare.

A thermolabile variant of the MTHFR gene has been identified and found to be a major cause of mild to moderate hyperhomocysteinemia. The mutation is highly prevalent: approximately 12% of the white population is homozygote. Homozygotes have approximately 25% (2.6 μmol/L) higher total homocysteine than wild types. Given the large contribution of thermolabile MTHFR to the incidence of hyperhomocysteinemia in the general population, studies to estimate the cardiovascular risk attributable to thermolabile MTHFR have had surprising results in light of the large amount of epidemiological data linking mild to moderate homocysteinemia with cardiovascular disease. Meta-analysis of studies that examine the relationship between thermolabile MTHFR and total homocysteine in patients with and without cardiovascular disease has shown that although this mutation is a major cause of hyperhomocysteinemia, it is not associated with increased cardiovascular risk (20). A similar lack of association has been observed in studies of thermolabile MTHFR and cerebrovascular disease (21,22).

One likely explanation for this lack of association is that the phenotypic expression of the thermolabile MTHFR mutation may vary according to serum folate levels, being more pronounced in populations characterized by low serum folate levels. A recent meta-analysis by Klerk et al. investigating the mutation's role in the development of coronary heart disease provides evidence in support of this. Overall, homozygous MTHFR individuals were at increased risk for coronary heart disease (CHD) (OR 1.16, 95% CI 1.05–1.28). However, there was significant variation across geographic boundaries with increased risk observed in European (OR 1.14, 95% CI, 1.01–1.28) but not North American populations (OR 0.87, 95% CI 0.73–1.05), where dietary folate fortification protocols implemented by federal governments may have resulted in higher serum folate levels (23).

Nutritional status plays a key role in determining circulating homocysteine levels. For example, approximately two-thirds of the cases of elevated homocysteine in the elderly population may be attributed to B6, B12, or folate deficiency (24). Vitamin B12 and folate are essential co-factors for enzymes involved in the remethylation pathway of homocysteine metabolism. Examination of the Framingham cohort reveals a strong inverse correlation between serum folate and fasting homocysteine level and a weaker yet still significant inverse correlation between vitamin B12 and fasting homocysteine (19). On the other hand, vitamin B6 deficiency disturbs the activity of the transsulfuration pathway of homocysteine metabolism, leading to aberrantly elevated post-methionine load homocysteine levels, not fasting ones. Studies in rats confirm the interactions between vitamin B12, folate and fasting homocysteine, and between vitamin B-6 and post-methionine load homocysteine (25).

HOMOCYSTEINE AND ATHEROTHROMBOSIS: PATHOPHYSIOLOGIC MECHANISMS

The argument that elevated homocysteine is a risk factor for atherothrombosis can be strengthened if a direct, pathophysiologic relationship between homocysteine and atherothrombosis can be elucidated by laboratory investigation. To establish clinical "meaning" by the criteria of evidence-based medicine, it is enough to demonstrate that a positive correlation between a variable and a disease exists and that modification of this variable attenuates or negates this correlation. However, when such information is not fully available, demonstrating a plausible causal mechanism for the association may strengthen the hypothesis.

Homocysteine and Atherothrombosis

Homocysteine has been associated with both atherosclerosis and thrombosis; mild to moderately elevated homocysteine is correlated with peripheral vascular disease, carotid artery stenosis (26), coronary artery disease as assessed by angiography, and large and small vessel cerebrovascular disease (22,27), while it also is associated with venous thromboembolism (28) and acute myocardial infarction. Ex vivo studies of homocysteine show that the molecule may indeed possess a number of atherogenic and thrombogenic properties that could explain some of these correlations. In culture, homocysteine is directly toxic to endothelial cells (29); stimulates vascular smooth muscle cell (VSMC) DNA synthesis and proliferation (30); increases extracellular superoxide dismutase (31); may promote the oxidation of low-density lipoprotein (32,33); increases collagen deposition (34); and impairs nitric oxide (NO) dependent vasodilation (35). It has also been proposed to play a role in lipid accumulation via induction of 3-hydroxy-3-methylglutaryl coenzyme A (HMG-CoA) reductase mRNA synthesis (36). These properties could create an environment of oxidative stress to facilitate the progression of atherosclerosis and the formation of unstable plaques.

In terms of thrombosis, homocysteine in vitro enhances endothelial-cell associated factor V activity (37) and impairs inactivation of factor Va by activated protein C (38); inhibits the binding of anti-thrombin III to the endothelium (39); reduces endothelial binding sites for tissue plasminogen activator (40); decreases cell surface thrombomodulin and protein-C activation (41); induces endothelial tissue factor activity (42); and stimulates platelet activation and aggregation in rats (43).

Homocysteine and Restenosis

Recent studies also postulate a role of homocysteine in restenosis following balloon angioplasty and stenting (44). Restenosis is a major limiting factor in the long-term success of percutaneous coronary intervention (PCI) with plain old balloon angioplasty (POBA) or coronary stenting. In POBA, restenosis is thought to occur from a combination of elastic recoil, negative arterial remodeling, and neointimal hyperplasia (45). In stented lesions, elastic recoil and negative remodeling are limited, and restenosis depends more critically on the degree of neointimal hyperplasia. Neointimal hyperplasia and vascular remodeling is likely a complex response to arterial injury. Circulating homocysteine could exacerbate restenosis by promoting this injury response, possibly through its oxidant and thrombogenic properties, its toxic effects on the endothelial cells and endothelial function, and its stimulatory effects on smooth muscle proliferation.

Animal data supports a possible role of homocysteine in the pathogenesis of restenosis after balloon angioplasty; diet-induced mild to moderate hyperhomocysteinemia in the rat carotid artery balloon-injury model attenuated re-endothelialization after injury and enhanced neointimal formation (46). Folate administration diminished this neointimal response. Continuous intraperitoneal infusion of homocysteine in rats after carotid artery balloon injury also increased intimal hyperplasia compared to controls (47). Recent clinical data also provide support to the notion that homocysteine may impact restenosis associated with

PCI. A small, prospective angiographic study showed no relationship between baseline homocysteine level and the incidence of restenosis at 6 months after POBA stenting; however, the majority of patients had baseline homocysteine levels within the normal range (mean 10.1 ± 3.7 µmol/L) (48). Homozygosity of the thermolabile mutant of the MTHFR was associated with greater target lesion restenosis by angiography and greater intimal hyperplasia area by intravascular ultrasound at 6 months after Palmaz-Shatz stent placement (49). Interestingly, in this study there was no significant difference in total homocysteine levels between MTHFR genotypes. This relationship between thermolabile MTHFR and restenosis was not found in a prospective angiographic study of POBA and stenting (1). Thus, the clinical evidence that homocysteine may play an important role in restenosis is not entirely consistent.

Homocysteine and Endothelial Dysfunction

A number of in vivo studies have analyzed the relationship between homocysteine levels and endothelial dysfunction in healthy volunteers and in patients with cardiovascular disease. The normal endothelium regulates local vascular tone and growth, thrombosis and thrombolysis, leukocyte adhesion, and platelet aggregation. It does so by releasing various factors, including but not limited to NO, Von Willebrand factor, prostacyclin, and interleukins (50). There is evidence that endothelial injury initiates atherosclerosis, and that areas of atherosclerosis demonstrate endothelial dysfunction, manifested by abnormalities in endothelin-dependent relaxation. These abnormalities are likely due to decreased bioavailability of NO. Furthermore, decreased NO has been associated with increased platelet aggregation, leukocyte adhesion, and vascular smooth muscle cell proliferation (51), all of which contribute to the atherothrombotic cascade.

There is laboratory evidence that homocysteine may deplete vascular stores of NO. Sulfhydryl compounds in general form reactive oxygen species by auto-oxidation; some of these species (O2-) combine with NO to form peroxynitrite (ONOO-) and thereby decrease NO bioavailability (52). Furthermore, at a concentration of 50 µmol/L, homocysteine uniquely inhibits the activity and production of glutathione peroxidase, an enzyme that prevents NO inactivation through its anti-oxidant activity (53).

In vivo data show that homocysteine may promote endothelial dysfunction, and that this dysfunction may arise from changes in NO bioavailability due to oxidative stress. Flow-mediated vasodilatation (FMVD), a marker of endothelial function, is significantly less in elderly hyperhomocysteinemic subjects (mean fasting tHcy 19.2 ± 0.8 µmol/L) without clinically evident atherosclerosis than in age- and sex-matched controls (54). The acute hyperhomocysteinemia induced by an oral methionine load significantly impairs FMVD in healthy subjects (55). One week pretreatment with the anti-oxidant vitamin C prior to the oral methionine load prevents this impairment without any change in peak post-load homocysteine levels (56), which supports the hypothesis that homocysteine decreases NO bioavailability via free radical formation. Furthermore, markers of coagulation and platelet aggregation increase after an oral methionine load in healthy patients, and this increase is blocked by pre-administration of vitamin E and vitamin C (57). In men with known CHD, 8 weeks of treatment with folate and B12 significantly improves FMVD compared to placebo; although total homocysteine levels also improve, after controlling for possible confounders, the improvement correlates independently only with the reduction in free homocysteine (58). This improvement occurs in patients with baseline total homocysteine in both the normal and abnormal range.

What conclusions about homocysteine and atherothrombosis can be drawn from these studies? First, one's interpretation must be guarded because endothelial dysfunction is a surrogate endpoint. No longitudinal study has shown that healthy patients with endothelial dysfunction will develop significant atherosclerosis, although there is other evidence that they are linked (50). The perils of using surrogate endpoints to establish risk, therapy, and outcome are reflected throughout the medical literature, most notably with the paradoxical association between estrogen and low-density lipoprotein (LDL) and endothelial dysfunction, as compared to estrogen and cardiovascular outcomes.

Second, the dysfunction induced by acute hyperhomocysteinemia in healthy volunteers may not be physiologically relevant in patients with chronic, mild-to-moderate hyperhomocysteinemia. The temporal perturbations in homo-cysteine concentration induced by a regular diet would be much smaller then that induced by the single large methionine bolus of the oral load. However, there is evidence that FMVD can be significantly impaired in healthy volunteers after oral doses one-tenth of that of the standard methionine load (59). Theoretically, then, chronic intake of a diet high in methionine (e.g., red meat) may promote chronic endothelial dysfunction via elevated homocysteine concentration, leading in time to clinical atherosclerosis.

Third, the beneficial effects of anti-oxidants vitamin C and E on endothelial dysfunction and coagulation parameters after a methionine load support the hypothesis that oxidative stress contributes to the pathogenesis of cardiovascular disease. However, in patients at high risk for cardiovascular events, vitamin E supplementation has no effect on cardiovascular outcomes (60).

In regard to the relative endothelial dysfunction found in patients with mild hyperhomocysteinemia *without clinical manifestations* of atherosclerosis, this association may not be causal but simply reflect that endothelial dysfunction and plasma homocysteine are co-markers of risk, reflecting the sub clinical atherosclerosis burden. Homocysteine elevation may be a response to, not a cause of, endothelial dysfunction (61).

The improvement in endothelial function in patients with coronary artery disease after supplementation with folate and B12 lends greater support to homocysteine as a true cardiovascular risk factor, in that modification of the homocysteine concentration favorably alters a surrogate cardiovascular endpoint. However, the significant correlation that was observed was between improvement of endothelial function and free homocysteine, and this improvement was seen even in patients with normal total homocysteine levels. This makes theoretical sense since the free homocysteine concentration better represents the biologically active component of total body homocysteine. Although this finding is from a single study, it may mean that the monitoring of total homocysteine reduction will be an insensitive measure of response to treatment in prospective trials that examine cardiovascular outcomes after vitamin supplementation. Indeed, supplementation with B vitamins may result in a more pronounced reduction in total homocysteine than free homocysteine (62). Folate may also improve endothelial function in individuals with coronary artery disease through mechanisms independent of homocysteine lowering (63).

In summary, the studies of homocysteine and endothelial dysfunction in humans reinforce the association, but not the causal relation, between homocysteine elevation and atherothrombosis.

The standard weakness of extrapolating ex vivo findings to in vivo actions limits the application of this data to homocysteine's potential pathophysiologic role. Compounding this limitation, these studies use concentrations of homocysteine ranging as high as 10 mmol/L, which is orders of magnitude higher than that found circulating in vivo. The lowest concentration in these studies is 0.1 mM/L, which, although found in patients with homocystinuria, is more than 5-fold higher than the concentration associated with increased atherothrombotic risk in the general population. These studies thus act merely as starting points for further in vivo investigation.

SIGNIFICANCE OF HOMOCYSTEINE CONCENTRATION IN ACUTE ATHEROTHROMBOTIC EVENTS

The possible actions of homocysteine—promotion of endothelial dysfunction, enhanced tissue factor production, increased factor V activity, reduced tissue plasminogen activator and anti-thrombin III binding, and stimulation of platelet activation and aggregation—are all pathophysiologic mechanisms contributing to the thrombus formation that occurs during unstable plaque rupture. Through these pro-thrombotic effects, an elevated homocysteine concentration may potentially cause increased myocardial injury and portend a worse outcome. Theoretically, then, the homocysteine level measured during an acute event itself—for example, in the emergency department for chest pain—may possibly have prognostic significance.

There is data to suggest that homocysteine may contribute to the degree of myocardial damage. Homocysteine concentrations correlate with plasma markers of thrombosis (64) and peak troponin T (65) in patients presenting with acute coronary syndromes. Also in these patients, elevated total homocysteine levels on admission are correlated with higher peak cardiac troponin T (65). However, the data regarding an association between short-term outcomes and admission homocysteine are inconsistent, although it does appear that elevated total homocysteine on admission for acute coronary syndromes may predict long-term events (66,67).

EPIDEMIOLOGICAL EVIDENCE FOR HOMOCYSTEINE AND ATHEROTHROMBOTIC DISEASE

Retrospective Analysis

McCully first noted the association between homocystinuria and the incidence of accelerated atherosclerosis and thromboembolism (68) through post-mortem examination of patients suffering from varied inborn errors of metabolism that all led to severe hyperhomocysteinemia. A large number of retrospective studies suggest an association between elevated homocysteine levels and atherothrombotic disease including peripheral vascular disease, cerebrovascular disease, and coronary artery disease. However, elevated fasting homocysteine levels have also been shown to be associated with such traditional markers of cardiovascular risk as male gender, advancing age, smoking, high cholesterol, high blood pressure, renal dysfunction, and sedentary lifestyle (10). Thus, an independent relationship of homocysteine with cardiovascular risk is difficult to establish.

The association between homocysteine and peripheral vascular disease in retrospective case-control studies is well established. One meta-analysis suggested an overall odds ratio of 6.8 (95% CI, 2.9–15.8) for peripheral vascular disease and elevated homocysteine (69). In a study of an elderly population taken from the Framingham cohort, elevated homocysteine concentrations were associated with extra-cranial carotid artery stenosis $\geq 25\%$, with an odds ratio of 2.0 in patients in the highest quartile (≥ 14.4 μmol/L) compared to those in lowest (≤ 9.1 μmol/L) (26). In addition, carotid intimal-medial thickness, a surrogate marker for cardiovascular risk, is significantly correlated to plasma homocysteine level (70,71). In nine retrospective case-control studies involving over 1700 patients, the estimated odds ratio for cerebrovascular disease was 2.5 (95% CI, 2.0–3.0) (69). A recent large meta-analysis of 30 studies from 1966 and 1999, the Homocysteine Studies Collaboration, revealed an odds ratio of 0.86 (95% CI, 0.73–1.01) for stroke for 25% lower homocysteine concentrations (72), equivalent to values post-folate supplementation (Table 1) (74). There is some evidence that homocysteine-associated events might be ischemic, not cardioembolic, in nature, caused by large vessel atherosclerosis and/or cerebral microangiopathy (22,27,75).

Retrospective studies have also demonstrated a strong, consistent association between homocysteine and coronary artery disease. Using 15 cross-sectional and case-control studies involving over 4200 individuals, Boushey et al. estimated an odds ratio for a 5 μmol/L increase in fasting total homocysteine of 1.6 in men and 1.8 in women (69). The Homocysteine Studies Collaboration recently compiled evidence from 30 studies and showed an odds ratio of 0.67 (95% CI, 0.62–0.71) for ischemic heart disease (IHD) for 25% lower homocysteine concentrations (Table 1) (72).

Table 1 Summary of Meta-Analyses Studying Relationship of Serum Homocysteine and Ischemic Heart Disease/Stroke

Source	Study types (of studies[a])	Sample size	Variable	Relative risk (95% CI)
Wald et al. 2002 (73)	Retrospective (based on + MTHFR mutation) (72)	16,849	MTHFR +	1.21 (1.06–1.39): IHD
				1.31 (0.80–2.15): Stroke
			+5µmol/L sHcy[b]	1.42 (1.11–1.84): IHD
				1.65 (0.66–4.13): Stroke
	Prospective (20)	3,820	+5µmol/L sHcy[b]	1.23 (1.14–1.32): IHD
				1.42 (1.21–1.66): Stroke
Homocysteine Studies Collaboration, 2002 (72)	Retrospective (18)	7,761	−3µmol/L sHcy[a]	0.67 (0.62–0.71): IHD
				0.86 (0.73–1.01): Stroke
	Prospective (12)	9,025	−3µmol/L sHcy[a]	0.83 (0.77–0.89): IHD
				0.77 (0.66–0.90): Stroke

[a] Denotes a 3µmol/L (25%) decrease in sHcy concentration between study groups.
[b] Signifies a 5µmol/L increase in sHcy concentration between study groups.
Abbreviations: sHcy, serum homocysteine; IHD, ischemic heart disease; MTHFR, methylene tetrahydrofolate reductase; CI, confidence interval.

A meta-analysis of studies investigating the relationship between homocysteine and venous thrombosis showed a pooled estimate of the odds ratio of 2.5 (95% CI, 1.8–3.5) for a fasting homocysteine level greater than the 95% percentile, and 2.6 (95% CI, 1.6–4.4) for an elevated post-methionine load homocysteine level (76).

Prospective Analysis

In contrast to the strong and consistent retrospective epidemiological data that mild to moderate hyperhomocysteinemia is associated with a wide spectrum of atherothrombosis, the evidence gathered from prospective studies is rather inconsistent (77). With respect to coronary artery disease, the Physicians' Health Study showed a relative risk of 3.4 for myocardial infarction (MI) in subjects with elevated homocysteine at a 5-year follow-up, but the relationship was no longer significant at 7.5 years (77); in the Multiple Risk Factor Intervention Trial, there was no association detected between homocysteine concentration and heart disease, and homocysteine was weakly associated with C-reactive protein, an inflammatory marker (78); in the Atherosclerosis Risk in Communities Study, total homocysteine was not correlated with the incidence of CHD after accounting for other risk factors (79); and there was no association between plasma homocysteine quartile and the risk of coronary events among cases and controls from a healthy cohort in the Kuopio Ischemic Heart Disease Risk Factor Study (80). In contrast, the British United Provident Association Study found that the relative risk for mortality from IHD was 2.9 when comparing the highest and lowest quartiles of homocysteine concentration (> 15.1 and < 10.1), and that there was a continuous dose-response relationship between homocysteine and coronary mortality (81). However, this odds ratio was adjusted for systolic blood pressure and apolipoprotein B, but not for other cardiovascular risk factors. Both a Norwegian study (82) and the Tromso health study (83) showed a graded relationship between mortality and homocysteine concentration.

Prospective studies of homocysteine and cerebrovascular disease provide inconsistent data as well. A nested case-control study of individuals within the British Regional Heart Study cohort—a group of patients ages 40–59 randomly selected from 24 towns in Britain—showed a graded increase in the relative risk of stroke in ascending quartiles of total homocysteine concentration, with an odds ratio of 2.8 in the fourth quartile in relation to the first (84). These patients had no history of stroke at baseline. In a prospective examination of elderly people in the Framingham cohort without history of stroke, individuals with non-fasting total homocysteine concentrations in the highest quartile had a relative risk of 1.82 (95% CI, 1.14–1.92) for stroke over 9.9 years of follow-up compared to individuals in the lowest quartile (85). This association is supported by a cohort study of elderly nursing home patients, which showed by Cox regression analysis a risk ratio for new stroke of 1.079 (95% CI, 1.038–1.121) for each micromole increase in plasma homocysteine in 31 months of follow-up (86). In a Dutch cohort study, high baseline levels of homocysteine were associated with a higher baseline prevalence of stroke, and were associated prospectively with an increased incidence of stroke in normotensive, but not hypertensive, subjects (87). However, in the healthy males (mean age, 59 years) of the Physicians' Health Study, the association between plasma homocysteine concentration and cerebrovascular events was not significant (88). A similar negative finding was reported in a Finnish population-based study of individuals between the ages of 40 and 64 years (89). Two large meta-analyses of prospective studies have recently been published. The Homocysteine Studies Collaboration took data from 30 studies between 1966 and 1999 and the results showed an odds ratio of 0.83 (95% CI, 0.77–0.89) for IHD and 0.77 (95% CI, 0.66–0.90), for stroke (Table 1) (72). Another large meta-analysis of 72 studies by Wald et al. used populations with MTHFR mutation to determine odds ratios in response to the standard of 5 µmol/L increase of serum homocysteine (SHcy) (Table 1). The results indicate an odds ratios of 1.23 (95% CI, 1.14–1.32) for IHD, and 1.42 (95% CI, 1.21–1.66) for stroke (73).

The inconsistent results of prospective studies relating homocysteine with atherothrombosis stand in contrast to the strong evidence from retrospective studies. The discrepant findings may be due to several factors:

Confounding bias—The strong association between homocysteine and traditional cardiovascular risk factors (10) raises the possibility that an element of confounding contributes to the retrospective association of homocysteine and atherosclerosis.

Sampling bias—Homocysteine concentrations have been shown to rise up to nearly 40% in the days to months following an acute atherothrombotic event

(12,54). Thus, the sampling of homocysteine concentration in retrospective studies in the days to months after an event could well overestimate the association between homocysteine and risk. In contrast, the deterioration of stored samples could contribute to the lack of significant association found in the prospective studies. The analysis of samples stored over a decade, however, does not support this possibility (90).

Elevated homocysteine as a marker of disease—An alternative explanation for the strong, retrospective association between homocysteine and athero-thrombosis is that an elevated homocysteine concentration is a measure of the subject's total atherothrombotic burden and may reflect chronic tissue injury (61). Some studies show higher homocysteine levels with greater degrees of atherosclerosis (91). An association between homocysteine and disease also may be seen in prospective studies if "healthy" cases have "subclinical" atherosclerosis and elevated homocysteine at the time of blood sampling (92).

Lack of power—Prospective studies lack sufficient power because of small sample sizes, generally healthy subjects with lower mean total homocysteine levels, and a low incidence of disease. For example, the Finnish study of cerebrovascular events (89) had a mean homocysteine of 9.0 µmol/L, lower than that of most of the retrospective studies. More recent meta-analyses have achieved a higher statistical power by being able to analyze multiple study populations. This power has enabled a highly significant association to be made between SHcy concentration and IHD as well as stroke (73). However, to fulfill the requirement of a risk factor, the ability to decrease this risk must be provided by prospective therapeutic interventional trials targeting homocysteine levels.

DOES REDUCTION OF ELEVATED HOMOCYSTEINE IMPACT ATHEROTHROMBOTIC DISEASE?

Therapeutic Options for Lowering Elevated Homocysteine

As noted previously, homocysteine concentration is inversely related to the levels of vitamin B12, folate, and to a lesser extent, vitamin B6 (24). The elevated homocysteine in patients with thermolabile MTHFR is manifested predominantly in those with low serum folate (20). One meta-analysis of vitamin supplemen-tation in patients with mild to moderate hyperhomocysteinemia reports that folate supplementation in doses of 0.5 to 5 mg/day significantly reduces total homocysteine concentration (74). A greater degree of reduction is observed in those with higher pretreatment homocysteine concentration (top quintile, approximately 40% proportional reduction) and in those with lower pretreatment folate concentration. After standardization to the approximate average concentrations for Western populations, treatment with folate lowers homo-cysteine concentrations by 25% (CI 23% to 28%). Supplementation with vitamin B-12 (dosage 0.02–1 mg/day, mean 0.5 mg) produces a small additional effect of about 7% (93). Vitamin B6 treatment alone does not lower fasting total homocysteine concentrations but does reduce post-methionine load concentrations, although not as much as in combination with folate (94). This finding is consistent with the role of vitamin B6 as a co-factor in the transsulfuration pathway of homocysteine to cysteine. Betaine-dependent remethylation of homocysteine to methionine occurs in the liver. Betaine supplementation in patients with homocystinuria significantly decreases total homocysteine concentration (95). In healthy patients, betaine supplementation significantly reduces fasting homocysteine, but to a far lesser degree than folate (96). Choline, a precursor to Betaine, can serve as a dietary supplement in phosphatidylcholine. This may act as another mechanism to decrease fasting and post-methionine load homocysteine concentrations in serum (97).

Vitamin supplementation may have benefits independent from homocysteine reduction. For example, folate, by stimulating tetrahydrobiopterin regeneration (98) and counteracting homocysteine inhibition of eNOS (99,100), may improve NO availability. In addition, vitamin B6, via its effects on the glutathione anti-oxidation system (101), could assuage the oxidant stress associated with hyperhomocysteinemia (102).

Table 2 summarizes the evidence base of homocysteine-lowering intervention on cardiovascular outcomes.

Impact on Surrogate Outcomes

Several lines of evidence suggest that vitamin supplementation in patients with elevated homocysteine affects surrogate clinical endpoints (Table 2). As noted previously, homocysteine-lowering with folate and vitamin B12 treatment improves endothelial dysfunction in subjects with coronary heart disease (58). Vitamin treatment decreases the incidence of positive stress electrocardiograms in relatives of patients with mild to moderately elevated homocysteine (107). Patients treated with a combination of folate, vitamin B-12, and vitamin B6 show a significant regression in carotid plaque area, even in those with a homocysteine concentration less than 14 µmol/L (108). A recent trial by Marcucci et al. demonstrated a significant benefit of therapeutic correction of hyperhomocysteinemia in renal transplant patients who are at high risk for cardiovascular disease. These high-risk patients were randomly assigned to receive vitamin supplementation (folic acid 5 mg/day, vitamin B6 50 mg/day, vitamin B12 400 µg) or placebo. Carotid intima-media thickness (cIMT) was evaluated after 6 months via ultrasound to serve as a surrogate marker for cardiovascular disease. Patients in the treatment group were found to have a mean cIMT decrease of $32 \pm 13\%$, while in the control group cIMT increased by a mean of $23 \pm 21\%$ (Table 2) (106). This significant discrepancy adds support to the hypothesis that homocysteine may be an important risk factor for cardiovascular disease.

In contrast to the positive studies, a recent study failed to demonstrate any beneficial effect of homocysteine-lowering on inflammatory markers that have been implicated in atherothrombosis. In a double-blind, randomized, placebo-controlled

Table 2   Summary of Randomized Controlled Trials Investigating the Impact of Homocysteine-Lowering Therapy on Cardiovascular Outcomes

Study	Sample size	Study duration	Treatment groups	Outcomes relative risk (95% CI)
Vascular disease: Schnyder et al. 2001 (44)	272 281	6 months	1 mg FA, 10 mg B6, 0.4 mg B12 versus placebo	**0.46 (0.28–0.73): Restenosis** 0.52 (0.28–0.98): MACE 0.48 (0.25–0.94): TLR
Schnyder et al. 2002 (103) (The Swiss heart study)	272 281	1 year	1 mg FA, 10 mg B6, 0.4 mg B12 versus placebo (x 6 months)	**0.68 (0.48–0.96): MACE** 0.62 (0.40–0.97): TLR 0.60 (0.24–1.51): Nonfatal MI 0.52 (0.13–2.04): cardiac death 0.54 (0.16–1.70): mortality
Lange et al. 2004 (104)	316 320	6 months	1 mg FA, 5 mg B6, 1 mg B12 IV[a] x1 + 1.2 mg FA, 48 mg B6, 60µg B12 versus placebo	**1.30 (1.0–1.69): Restenosis** 1.5 (1.0–2.3): MACE
Toole et al. 2004 (105) (The VISP trial)	1827 1853	2 years	2.5 mg FA, 25 mg B6, 0.4 mg B12 versus 0.02 mg FA, 0.2 mg B6, 6 µg B12	**1.0 (0.8–1.3): Recurrent stroke** 0.9 (0.7–1.2): MACE 0.9 (0.7–1.1): mortality
Renal disease: Marcucci et al. 2003 (106)	25 28	6 months	5 mg FA, 50 mg B6, 4 mg B12 versus placebo	32+13% decrease in CIMT 23+21% increase in CIMT
Nonpatient population: Vermeulen et al. 2000 (107)	78 80	2 years	5 mg FA, 250 mg B6 versus placebo	0.9 (0.6–1.3): ABI 1.0 (0.3–4.1): PAD 0.9 (0.5–1.6): carotid stenosis 0.4 (0.2–0.9)+stress ECG

[a] An initial intravenous (IV) bolus dose of vitamins was followed by oral maintenance therapy.
Abbreviations: CI, confidence interval; FA, folic acid; B6 and B12, vitamin B6 and vitamin B12; MACE, major adverse cardiac events (cardiac-cause death, nonfatal MI, revascularization); TLR, target lesion revascularization; TVR, target vessel revascularization; CIMT, carotid intima: media thickness; ABI, ankle-brachial index; PAD, peripheral arterial disease; ECG, electrocardiogram. Primary endpoints are shown in bold fonts.

trial among 381 men and 159 postmenopausal women with homocysteine concentrations of 13 µmol/L at screening, the effect of folic acid supplementation (0.8 mg/d) versus placebo for 1 year was investigated on inflammatory markers— serum concentrations of C-reactive protein, soluble intercellular adhesion molecule-1, oxidized low-density lipoprotein, and autoantibodies against oxidized LDL (109). Despite a 4-fold increase in serum folate and a 25% reduction in homocysteine levels, no changes in plasma concentrations of the inflammatory markers were observed with treatment.

Impact on Clinical Outcomes

The evidence that vitamin supplementation reduces cardiovascular clinical outcomes in patients with elevated homocysteine is incomplete and inconsistent. One recent large, multicenter, double-blind randomized active control study, the Vitamin Intervention for Stroke Prevention (VISP) trial, failed to demonstrate significant risk reduction in recurrent stroke (primary endpoint) or CHD events (secondary endpoint) in high-risk individuals in response to high-dose homocysteine-lowering therapy for 2 years (Table 2) (105). However, this trial was not placebo-controlled but, rather, a head-to-head comparison of daily high-dose vitamin formulations (folic acid 2.5 mg, vitamin B6 25 mg, vitamin B12 0.4 mg) against low-dose daily formulations (folic acid 20 µg, vitamin B6 200 µg, and vitamin B12 6 µg).

Several studies have investigated the effect of homocysteine lowering on restenosis following percutaneous coronary intervention (PCI). A prospective, double-blinded, randomized clinical trial of folate (1 mg/day), vitamin B6 (10 mg/day), and vitamin B12 (400 µg/day) therapy in 205 patients after coronary angioplasty and/or stenting provides the most compelling evidence for the role of homocysteine in post-angioplasty restenosis (Table 2) (44). These patients had baseline normal-to-mild hyperhomocysteinemia (11.1 ± 4.3 µmol/L). Combination therapy with folate, vitamin B12, and vitamin B6 provided a statistically significant 18% absolute risk reduction (19.6% vs. 37.6%, $p = 0.01$) in the primary endpoint of angiographic restenosis (defined as a stenosis of > 50% at 6-month follow-up). This benefit was primarily observed in patients undergoing angioplasty (10.3% vs. 41.9%, $p < 0.001$), but not stenting (20.6 vs. 29.9%, $p = 0.32$).

The Swiss Heart Study was a randomized, controlled trial that aimed to evaluate the impact of homocysteine-lowering therapy on clinical outcomes (major adverse cardiac outcomes) in 553 patients treated with angioplasty with or without stenting (Table 2) (103). Although homocysteine-lowering therapy did show significant risk reduction in overall adverse outcomes, the benefit was driven primarily by a reduced rate of target lesion revascularization with no significant impact on nonfatal MI or death (103).

In a recent placebo-controlled trial, Lange et al. examined the effect of vitamin therapy at higher doses (folic acid 1.2 mg, vitamin B6 48 mg, vitamin B12 0.06 mg) following an initial intravenous bolus loading dose, on 636 patients following successful coronary stenting with bare-metal stents (Table 2) (104).

The multi-vitamin therapy successfully reduced SHcy levels, but contrary to the previous results by Schnyder et al., the folate therapy actually resulted in significantly increased restenosis and target vessel revascularization rates at 6 months, although clinical endpoints were not affected. The divergent findings of the two studies may be reconciled by considering differences with respect to treatment dose (intravenous loading dose plus higher folate and vitamin B6 maintenance dose in the Lange study), mode of PCI (100% stenting vs nearly 50% in the Schnyder study), lesion length (shorter in Lange et al.), patient population (higher risk in the Schnyder study—more smokers, diabetics and, previous history of myocardial infarction), SHcy levels (lower baseline levels in Schnyder et al.), and angiographic follow-up (only 76% follow-up in Lange et al.). While the risk of high-dose homocysteine-lowering therapy in post-stent patients is of some concern, this is unlikely to have an impact on the overall incidence of coronary restenosis in clinical practice in the United States given the widespread adoption of drug-eluting stents (nearly 85% of all PCIs).

In summary, the evidence generated from intervention studies is inconsistent. More reliable evidence is needed to recommend routine homocysteine-lowering therapy for modifying atherothrombotic vascular risk. Several large-scale studies are currently underway in the United States, Canada, and Europe to examine the effects of lowering blood homocysteine levels on the incidence of heart attacks and/or strokes: the Norwegian Vitamin Interventional Trial (NORVIT), the Western Norway B-vitamin Intervention Trial (WENBIT), the Study of Effectiveness of Additional Reduction in Cholesterol and Homocysteine (SEARCH), the Prevention with a Combined Inhibitor and Folate in Coronary Heart Disease (PACIFIC) Trial, the Vitamins to Prevent Stroke (VITATOPS), etc. One will have to wait for these trial data to accrue before one can confirm or refute the homocysteine hypothesis in atherothrombosis.

CONCLUSION

Severe elevation of homocysteine concentration in patients with homocystinuria leads to a high incidence of premature atherothrombotic events. In vitro and in vivo studies demonstrate a plethora of biologically plausible mechanisms that implicate homocysteine in promoting atherosclerotic and thrombotic vascular disease. Numerous observational studies have also reported on the association between mild to moderately elevated homocysteine levels and vascular risk in both the general population and in those with preexisting vascular disease. In general, the risk for vascular disease is small with prospective, longitudinal studies reporting substantially weaker associations between homocysteine and atherothrombotic vascular disease than retrospective case-control and cross-sectional studies. It is unclear whether a causal relationship exists between homocysteine and cardiovascular risk, if homocysteine is related to other confounding cardiovascular risk factors, or if homocysteine is a marker of existing disease burden. Routine screening for elevated homocysteine is not yet recommended (1,104). However, screening may be advisable for individuals who manifest atherothrombotic disease that is out of proportion to their traditional risk factors or who have a family history of premature atherosclerotic disease. Vitamin supplementation with folate, B6, and B12 significantly lowers homocysteine concentration and has also been shown to alter surrogate cardiovascular endpoints. Although there is incomplete evidence that vitamin supplementation reduces cardiovascular risk, treatment with low doses is safe and inexpensive. Whether homocysteine is causative in the pathogenesis of atherothrombotic vascular disease will have to await the completion of a number of large, randomized controlled trials studying the effect of homocysteine-lowering vitamins on cardiovascular end points. Until then, the status of homocysteine as a risk factor remains unresolved.

REFERENCES

1. Malinow MR, Bostom AG, Krauss RM. Homocyst(e)ine, diet, and cardiovascular diseases: a statement for healthcare professionals from the Nutrition Committee, American Heart Association. Circulation 1999; 99:178–182.
2. Welch GN, Loscalzo J. Homocysteine and atherothrombosis. N Engl J Med 1998; 338:1042–1050.
3. Mudd SH, Finkelstein JD, Refsum H, et al. Homocysteine and its disulfide derivatives: a suggested consensus terminology. Arterioscler Thromb Vasc Biol 2000; 20:1704–1706.
4. Mansoor MA, Ueland PM, Aarsland A, Svardal AM. Redox status and protein binding of plasma homocysteine and other aminothiols in patients with homocystinuria. Metabolism 1993; 42:1481–1485.
5. Tzakas PAN, Langman LJ, Evrovsky J, Cole DEC. The importance of serum proteins in the interpretation of total homocysteine. Clin Biochem 2000; 33:240–241.
6. Guttormsen AB, Schneede J, Fiskerstrand T, Ueland PM, Refsum HM. Plasma concentrations of homocysteine and other aminothiol compounds are related to food intake in healthy human subjects. J Nutr 1994; 124:1934–1941.
7. Ubbink JB, Vermaak WJ, van der Merwe A, Becker PJ. The effect of blood sample aging and food consumption on plasma totalhomocysteine levels. Clin Chim Acta 1992; 207:119–128.
8. Andersson A, Isaksson A, Hultberg B. Homocysteine export from erythrocytes and its implication for plasma sampling. Clin Chem 1992; 38:1311–1315.
9. From the Centers for Disease Control and Prevention. Assessment of laboratory tests for plasma homocysteine–selected laboratories, July-September 1998. JAMA 1999; 282:2112–2113.
10. Nygard O, Vollset SE, Refsum H, et al. Total plasma homocysteine and cardiovascular risk profile. the hordaland homocysteine Study. JAMA 1995; 274:1526–1533.
11. Auer J, Eber B. Homocysteine and fibrinolysis in acute occlusive coronary events. Lancet 1999; 354:1474–1475.

12. Egerton W, Silberberg J, Crooks R, Ray C, Xie L, Dudman N. Serial measures of plasma homocyst(e)ine after acute myocardial infarction. Am J Cardiol 1996; 77:759–761.

13. Landgren F, Israelsson B, Lindgren A, Hultberg B, Andersson A, Brattstrom L. Plasma homocysteine in acute myocardial infarction: homocysteine-lowering effect of folic acid. J Intern Med 1995; 237:381–388.

14. Lindgren A, Brattstrom L, Norrving B, Hultberg B, Andersson A, Johansson BB. Plasma homocysteine in the acute and convalescent phases after stroke. Stroke 1995; 26:795–800.

15. Bostom AG, Jacques PF, Nadeau MR, Williams RR, Ellison RC, Selhub J. Post-methionine load hyperhomocysteinemia in persons with normal fasting total plasma homocysteine: initial results from the NHLBI Family Heart Study. Atherosclerosis 1995; 116:147–151.

16. Girelli D, Olivieri O, Russo C, Corrocher R. Is the Oral Methionine Loading Test Insensitive to the Remethylation Pathway of Homocysteine? Blood 1999; 93:1118–1120.

17. Silberberg J, Crooks R, Fryer J, et al. Gender differences and other determinants of the rise in plasma homocysteine after L-methionine loading. Atherosclerosis 1997; 133:105–110.

18. Graham IM, Daly LE, Refsum HM, et al. Plasma homocysteine as a risk factor for vascular disease. the european concerted action project. JAMA 1997; 277:1775–1781.

19. Tsai MY, Welge BG, Hanson NQ, et al. Genetic causes of mild hyperhomocysteinemia in patients with premature occlusive coronary artery diseases. Atherosclerosis 1999; 143:163–170.

20. Brattstrom L, Wilcken DE, Ohrvik J, Brudin L. Common methylenetetrahydrofolate reductase gene mutation leads to hyperhomocysteinemia but not to vascular disease: the result of a meta-analysis. Circulation 1998; 98:2520–2526.

21. Markus H, Ali N, Swaminathan R, Sankaralingam A, Molloy J, Powell J. A common polymorphism in the methylenetetrahydrofolate reductase gene, homocysteine, and ischemic cerebrovascular disease. Stroke 1997; 28:1739–1743.

22. Eikelboom JW, Hankey GJ, Anand SS, Lofthouse E, Staples N, Baker RI. Association between high homocyst(e)ine and ischemic stroke due to large- and small-artery disease but not other etiologic subtypes of ischemic stroke. Stroke 2000; 31:1069–1075.

23. Klerk M, Verhoef P, Clarke R, et al. MTHFR 677C->T polymorphism and risk of coronary heart disease: a meta-analysis. JAMA 2002; 288:2023–2031.

24. Selhub J, Jacques PF, Wilson PW, Rush D, Rosenberg IH. Vitamin status and intake as primary determinants of homocysteinemia in an elderly population. JAMA 1993; 270:2693–2698.

25. Miller JW, Nadeau MR, Smith D, Selhub J. Vitamin B-6 deficiency vs folate deficiency: comparison of responses to methionine loading in rats. Am J Clin Nutr 1994; 59:1033–1039.

26. Selhub J, Jacques PF, Bostom AG, et al. Association between plasma homocysteine concentrations and extracranial carotid-artery stenosis. N Engl J Med 1995; 332:286–291.

27. Evers S, Koch HG, Grotemeyer KH, Lange B, Deufel T, Ringelstein EB. Features, symptoms, and neurophysiological findings in stroke associated with hyperhomocysteinemia. Arch Neurol 1997; 54:1276–1282.

28. den Heijer M, Koster T, Blom HJ, et al. Hyperhomocysteinemia as a risk factor for deep-vein thrombosis. N Engl J Med 1996; 334:759–762.

29. Wall RT, Harlan JM, Harker LA, Striker GE. Homocysteine-induced endothelial cell injury in vitro: a model for the study of vascular injury. Thromb Res 1980; 18:113–121.

30. Tsai JC, Wang H, Perrella MA, et al. Induction of cyclin A gene expression by homocysteine in vascular smooth muscle cells. J Clin Invest 1996; 97:146–153.

31. Wang XL, Duarte N, Cai H, et al. Relationship between total plasma homocysteine, polymorphisms of homocysteine metabolism related enzymes, risk factors and coronary artery disease in the Australian hospital-based population. Atherosclerosis 1999; 146:133–140.

32. Heinecke JW, Kawamura M, Suzuki L, Chait A. Oxidation of low density lipoprotein by thiols: superoxide-dependent and-independent mechanisms. J Lipid Res 1993; 34:2051–2061.

33. Parthasarathy S. Oxidation of low-density lipoprotein by thiol compounds leads to its recognition by the acetyl LDL receptor. Biochim Biophys Acta 1987; 917:337–340.

34. Majors A, Ehrhart LA, Pezacka EH. Homocysteine as a risk factor for vascular disease: enhanced collagen production and accumulation by smooth muscle cells. Arterioscler Thromb Vasc Biol 1997; 17:2074–2081.

35. Tawakol A, Forgione MA, Stuehlinger M, et al. Homocysteine impairs coronary microvascular dilator function in humans. J Am Coll Cardiol 2002; 40:1051–1058.

36. Woo CW, Siow YL, Pierce GN, Choy PC, Minuk GY, Mymin D, Karmin O. Hyperhomocysteinemia induces hepatic cholesterol biosynthesis and lipid accumulation via activation of transcription factors. Am J Physiol Endocrinol Metab 2005; 288:E1002–E1010.

37. Rodgers GM, Kane WH. Activation of endogenous factor V by a homocysteine-induced vascular endothelial cell activator. J Clin Invest 1986; 77:1909–1916.

38. Undas A, Williams EB, Butenas S, Orfeo T, Mann KG. Homocysteine inhibits inactivation of factor Va by activated protein C. J Biol Chem 2000.

39. Nishinaga M, Ozawa T, Shimada K. Homocysteine, a thrombogenic agent, suppresses anticoagulant heparan sulfate expression in cultured porcine aortic endothelial cells. J Clin Invest 1993; 92:1381–1386.

40. Hajjar KA. Homocysteine-induced modulation of tissue plasminogen activator binding to its endothelial cell membrane receptor. J Clin Invest 1993; 91:2873–2879.

41. Lentz SR, Sadler JE. Inhibition of thrombomodulin surface expression and protein C activation by the thrombogenic agent homocysteine. J Clin Invest 1991; 88:1906–1914.

42. Fryer RH, Wilson BD, Gubler DB, Fitzgerald LA, Rodgers GM. Homocysteine, a risk factor for premature vascular disease and thrombosis, induces tissue factor activity in endothelial cells. Arterioscler Thromb 1993; 13:1327–1333.

43. Ungvari Z, Sarkadi-Nagy E, Bagi Z, Szollar L, Koller A. Simultaneously increased TxA(2) activity in isolated arterioles and platelets of rats with hyperhomocysteinemia. Arterioscler Thromb Vasc Biol 2000; 20:1203–1208.

44. Schnyder G, Roffi M, Pin R, et al. Decreased rate of coronary restenosis after lowing of plasma homocystein levels. N Engl J Med 2001; 345:1593–1600.

45. Moscucci M, Muller DWM. Restenosis. In: Freed M, Grines C, Safian RD, eds. The New Manual of Interventional Cardiology. 3rd ed. Bloomington, Michigan: Physician's Press, 1997:423–438.

46. Morita H, Kurihara H, Yoshida S, et al. Diet-induced hyperhomocysteinemia exacerbates neointima formation in rat carotid arteries after balloon injury. Circulation 2001; 103:133–139.
47. Chen C, Surowiec SM, Morsy AH, Ma M. Intraperitoneal infusion of homocysteine increases intimal hyperplasia in balloon-injured rat carotid arteries. Atherosclerosis 2002; 160:103–114.
48. Miner SE, Hegele RA, Sparkes J, et al. Homocysteine, lipoprotein(a), and restenosis after percutaneous transluminal coronary angioplasty: a prospective study. Am Heart J 2000; 140:272–278.
49. Kosokabe T, Okumura K, Sone T, et al. Relation of a Common Methylenetetrahydrofolate Reductase Mutation and Plasma Homocysteine With Intimal Hyperplasia After Coronary Stenting. Circulation 2001; 103:2048–2054.
50. Celermajer DS. Endothelial dysfunction: does it matter? Is it reversible? J Am Coll Cardiol 1997; 30:325–333.
51. Cooke JP, Tsao PS. Is nitric oxide (NO) an endogenous antiatherogenic molecule? Arterioscler Thromb 1994; 14:653–655.
52. Loscalzo J. The oxidant stress of hyperhomocyst(e)inemia. J Clin Invest 1996; 98:5–7.
53. Upchurch GR, Welch GN, Freedman JE, Loscalzo J. Homocyst(e)ine attenuates endothelial glutathione peroxidase and thereby potentiates peroxide-mediated injury. Circulation 1995; 92:I-228.
54. Tawakol A, Omland T, Gerhard M, Wu JT, Creager MA. Hyperhomocyst(e)inemia is associated with impaired endothelium-dependent vasodilation in humans. Circulation 1997; 95:1119–1121.
55. Bellamy MF, McDowell IF, Ramsey MW, et al. Hyperhomocysteinemia after an oral methionine load acutely impairs endothelial function in healthy adults. Circulation 1998; 98:1848–1852.
56. Chambers JC, McGregor A, Jean-Marie J, Obeid OA, Kooner JS. Demonstration of rapid onset vascular endothelial dysfunction after hyperhomocysteinemia: an effect reversible with vitamin C therapy. Circulation 1999; 99:1156–1160.
57. Nappo F, De Rosa N, Marfella R, et al. Impairment of endothelial functions by acute hyperhomocysteinemia and reversal by antioxidant vitamins. JAMA 1999; 281:2113–2118.
58. Chambers JC, Ueland PM, Obeid OA, Wrigley J, Refsum H, Kooner JS. Improved vascular endothelial function after oral B vitamins: An effect mediated through reduced concentrations of free plasma homocysteine. Circulation 2000; 102:2479–2483.
59. Chambers JC, Obeid OA, Kooner JS. Physiological increments in plasma homocysteine induce vascular endothelial dysfunction in normal human subjects. Arterioscler Thromb Vasc Biol 1999; 19:2922–2927.
60. Yusuf S, Dagenais G, Pogue J, Bosch J, Sleight P. Vitamin E supplementation and cardiovascular events in high-risk patients. the heart outcomes prevention evaluation study investigators. N Engl J Med 2000; 342:154–160.
61. Dudman NP. An alternative view of homocysteine. Lancet 1999; 354:2072–2074.
62. Bronstrup A, Hages M, Pietrzik K. Lowering of homocysteine concentrations in elderly men and women. Int J Vitam Nutr Res 1999; 69:187–193.
63. Doshi SN, McDowell IF, Moat SJ, et al. Folic acid improves endothelial function in coronary artery disease via mechanisms largely independent of homocysteine lowering. Circulation 2002; 105:22–26.

64. Al-Obaidi MK, Philippou H, Stubbs PJ, et al. Relationships between homocysteine, factor VIIa, and thrombin generation in acute coronary syndromes. Circulation 2000; 101:372–377.

65. Al-Obaidi MK, Stubbs PJ, Collinson P, Conroy R, Graham I, Noble MI. Elevated homocysteine levels are associated with increased ischemic myocardial injury in acute coronary syndromes. J Am Coll Cardiol 2000; 36:1217–1222.

66. Omland T, Samuelsson A, Hartford M, et al. Serum homocysteine concentration as an indicator of survival in patients with acute coronary syndromes. Arch Intern Med 2000; 160:1834–1840.

67. Stubbs PJ, Al-Obaidi MK, Conroy RM, et al. Effect of plasma homocysteine concentration on early and late events in patients with acute coronary syndromes. Circulation 2000; 102:605–610.

68. McCully KS. Vascular pathology of homocysteinemia: implications for the pathogenesis of arteriosclerosis. Am J Pathol 1969; 56:111–128.

69. Boushey CJ, Beresford SA, Omenn GS, Motulsky AG. A quantitative assessment of plasma homocysteine as a risk factor for vascular disease. probable benefits of increasing folic acid intakes. JAMA 1995; 274:1049–1057.

70. Tsai MY, Arnett DK, Eckfeldt JH, Williams RR, Ellison RC. Plasma homocysteine and its association with carotid intimal-medial wallthickness and prevalent coronary heart disease: NHLBI Family Heart Study. Atherosclerosis 2000; 151:519–524.

71. Eikelboom JW, Lonn E, Genest J, Jr., Hankey G, Yusuf S. Homocyst(e)ine and cardiovascular disease: a critical review of the epidemiologic evidence. Ann Intern Med 1999; 131:363–375.

72. The Homocysteine Studies Collaboration. Homocysteine and risk of ischemic heart disease and stroke: a meta-analysis. JAMA 2002; 288:2015–2022.

73. Wald DS, Law M, Morris JK. Homocysteine and cardiovascular disease: evidence on causality from a meta-analysis. BMJ 2002; 325:1202.

74. Homocysteine Lowering Trialists' Collaboration. Lowering blood homocysteine with folic acid based supplements: meta-analysis of randomised trials. BMJ 1998; 316:894–898.

75. Fassbender K, Mielke O, Bertsch T, Nafe B, Froschen S, Hennerici M. Homocysteine in cerebral macroangiography and microangiopathy. Lancet 1999; 353:1586–1587.

76. den Heijer M, Rosendaal FR, Blom HJ, Gerrits WB, Bos GM. Hyperhomocysteinemia and venous thrombosis: a meta-analysis. Thromb Haemost 1998; 80:874–877.

77. Christen WG, Ajani UA, Glynn RJ, Hennekens CH. Blood levels of homocysteine and increased risks of cardiovascular disease: causal or casual? Arch Intern Med 2000; 160:422–434.

78. Evans RW, Shaten BJ, Hempel JD, Cutler JA, Kuller LH. Homocyst(e)ine and risk of cardiovascular disease in the Multiple Risk Factor Intervention Trial. Arterioscler Thromb Vasc Biol 1997; 17:1947–1953.

79. Folsom AR, Nieto FJ, McGovern PG, et al. Prospective study of coronary heart disease incidence in relation to fasting total homocysteine, related genetic polymorphisms, and B vitamins: the Atherosclerosis Risk in Communities (ARIC) study. Circulation 1998; 98:204–210.

80. Voutilainen S, Lakka TA, Hamelahti P, Lehtimaki T, Poulsen HE, Salonen JT. Plasma total homocysteine concentration and the risk of acute coronary events: the Kuopio Ischaemic Heart Disease Risk Factor Study. J Intern Med 2000; 248:217–222.

81. Wald NJ, Watt HC, Law MR, Weir DG, McPartlin J, Scott JM. Homocysteine and ischemic heart disease: results of a prospective study with implications regarding prevention. Arch Intern Med 1998; 158:862–867.

82. Nygard O, Nordrehaug JE, Refsum H, Ueland PM, Farstad M, Vollset SE. Plasma homocysteine levels and mortality in patients with coronary artery disease. N Engl J Med 1997; 337:230–236.

83. Arnesen E, Refsum H, Bonaa KH, Ueland PM, Forde OH, Nordrehaug JE. Serum total homocysteine and coronary heart disease. Int J Epidemiol 1995; 24:704–709.

84. Perry IJ, Refsum H, Morris RW, Ebrahim SB, Ueland PM, Shaper AG. Prospective study of serum total homocysteine concentration and risk of stroke in middle-aged British men. Lancet 1995; 346:1395–1398.

85. Bostom AG, Rosenberg IH, Silbershatz H, et al. Nonfasting plasma total homocysteine levels and stroke incidence in elderly persons: the framingham study. Ann Intern Med 1999; 131:352–355.

86. Aronow WS, Ahn C, Gutstein H. Increased plasma homocysteine is an independent predictor of new atherothrombotic brain infarction in older persons. Am J Cardiol 2000; 86:585–586.

87. Stehouwer CD, Weijenberg MP, van den Berg M, Jakobs C, Feskens EJ, Kromhout D. Serum homocysteine and risk of coronary heart disease and cerebrovascular disease in elderly men: a 10-year follow-up. Arterioscler Thromb Vasc Biol 1998; 18:1895–1901.

88. Verhoef P, Hennekens CH, Malinow MR, Kok FJ, Willett WC, Stampfer MJ. A prospective study of plasma homocyst(e)ine and risk of ischemic stroke. Stroke 1994; 25:1924–1930.

89. Alfthan G, Pekkanen J, Jauhiainen M, et al. Relation of serum homocysteine and lipoprotein(a) concentrations to atherosclerotic disease in a prospective Finnish population based study. Atherosclerosis 1994; 106:9–19.

90. Israelsson B, Brattström L, Refsum H. Homocysteine in frozen plasma samples: a short cut to establish hyperhomocysteinaemia as a risk factor for arteriosclerosis? Scand J Clin Lab Invest 1993; 53:465–469.

91. Nielsen NE, Brattstrom L, Hultberg B, Landgren F, Swahn E. Plasma total homocysteine levels in postmenopausal women with unstable coronary artery disease. Atherosclerosis 2000; 151:423–431.

92. Kuller LH, Evans RW. Homocysteine, vitamins, and cardiovascular disease. Circulation 1998; 98:196–199.

93. Clarke R, Armitage J. Vitamin supplements and cardiovascular risk: review of the randomized trials of homocysteine-lowering vitamin supplements. Semin Thromb Hemost 2000; 26:341–348.

94. van der Griend R, Biesma DH, Haas FJ, et al. The effect of different treatment regimens in reducing fasting and postmethionine-load homocysteine concentrations. J Intern Med 2000; 248:223–229.

95. Wilcken DE. The natural history of vascular disease in homocystinuria and the effects of treatment. J Inherit Metab Dis 1997; 20:295–300.

96. Brouwer IA, Verhoef P, Urgert R. Betaine supplementation and plasma homocysteine in healthy volunteers. Arch Intern Med 2000; 160:2546–2547.

97. Olthof MR, Brink EJ, Katan MB, Verhoef P. Choline supplemented as phosphatidylcholine decreases fasting and postmethionine-loading plasma homocysteine concentrations in healthy men. Am J Clin Nutr 2005; 82:111–117.

98. Verhaar MC, Wever RM, Kastelein JJ, van Dam T, Koomans HA, Rabelink TJ. 5-methyltetrahydrofolate, the active form of folic acid, restores endothelial function in familial hypercholesterolemia. Circulation 1998; 97:237–241.

99. Wever RMF, van Dam T, van Rijn HJM, de Groot FG, Rabelink TJ. Tetrahydrobiopterin regulates superoxide and nitric oxide generation by recombinant endothelial nitric oxide synthase. Biochem Biophys Res Commun 1997; 237:340–344.

100. Zhang X, Li H, Jin H, Ebin Z, Brodsky S, Goligorsky MS. Effects of homocysteine on endothelial nitric oxide production. Am J Physiol 2000; 279:671–678.

101. Cabrini L, Bergami R, Fiorentini D, Marchetti M, Landi L, Tolomelli B. Vitamin B6 deficiency affects antioxidant defences in rat liver and heart. Biochem Mol Biol Int 1998; 46:689–697.

102. Mosharov E, Cranford MR, Banerjee R. The quantitatively important relationship between homocysteine metabolism and glutathione synthesis by the transsulfuration pathway and its regulation by redox changes. Biochemistry 2000; 39:13005–13011.

103. Schnyder G, Roffi M, Flammer Y, Pin R, Hess OM. Effect of homocyteine-lowering therapy with folic acid. vitamin B12, and vitamin B6 on clinical outcom after percutaneous coronary intervention. the swiss heart study: a randomized controlled trial. JAMA 2002; 288:973–979.

104. Lange H, Suryapranata H, DeLuca G, et al. Folate therapy and in-stent retenosis after coronary stenting. N Engl J Med 2004; 350:2673–2681.

105. Toole JF, Malinow M, Rene MD, et al. Lowering homocysteine in patients with ischemic stroke to prevent recurrent stroke myocardial infarction, and death: the vitamin intervention for stroke prevention (VISP) randomized controlled Trial. JAMA 2004; 291:565–575.

106. Marcucci R, Zanazzi M, Bertoni E, et al. Vitamin Supplementation reduces the progression of atherosclerosis in hyperhomo-cysteinemic renal-transplant recipients. Transplantation 2003; 75:1551–1555.

107. Vermeulen EG, Stehouwer CD, Twisk JW, et al. Effect of homocysteine-lowering treatment with folic acid plus vitamin B6 on progression of subclinical atherosclerosis: a randomised, placebo-controlled trial. Lancet 2000; 355:517–522.

108. Hackam DG, Peterson JC, Spence JD. What level of plasma homocyst(e)ine should be treated? Effects of vitamin therapy on progression of carotid atherosclerosis in patients with homocyst(e)ine levels above and below 14 micromol/L Am J Hypertens 2000; 13:105–110.

109. Durga J, van Tits LJ, Schouten EG, Kok FJ, Verhoef P. Effect of lowering of homocysteine levels on inflammatory markers: a randomized controlled trial. Arch Intern Med 2005; 165:1388–1394.

5

Inflammation, Inflammatory Markers, and Cardiovascular Risk

P. K. Shah

Atherosclerosis Research Center, Division of Cardiology and Department of Medicine, Cedars-Sinai Medical Center and David Geffen School of Medicine, University of California, Los Angeles, California, U.S.A.

INTRODUCTION

Several lines of evidence suggest that inflammatory processes play a critical role in the initiation, progression, and destabilization of atherosclerosis (1–6). Most of the known risk factors for atherosclerosis are believed to trigger inflammatory gene induction/activation in the arterial wall leading ultimately to recruitment, retention, and activation of mononuclear inflammatory cells (monocytes-macrophages, T-cells, mast cells, and dendritic cells) in the subendothelial space. These inflammatory cells contribute to the initiation, growth, and eventual disruption of atherosclerotic plaques leading to thrombosis and acute clinical vaso-occlusive events (1–6). These pathophysiologic underpinnings are supported by accumulating evidence that circulating markers of inflammation can provide important prognostic information across a wide spectrum of clinical settings in a broad array of patient populations, and that such information is often additive and incremental to that obtained from standard markers of cardiovascular risk (7,8). A series of experimental observations further raise the possibility that some of these inflammatory markers such as C-reactive protein (CRP) may not simply be markers but instead may also play a causal role in the pathophysiology of athero-thrombosis through a variety of putative biological actions (9–11).

ROLE OF INFLAMMATION IN ATHEROGENESIS, PLAQUE DISRUPTION, AND THROMBOSIS (FIG. 1)

Atherosclerosis-prone areas include sites of oscillating shear stress where atherogenic lipoproteins appear to be preferentially retained within the arterial wall leading to their oxidative modification and aggregation. According to the prevailing paradigm, a number of stimuli injure or activate vascular endothelium. These stimuli include oscillating shear stress, oxidative stress, elevated levels of atherogenic lipoproteins, modified lipoproteins, hyperglycemia, elevated levels of angiotensin II, low levels HDL, elevated levels of homocysteine, high blood pressure, possibly chronic infections, immune activation, and cigarette smoke. Endothelial activation leads to enhanced expression of several pro-inflammatory genes, which include leukocyte adhesion molecules such as VCAM-1 (vascular cell adhesion molecule) and ICAM-1 (intercellular adhesion molecule) and E-selectin, which in concert with chemokines such as MCP-1 (monocyte chemotactic protein) and interleukin-8, lead to subendothelial recruitment of mononuclear leukocytes (1,12). In the vessel wall, monocytes are exposed to other cytokines such as M-CSF (macrophage colony stimulating factor) induced by retained oxidatively modified lipoproteins, leading to differentiation of monocytes into macrophages. Macrophages ingest lipoproteins through their non-downregulatable scavenger receptors leading to formation of foam cells. Eventually, chemotactic factors and growth factors for smooth muscle cells are induced leading to accumulation of matrix synthesizing smooth muscle cells in the arterial intima leading to the formation of the fibrofatty lesion of atherosclerosis (1,12). Several experimental studies, using gene knockout strategies, have established a key relationship between inflammation and atherogenesis. Thus deficiency of MCP-1, interleukin-8, and M-CSF have been shown to inhibit atherogenesis despite severe hyperpelipidemia in murine models (1,12).

In the clinical setting of atherosclerotic vascular disease, the majority of acute and potentially serious ischemic manifestations are triggered by the superimposition of a thrombus on a disrupted atherosclerotic plaque (2–5,13,14). Atherosclerotic plaques containing a large lipid-rich core and active inflammation are believed to be vulnerable to disruption (so called vulnerable plaques). The integrity of the protective collagen-rich fibrous cap that normally segregates the deeper lipid-rich components of the advanced atherosclerotic plaque from circulating blood, is dependent upon the balance between matrix synthetic and degradative activities within the plaque. While smooth muscle cells synthesize matrix, inflammatory cells may contribute to matrix degradation. Disruption of the fibrous cap is believed to result from excessive matrix degrading activity within the plaque, attributed largely to a family of matrix degrading proteolytic enzymes such as MMP's (matrix degrading metalloproteinase) and other proteases, produced by the inflammatory cells (2–5,13,14). Inflammatory cells in the atherosclerotic plaque are also the major source of tissue factor, a key initiator of the coagulation cascade (2–5,13,14).

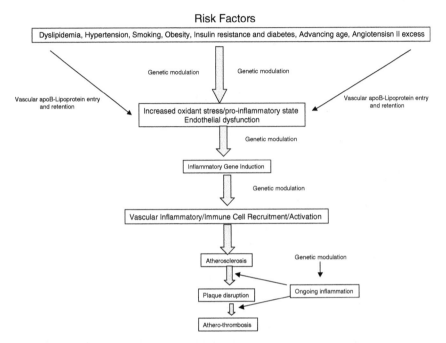

Figure 1   Role of inflammation in atherogenesis, plaque disruption, and thrombosis.

Thus lipid-rich regions of atherosclerotic plaque are impregnated with tissue factor derived from apoptotic inflammatory cells, accounting for its enhanced thrombogenicity (2–5,13,14). Taken together, a considerable amount of evidence implicates inflammation in initiation and destablization of atherosclerosis.

SYSTEMIC MARKERS OF INFLAMMATION AND CARDIOVASCULAR RISK

As the inflammatory paradigm of atherothrombosis is becoming a mainstream pathophysiologic concept, investigators have been examining the value of several systemic markers of ongoing inflammation as potential predictors of cardiovascular risk. These systemic markers include CRP, interleukin-6 (IL-6), tumor necrosis factor alpha, CD 40 ligand, myeloperoxidase, serum amyloid A, soluble cell adhesion molecules (VCAM-1 and ICAM-1, P-selectin), metalloproteinases such as MMP-9, pregnancy-associated protein (PAP), and lipoprotein-associated phospholipase A-2 (LP-PLA2), myeloperoxidase, and adipocytokines such as the anti-inflammatory cytokine adiponectin (Table 1) (7,8,15–28).

Table 1 Systemic Inflammatory Markers

C-reactive protein
Lipoprotein-associated phospholipase A-2
Interleukin-6, Interleukin-1
Pregnancy-associated protease
Matrix metalloproteinase-9
Soluble adhesion molecules: vascular cell adhesion molecule, intercellular adhesion
    molecule, P-selectin
CD 40 ligand
Tumor necrosis factor alpha
Myeloperosidase
Adiponectin (anti-inflammatory cytokine)

C-Reactive Protein (CPR)

Among the various markers, considerable attention has been devoted to circulating
levels of CRP as a risk indicator. CRP is an acute phase protein with a plasma half
life of 19 hours, named for its ability to precipitate the C-polysaccharide of
Pneumococcus. It is a member of the pentraxin family of calcium dependant
ligand-binding plasma proteins involved in the innate immune system produced
almost exclusively by liver in response to IL-6 after tissue injury, infection, or
other inflammatory stimuli. The human CRP molecule consists of five identical
non-glycosylated polypeptide chains each containing 206 amino acids (29). The
CRP levels in blood can be measured accurately and reproducibly down to very
low levels using recently developed high sensitivity assays. It is a stable molecule
with a long half life and does not exhibit circadian variation. Subjects in the
general population tend to have stable CRP levels characteristic for each
individual except for occasional increases associated with minor or subclinical
infections, trauma, or inflammation. Twin studies show a highly significant
genetic basis for CRP levels which is independent of age and body mass index.
The levels of CRP may also be regulated by genetic variations (30–32).

The precise mechanisms of CRP elevation in vascular disease are not well
understood and several potential mechanisms have been suggested, which include:
(1) increased release of IL-1 and IL-6 from inflammatory foci within atherosclerotic
plaque leading to hepatic overproduction of CRP; (2) myocyte damage resulting
from acute vascular occlusion resulting in an acute phase response; and (3) systemic
stimuli (such as chronic infections) that create chronic inflammation that leads to
increased CRP levels as well as to vascular inflammation.

C-Reactive Protein and Vascular Disease Risk in Subjects with No Known Vascular Disease or with Subclinical Vascular Disease

Several prospective studies have shown that, among individuals with no known
cardiovascular disease or known pre-clinical vascular disease, elevated CRP levels

measured by high sensitivity assays, are associated with an increased future risk of cardiovascular events (18,33–42). These predictive relationships were shown to persist even after correction for other known risk factors such as smoking status, lipoprotein profile, and fibrinogen levels and were also observed in women. Ridker and colleagues have recently demonstrated that the adverse prognostic value of elevated CRP levels is additive to that of lipoprotein variables (43).

The recent findings of the Reykjavik study (44), supplemented by a meta-analysis of all 22 prospective studies, have indicated that overall an elevated CRP provides only a modest incremental prognostic value over other traditional risk factors with an overall adjusted odds ratio of about 1.5 (95% CI: 1.25 to 1.68) for the highest third compared to the lowest third of CRP values (44). In contrast the corresponding odds ratio was 2.4 for elevated cholesterol and 1.9 for smoking (44). Recent studies have also suggested that CRP levels may not be an independent predictor of first cardiovascular events in elderly patients, which is in contrast to most studies that have involved middle-aged patients (45). Elevated CRP levels have also been noted with obesity, insulin resistance, type II diabetes (24,46–52), and depression (53). Elevated CRP and IL-6 levels were recently shown to predict an increased risk of future development of type II diabetes in the Women's Health Study (54).

C-Reactive Protein and Vascular Risk in Patients with Known Chronic Vascular Disease

Similarly, in a prospective European Trial involving 2121 patients with angina, elevated CRP levels at baseline were associated with an increased risk for future non-fatal myocardial infarction or sudden cardiac death with an odds ratio of 1.81 for patients in the fifth quintile of CRP (55).

C-Reactive Protein and Vascular Risk in Patients with Unstable Angina Syndromes

Following an initial description by Berk et al. in 1990, several studies involving patients with unstable angina/non-q myocardial infarction, elevated CRP was shown to be associated with increased short-term risk of recurrent ischemic events (56–60). Furthermore, the prognostic value appeared to be additive to that of cardiac specific troponin in the TIMI study and incremental to other risk factors including troponin-T in another study (59,60). In addition to short-term outcome, adverse prognostic implications of elevated CRP levels prior to discharge on long-term outcome was also shown (61–63). These findings have been contradicted by other studies that failed to observe any significant prognostic implications of an elevated CRP in patients with unstable angina.

C-Reactive Protein and Vascular Risk in Patients with Acute Myocardial Infarction

Acute myocardial infarction is associated with elevation of CRP levels, at least in part related to myocardial necrosis and a secondary inflammatory response.

Several studies in patients with acute myocardial infarction have shown that elevated CRP levels are associated with increased risk of cardiovascular complications including cardiac rupture and that successful reperfusion is associated with a fall in elevated CRP levels beyond that predictable on the basis of infarct size reduction (58,64–66).

C-Reactive Protein and Therapeutic Interventions

In as much as CRP levels are elevated in presence of modifiable risk factors such as obesity, insulin resistance, and cigarette smoking, emphasis on vigorous risk modification is appropriate in such cases to reduce the pro-inflammatory state and cardiovascular risk.

Elevated cardiovascular risk associated with elevated levels of CRP in apparently healthy subjects was shown to be attenuated by use of aspirin in the Physicians Health Study (18). The group in the lowest quartile of risk (based on CRP) had only a 14% relative risk reduction, whereas the group in the highest quartile of risk experienced a robust 56% relative risk reduction with aspirin. It is interesting to note that aspirin in conventional antithrombotic doses does not reduce circulating CRP levels. Several studies have shown that CRP levels fall with initiation of statin therapy, often independent of LDL lowering, consistent with their anti-inflammatory effects (67–70). Although some of the studies have suggested that the decrease in CRP with statins occurs independent of LDL lowering, additional studies are needed to definitively prove whether CRP lowering is or is not related to lipid (both LDL and non-LDL lipid fractions) modifying effects of statins. Furthermore, data from the secondary prevention CARES trial showed that pravastatin was most effective in reducing cardiovascular risk in the subgroup with elevated CRP levels (67). Most recently, retrospective analysis of the AFCAPS/TEXCAPS primary prevention trial also showed that increased cardiovascular risk associated with elevated CRP levels was reduced by statin therapy (lovastatin), even in subjects with average or below average cholesterol levels (71).

Since nearly half of all myocardial infarctions occur in subjects with average or below average cholesterol levels, these tantalizing observations if confirmed in prospective trials would provide a useful way of selecting a relatively high-risk subset of such individuals who could benefit from statin therapy despite average or below average cholesterol levels. Analysis of two recent trials of low (pravastatin, 40 mg) and high dose statin (atorvastatin, 80 mg) therapy in patients with established coronary heart disease showed that patients achieving a reduction in CRP levels had better overall clinical outcomes across all levels of LDL cholesterol, with the best outcomes achieved among patients with LDL below 70 mg/dl and CRP lowering to levels below 2 mg/L (72,73). These intriguing observations raise an interesting question: Should CRP monitoring supplement LDL monitoring in patients receiving statins or, for that matter, other risk modifying therapies? Answers to this question must await additional prospective trials such as the JUPITER trial, which is currently ongoing.

C-Reactive Protein and Pathogenesis of Athero-Thrombosis

It has been argued that downstream cellular effects of CRP may directly contribute to athero-thrombosis thus serving as a risk factor in addition to being a risk marker. Recent data suggest that CRP may be also produced by vascular wall cells where it may have pro-inflammatory effects and stimulate macrophage uptake of LDL, thereby contributing to the pathogenesis of athero-thrombosis (9,10,74–78). Immunoreactive CRP has been identified in atheromatous plaques and aggregated CRP binds to LDL, whereas native CRP binds to oxidized and aggregated LDL leading to complement activation (29,75,76,79–82). Complement activation, known to be potentially involved in atherogenesis, may be one potential mechanism by which CRP could contribute to atherogenesis. Other potential cellular mechanisms that may contribute to pro-atherogenic effects of CRP include its ability to stimulate LDL uptake by cells facilitating foam cell formation, induce tissue factor expression in monocytes in culture, and induce the expression of pro-inflammatory molecules in cell culture (77,83–85). Other investigators have attributed these pro-inflammatory effects of CRP in cell culture to contaminants such as azide and endotoxin present in the commercial preparations of CRP (29,86). Murine experiments have both supported as well as refuted pro-atherogenic effects of over-expression of CRP (87–91). Thus, the issue of pro-atherothrombotic effects of CRP and their relevance to human disease remains uncertain and further investigation of this intriguing concept is warranted.

Inflammatory Markers Other than C-Reactive Protein: Lipoprotein-Associated Phospholipase A-2 as a Risk Marker

Although CRP has been the most studied of systemic inflammatory markers, other proteins that are involved in inflammatory cascades such as IL-6, serum amyloid A, and soluble leucocyte adhesion molecules such as VACM-1 and ICAM-1, P-selectin, PAP, and Lp-PLA2, myeloperoxidase, and adiponectin have also been evaluated as potential biomarkers of vascular risk.

Lipoprotein-Associated Phospholipase A-2 as a Risk Marker

Among these markers, Lp-PLA2 has undergone fairly extensive evaluation as a risk marker as well as a potential risk factor for cardiovascular events (92). Lp-PLA2 (also known as platelet activating factor acetylhydrolase or PAF-AH) is a subtype of the phospholipase A2 superfamily that hydrolyzes phospholipids. Recent epidemiologic data have suggested that Lp-PLA2 levels using an immunoassay for its mass (PLAC test) may identify individuals at increased risk for cardiovascular events including stroke (92). An analysis of data from the primary prevention statin trial, the West of Scotland Coronary Prevention Study (WOSCOPS), demonstrated a modestly increased risk associated with increasing levels of Lp-PLA-2 after multivariate analysis that was independent of CRP, fibrinogen, white cell count, and classical risk factors including smoking (93). Similar results were observed in the ARIC (atherosclerosis risk in communities) study where both elevated CRP and Lp-PLA2 independently and additively contributed to increased risk for cardiovascular events with hazard ratios ranging from 1.78 for Lp-PLA2 elevation, to 2.53 for CRP elevation, and to 2.95 for the combined elevation of Lp-PLA2 and CRP (94,95). Similar results were observed in the MONICA (monitoring trends and determinants in cardiovascular disease) cohort study (96) and the Rotterdam study (97). A smaller prospective nested case control study, however, failed to show a relationship between Lp-PLA2 and cardiovascular events after multivariate adjustment (98).

Several small prospective studies have also identified a modest relationship between the angiographic or electron beam computed tomographic evidence of coronary artery disease and Lp-PLA2 levels (92). Elevated levels of Lp-PLA2 have also been noted in a relatively small cohort of patients with acute coronary syndromes where an elevated level of Lp-PLA2 has been linked to increased cardiovascular risk (92).

Lipoprotein-Associated Phospholipase A-2 as a Contributor to Atherothrombosis

As in the case of CRP, it remains unclear whether Lp-PLA2 has pro-atherothrombotic effects in addition to being a marker of inflammation. In mice, Lp-PLA2 is mostly associated with HDL and experimental observations suggest an anti-atherogenic role for Lp-PLA2 in mice (92). However in humans, Lp-PLA2 is mostly associated with LDL and pro-atherogenic effects have been attributed to it, leading to the development of inhibitors of Lp-PLA2 activity as potential anti-atherosclerotic agents; these inhibitors are currently undergoing clinical evaluation (92). As in the case of CRP, statin therapy has also been shown to reduce Lp-PLA2 levels (92).

Adiponectin (An Adipose Tissue Derived Anti-Inflammatory Cytokine) and Cardiovascular Risk

Recently, a novel circulating cytokine, derived predominantly from adipocytes, called adipnectin, has been described (99). Adiponectin has anti-inflammatory, insulin-sensitizing effects and athero-protective actions (99). Circulating levels of adiponectin are generally reduced in obesity and metabolic syndrome and appear to be inversely related to future risk of myocardial infarction in healthy subjects largely independent of lipids, CRP, and other known risk factors (17). Additional studies are needed to define the role of this novel anti-inflammatory cytokine in cardiovascular disease protection and risk prediction.

CONCLUSION

A body of evidence implicates inflammation in the pathophysiology of athero-thrombosis and thus systemic markers of inflammation could provide additional prognostic information in patients at risk for or with established disease. Extensive investigation of CRP has identified it as a lead candidate although other markers such as Lp-PLA2 and others could supplement or supplant CRP. The overall incremental value, over and above known risk factors, appears to be statistically significant but biologically modest in magnitude, perhaps belying the complex pathophysiology of atherothrombosis and the gaps in our knowledge. Continued investigation and refinements in biomarkers could, in the future, establish a clinically relevant role for inflammatory markers for prediction of risk and perhaps for monitoring the efficacy of therapy as well.

REFERENCES

1. Ross R. Atherosclerosis—an inflammatory disease. N Engl J Med 1999; 340:115–126.
2. Shah PK. Plaque disruption and thrombosis. Potential role of inflammation and infection. Cardiol Clin 1999; 17:271–281.
3. Shah PK. Plaque disruption and thrombosis: potential role of inflammation and infection. Cardiol Rev 2000; 8:31–39.
4. Shah PK. Insights into the molecular mechanisms of plaque rupture and thrombosis. Indian Heart J 2005; 57:21–30.
5. Shah PK. Mechanisms of plaque vulnerability and rupture. J Am Coll Cardiol 2003; 41:15S–22S.
6. Libby P, Ridker PM, Maseri A. Inflammation and atherosclerosis. Circulation 2002; 105:1135–1143.
7. Blake GJ, Ridker PM. C-reactive protein, subclinical atherosclerosis, and risk of cardiovascular events. Arterioscler Thromb Vasc Biol 2002; 22:1512–1513.
8. Blake GJ, Ridker PM. Inflammatory bio-markers and cardiovascular risk prediction. J Intern Med 2002; 252:283–294.
9. Pasceri V, Willerson JT, Yeh ET. Direct proinflammatory effect of C-reactive protein on human endothelial cells. Circulation 2000; 102:2165–2168.
10. Pasceri V, Cheng JS, Willerson JT, et al. Modulation of C-reactive protein-mediated monocyte chemoattractant protein-1 induction in human endothelial cells by anti-atherosclerosis drugs. Circulation 2001; 103:2531–2534.
11. Yeh ET. C-reactive protein is an essential aspect of cardiovascular risk factor stratification. Can J Cardiol 2004; 20:93B–96B.
12. Lusis AJ. Atherosclerosis. Nature 2000; 407:233–241.
13. Shah PK. Role of inflammation and metalloproteinases in plaque disruption and thrombosis. Vasc Med 1998; 3:199–206.
14. Shah PK. Pathophysiology of coronary thrombosis: role of plaque rupture and plaque erosion. Prog Cardiovasc Dis 2002; 44:357–368.
15. Fortuno A, Rodriguez A, Gomez-Ambrosi J, et al. Adipose tissue as an endocrine organ: role of leptin and adiponectin in the pathogenesis of cardiovascular diseases. J Physiol Biochem 2003; 59:51–60.

16. Ouchi N, Kihara S, Funahashi T, et al. Obesity, adiponectin and vascular inflammatory disease. Curr Opin Lipidol 2003; 14:561–566.

17. Pischon T, Girman CJ, Hotamisligil GS, et al. Plasma adiponectin levels and risk of myocardial infarction in men. JAMA 2004; 291:1730–1737.

18. Ridker PM, Cushman M, Stampfer MJ, et al. Inflammation, aspirin, and the risk of cardiovascular disease in apparently healthy men. N Engl J Med 1997; 336:973–979.

19. Kvasnicka J, Skrha J, Perusicova J, et al. Haemostasis, cytoadhesive molecules (sE-selectin and sICAM-1) and inflammatory markers in non-insulin dependent diabetes mellitus (NIDDM). Sb Lek 1998; 99:97–101.

20. Blake GJ, Ridker PM. C-reactive protein and other inflammatory risk markers in acute coronary syndromes. J Am Coll Cardiol 2003; 41:37S–42S.

21. Folsom AR, Rosamond WD, Shahar E, et al. Prospective study of markers of hemostatic function with risk of ischemic stroke. The atherosclerosis risk in communities (ARIC) study investigators. Circulation 1999; 100:736–742.

22. Kalela A, Ponnio M, Koivu TA, et al. Association of serum sialic acid and MMP-9 with lipids and inflammatory markers. Eur J Clin Invest 2000; 30:99–104.

23. Demerath E, Towne B, Blangero J, et al. The relationship of soluble ICAM-1, VCAM-1, P-selectin and E-selectin to cardiovascular disease risk factors in healthy men and women. Ann Hum Biol 2001; 28:664–678.

24. Weyer C, Yudkin JS, Stehouwer CD, et al. Humoral markers of inflammation and endothelial dysfunction in relation to adiposity and in vivo insulin action in Pima Indians. Atherosclerosis 2002; 161:233–242.

25. Elkind MS, Cheng J, Boden-Albala B, et al. Tumor necrosis factor receptor levels are associated with carotid atherosclerosis. Stroke 2002; 33:31–37.

26. Tracy RP. Hemostatic and inflammatory markers as risk factors for coronary disease in the elderly. Am J Geriatr Cardiol 2002; 11:93–100 see also 107.

27. Bayes-Genis A, Conover CA, Overgaard MT, et al. Pregnancy-associated plasma protein A as a marker of acute coronary syndromes. N Engl J Med 2001; 345:1022–1029.

28. Nambi V. The use of myeloperoxidase as a risk marker for atherosclerosis. Curr Atheroscler Rep 2005; 7:127–131.

29. Pepys MB, Hirschfield GM. C-reactive protein: a critical update. J Clin Invest 2003; 111:1805–1812.

30. Pankow JS, Folsom AR, Cushman M, et al. Familial and genetic determinants of systemic markers of inflammation: the NHLBI family heart study. Atherosclerosis 2001; 154:681–689.

31. Szalai AJ, Wu J, Lange EM, et al. Single-nucleotide polymorphisms in the C-reactive protein (CRP) gene promoter that affect transcription factor binding, alter transcriptional activity, and associate with differences in baseline serum CRP level. J Mol Med 2005; 83:440–447.

32. Zee RY, Ridker PM. Polymorphism in the human C-reactive protein (CRP) gene, plasma concentrations of CRP, and the risk of future arterial thrombosis. Atherosclerosis 2002; 162:217–219.

33. Kuller LH, Tracy RP, Shaten J, et al. Relation of C-reactive protein and coronary heart disease in the MRFIT nested case-control study. Multiple risk factor intervention trial. Am J Epidemiol 1996; 144:537–547.

34. Koenig W, Sund M, Frohlich M, et al. C-reactive protein, a sensitive marker of inflammation, predicts future risk of coronary heart disease in initially healthy

middle-aged men: results from the MONICA (monitoring trends and determinants in cardiovascular disease) Augsburg cohort study, 1984 to 1992. Circulation 1999; 99:237–242.

35. Ridker PM, Hennekens CH, Buring JE, et al. C-reactive protein and other markers of inflammation in the prediction of cardiovascular disease in women. N Engl J Med 2000; 342:836–843.

36. Ridker PM, Haughie P. Prospective studies of C-reactive protein as a risk factor for cardiovascular disease. J Investig Med 1998; 46:391–395.

37. Tracy RP, Psaty BM, Macy E, et al. Lifetime smoking exposure affects the association of C-reactive protein with cardiovascular disease risk factors and subclinical disease in healthy elderly subjects. Arterioscler Thromb Vasc Biol 1997; 17:2167–2176.

38. Tracy RP, Lemaitre RN, Psaty BM, et al. Relationship of C-reactive protein to risk of cardiovascular disease in the elderly. Results from the cardiovascular health study and the rural health promotion project. Arterioscler Thromb Vasc Biol 1997; 17:1121–1127.

39. Danesh J, Whincup P, Walker M, et al. Low grade inflammation and coronary heart disease: prospective study and updated meta-analyses. BMJ 2000; 321:199–204.

40. Ridker PM, Stampfer MJ, Rifai N. Novel risk factors for systemic atherosclerosis: a comparison of C-reactive protein, fibrinogen, homocysteine, lipoprotein(a), and standard cholesterol screening as predictors of peripheral arterial disease. JAMA 2001; 285:2481–2485.

41. Rost NS, Wolf PA, Kase CS, et al. Plasma concentration of C-reactive protein and risk of ischemic stroke and transient ischemic attack: the Framingham study. Stroke 2001; 32:2575–2579.

42. Ridker PM. High-sensitivity C-reactive protein: potential adjunct for global risk assessment in the primary prevention of cardiovascular disease. Circulation 2001; 103:1813–1818.

43. Ridker PM, Glynn RJ, Hennekens CH. C-reactive protein adds to the predictive value of total and HDL cholesterol in determining risk of first myocardial infarction. Circulation 1998; 97:2007–2011.

44. Danesh J, Wheeler JG, Hirschfield GM, et al. C-reactive protein and other circulating markers of inflammation in the prediction of coronary heart disease. N Engl J Med 2004; 350:1387–1397.

45. Kistorp C, Raymond I, Pedersen F, et al. N-terminal pro-brain natriuretic peptide, C-reactive protein, and urinary albumin levels as predictors of mortality and cardiovascular events in older adults. JAMA 2005; 293:1609–1616.

46. Temelkova-Kurktschiev T, Siegert G, Bergmann S, et al. Subclinical inflammation is strongly related to insulin resistance but not to impaired insulin secretion in a high risk population for diabetes. Metabolism 2002; 51:743–749.

47. Yudkin JS, Kumari M, Humphries SE, et al. Inflammation, obesity, stress and coronary heart disease: is interleukin-6 the link? Atherosclerosis 2000; 148:209–214.

48. Yudkin JS, Juhan-Vague I, Hawe E, et al. Low-grade inflammation may play a role in the etiology of the metabolic syndrome in patients with coronary heart disease: the HIFMECH study. Metabolism 2004; 53:852–857.

49. vThor M, Yu A, Swedenborg J. Markers of inflammation and hypercoagulability in diabetic and nondiabetic patients with lower extremity ischemia. Thromb Res 2002; 105:379–383.

50. Visser M, Bouter LM, McQuillan GM, et al. Elevated C-reactive protein levels in overweight and obese adults. JAMA 1999; 282:2131–2135.
51. Festa A, D'Agostino R, Jr., Howard G, et al. Chronic subclinical inflammation as part of the insulin resistance syndrome: the insulin resistance atherosclerosis study (IRAS). Circulation 2000; 102:42–47.
52. Barzilay JI, Abraham L, Heckbert SR, et al. The relation of markers of inflammation to the development of glucose disorders in the elderly: the cardiovascular health study. Diabetes 2001; 50:2384–2389.
53. Shimbo D, Chaplin W, Crossman D, et al. Role of depression and inflammation in incident coronary heart disease events. Am J Cardiol 2005; 96:1016–1021.
54. Pradhan AD, Manson JE, Rifai N, et al. C-reactive protein, interleukin 6, and risk of developing type 2 diabetes mellitus. JAMA 2001; 286:327–334.
55. Haverkate F, Thompson SG, Pyke SD, et al. Production of C-reactive protein and risk of coronary events in stable and unstable angina. Lancet 1997; 349:462–466.
56. Berk BC, Weintraub WS, Alexander RW. Elevation of C-reactive protein in "active" coronary artery disease. Am J Cardiol 1990; 65:168–172.
57. Liuzzo G, Biasucci LM, Gallimore JR, et al. The prognostic value of C-reactive protein and serum amyloid a protein in severe unstable angina. N Engl J Med 1994; 331:417–424.
58. Morrow DA, Rifai N, Antman EM, et al. C-reactive protein is a potent predictor of mortality independently of and in combination with troponin T in acute coronary syndromes: a TIMI 11A substudy. Thrombolysis in myocardial infarction. J Am Coll Cardiol 1998; 31:1460–1465.
59. Heeschen C, Hamm CW, Bruemmer J, et al. Predictive value of C-reactive protein and troponin T in patients with unstable angina: a comparative analysis. CAPTURE investigators. Chimeric c7E3 antiPlatelet therapy in unstable angina REfractory to standard treatment trial. J Am Coll Cardiol 2000; 35:1535–1542.
60. Lindahl B, Toss H, Siegbahn A, et al. Markers of myocardial damage and inflammation in relation to long-term mortality in unstable coronary artery disease. FRISAC study group. Fragmin during instability in coronary artery disease. N Engl J Med 2000; 343:1139–1147.
61. Biasucci LM, Colizzi C, Rizzello V, et al. Role of inflammation in the pathogenesis of unstable coronary artery diseases. Scand J Clin Lab Invest Suppl 1999; 230:12–22.
62. Ferreiros ER, Boissonnet CP, Pizarro R, et al. Independent prognostic value of elevated C-reactive protein in unstable angina. Circulation 1999; 100:1958–1963.
63. Bazzino O, Ferreiros ER, Pizarro R, et al. C-reactive protein and the stress tests for the risk stratification of patients recovering from unstable angina pectoris. Am J Cardiol 2001; 87:1235–1239.
64. Mulvihill NT, Foley JB, Murphy RT, et al. Risk stratification in unstable angina and non-Q wave myocardial infarction using soluble cell adhesion molecules. Heart 2001; 85:623–627.
65. Retterstol L, Eikvar L, Bohn M, et al. C-reactive protein predicts death in patients with previous premature myocardial infarction–a 10 year follow-up study. Atherosclerosis 2002; 160:433–440.
66. Ridker PM, Rifai N, Pfeffer MA, et al. Inflammation, pravastatin, and the risk of coronary events after myocardial infarction in patients with average cholesterol levels. Cholesterol and recurrent events (CARE) investigators. Circulation 1998; 98:839–844.

67. Ridker PM, Rifai N, Pfeffer MA, et al. Long-term effects of pravastatin on plasma concentration of C-reactive protein. The cholesterol and recurrent events (CARE) investigators. Circulation 1999; 100:230–235.
68. Albert MA, Danielson E, Rifai N, et al. Effect of statin therapy on C-reactive protein levels: the pravastatin inflammation/CRP evaluation (PRINCE): a randomized trial and cohort study. JAMA 2001; 286:64–70.
69. Jialal I, Stein D, Balis D, et al. Effect of hydroxymethyl glutaryl coenzyme a reductase inhibitor therapy on high sensitive C-reactive protein levels. Circulation 2001; 103:1933–1935.
70. Ridker PM, Rifai N, Lowenthal SP. Rapid reduction in C-reactive protein with cerivastatin among 785 patients with primary hypercholesterolemia. Circulation 2001; 103:1191–1193.
71. Ridker PM, Rifai N, Clearfield M, et al. Measurement of C-reactive protein for the targeting of statin therapy in the primary prevention of acute coronary events. N Engl J Med 2001; 344:1959–1965.
72. Ridker PM, Cannon CP, Morrow D, et al. C-reactive protein levels and outcomes after statin therapy. N Engl J Med 2005; 352:20–28.
73. Nissen SE, Tuzcu EM, Schoenhagen P, et al. Statin therapy, LDL cholesterol, C-reactive protein, and coronary artery disease. N Engl J Med 2005; 352:29–38.
74. Yasojima K, Schwab C, McGeer EG, et al. Generation of C-reactive protein and complement components in atherosclerotic plaques. Am J Pathol 2001; 158:1039–1051.
75. Torzewski J, Torzewski M, Bowyer DE, et al. C-reactive protein frequently colocalizes with the terminal complement complex in the intima of early atherosclerotic lesions of human coronary arteries. Arterioscler Thromb Vasc Biol 1998; 18:1386–1392.
76. Torzewski M, Rist C, Mortensen RF, et al. C-reactive protein in the arterial intima: role of C-reactive protein receptor-dependent monocyte recruitment in atherogenesis. Arterioscler Thromb Vasc Biol 2000; 20:2094–2099.
77. Zwaka TP, Hombach V, Torzewski J. C-reactive protein-mediated low density lipoprotein uptake by macrophages: implications for atherosclerosis. Circulation 2001; 103:1194–1197.
78. Koenig W, Torzewski J. C-reactive protein and atherosclerosis: quo vadis? Ital Heart J 2001; 2:801–803.
79. Chang MK, Binder CJ, Torzewski M, et al. C-reactive protein binds to both oxidized LDL and apoptotic cells through recognition of a common ligand: phosphorylcholine of oxidized phospholipids. Proc Natl Acad Sci USA 2002; 99:13043–13048.
80. de Beer FC, Soutar AK, Baltz ML, et al. Low density lipoprotein and very low density lipoprotein are selectively bound by aggregated C-reactive protein. J Exp Med 1982; 156:230–242.
81. Bhakdi S, Torzewski M, Klouche M, et al. Complement and atherogenesis: binding of CRP to degraded, nonoxidized LDL enhances complement activation. Arterioscler Thromb Vasc Biol 1999; 19:2348–2354.
82. Zhang YX, Cliff WJ, Schoefl GI, et al. Coronary C-reactive protein distribution: its relation to development of atherosclerosis. Atherosclerosis 1999; 145:375–379.
83. Hundt M, Zielinska-Skowronek M, Schmidt RE. Lack of specific receptors for C-reactive protein on white blood cells. Eur J Immunol 2001; 31:3475–3483.

84. Saeland E, van Royen A, Hendriksen K, et al. Human C-reactive protein does not bind to FcgammaRIIa on phagocytic cells. J Clin Invest 2001; 107:641–643.
85. Cermak J, Key NS, Bach RR, et al. C-reactive protein induces human peripheral blood monocytes to synthesize tissue factor. Blood 1993; 82:513–520.
86. Pepys MB, Hawkins PN, Kahan MC, et al. Proinflammatory effects of bacterial recombinant human C-reactive protein are caused by contamination with bacterial products, not by C-reactive protein itself. Circ Res 2005; 97:e97–e103.
87. Hirschfield GM, Gallimore JR, Kahan MC, et al. Transgenic human C-reactive protein is not proatherogenic in apolipoprotein E-deficient mice. Proc Natl Acad Sci USA 2005; 102:8309–8314.
88. Trion A, de Maat MP, Jukema JW, et al. No effect of C-reactive protein on early atherosclerosis development in apolipoprotein E*3-leiden/human C-reactive protein transgenic mice. Arterioscler Thromb Vasc Biol 2005; 25:1635–1640.
89. Danenberg HD, Szalai AJ, Swaminathan RV, et al. Increased thrombosis after arterial injury in human C-reactive protein-transgenic mice. Circulation 2003; 108:512–515.
90. Paul A, Ko KW, Li L, et al. C-reactive protein accelerates the progression of atherosclerosis in apolipoprotein E-deficient mice. Circulation 2004; 109:647–655.
91. Schwedler SB, Amann K, Wernicke K, et al. Native C-reactive protein increases whereas modified C-reactive protein reduces atherosclerosis in apolipoprotein E-knockout mice. Circulation 2005; 112:1016–1023.
92. Sudhir K. Clinical review: lipoprotein-associated phospholipase A2, a novel inflammatory biomarker and independent risk predictor for cardiovascular disease. J Clin Endocrinol Metab 2005; 90:3100–3105.
93. Packard CJ, O'Reilly DS, Caslake MJ, et al. Lipoprotein-associated phospholipase A2 as an independent predictor of coronary heart disease. N Engl J Med 2000; 343:1148–1155.
94. Ballantyne CM, Hoogeveen RC, Bang H, et al. Lipoprotein-associated phospholipase A2, high-sensitivity C-reactive protein, and risk for incident ischemic stroke in middle-aged men and women in the Atherosclerosis risk in communities (ARIC) study. Arch Intern Med 2005; 165:2479–2484.
95. Ballantyne CM, Hoogeveen RC, Bang H, et al. Lipoprotein-associated phospholipase A2, high-sensitivity C-reactive protein, and risk for incident coronary heart disease in middle-aged men and women in the atherosclerosis risk in communities (ARIC) study. Circulation 2004; 109:837–842.
96. Koenig W, Khuseyinova N, Lowel H, et al. Lipoprotein-associated phospholipase A2 adds to risk prediction of incident coronary events by C-reactive protein in apparently healthy middle-aged men from the general population: results from the 14-year follow-up of a large cohort from southern Germany. Circulation 2004; 110:1903–1908.
97. Oei HH, van der Meer IM, Hofman A, et al. Lipoprotein-associated phospholipase A2 activity is associated with risk of coronary heart disease and ischemic stroke: the Rotterdam study. Circulation 2005; 111:570–575.
98. Blake GJ, Dada N, Fox JC, et al. A prospective evaluation of lipoprotein-associated phospholipase A(2) levels and the risk of future cardiovascular events in women. J Am Coll Cardiol 2001; 38:1302–1306.
99. Hug C, Lodish HF. The role of the adipocyte hormone adiponectin in cardiovascular disease. Curr Opin Pharmacol 2005; 5:129–134.

6

Chronic Infections as Risk Factors for Atherothrombosis

P. K. Shah and Bojan Cercek

*Atherosclerosis Research Center, Division of Cardiology and Department
of Medicine, Cedars-Sinai Medical Center and David Geffen School of
Medicine, University of California, Los Angeles, California, U.S.A.*

INTRODUCTION

Atherothrombotic vascular disease is the leading cause of death in most of the western nations and predicted to become the leading cause of death in the world over the next decade. A number of risk factors have been identified that increase the risk of atherothrombosis and they include family history of premature vascular disease, dyslipidemia, smoking, hypertension, insulin resistance and diabetes mellitus, obesity, atherogenic diet, hyperhomocystenemia, estrogen deficiency, and lack of physical activity. However, these conventional risk factors do not account for all of the attributable risk of atherothrombotic vascular disease. A search for additional risk factors has led to the idea that chronic infections may be an important risk factor. Chronic infections as potential culprits in the vascular inflammatory response have received renewed interest since the critical role of inflammation in the evolution, progression, and destabilization of atherothrombosis has been recognized (1–3). From a historical perspective, the idea that infections may contribute to atherosclerosis was suggested by several authors around the beginning of the 20th century (4,5). In fact, in 1911, Frothingham stated that "The sclerosis of old age may simply be a summation of lesions arising from infectious or metabolic toxins" (6). Based on examination of 400,000 sections from 40 necropsy cases, Leary coined the term "abscess" to describe atheromatous plaques containing leucocyte infiltration (7). Based on recent seroepidemiologic data, human pathology, biological plausibility, experimental models, and pilot clinical trials, a potential causal link between chronic infections and atherothrombotic disease has received much attention in recent years (8–10).

VIRAL INFECTIONS AND ATHEROTHROMBOSIS

Experimental observations of Fabricant et al. suggested a link between cytomegalovirus (CMV) infection and atherosclerosis (11,12). In noncholesterolemic chickens, an avian herpes virus (Marek's disease virus) induced atherosclerotic lesions and increased cholesterol ester accumulation in aortic smooth muscle cells. Furthermore, virus-induced atherosclerosis could be prevented by a vaccine derived from turkey herpes virus (11,12). These early observations have been supported by experimental findings in rat models of atherosclerosis or accelerated allograft atherosclerosis (13) and in atherosclerosis-prone transgenic mice (14,15). CMV infection induces human arterial smooth muscle cell proliferation, possibly by inactivating p53, a pro-apoptotic tumor suppressor gene that stimulates cholesterol esters accumulation in smooth muscle cells and induces a prothrombotic phenotype in endothelial cells. These observations provide biologic plausibility to the potential causal link between CMV infection and atherothrombotic and proliferative vascular disease (16,17). However, seroepidemiologic data and data from direct examination of vascular tissue from humans have been less than persuasive for native atherosclerosis and negative or at best inconsistent for restenosis and transplant vasculopathy (18–25). Thus, data to definitively link CMV to atherosclerosis or restenosis are lacking. Other herpes viruses, hepatitis A and B virus, and the influenza virus have also been implicated in some but not in other studies. However, the evidence is indirect and far from established (26–28). Influenza epidemics were associated with significant increase in cardiovascular death (29) and in many patients the acute myocardial infarctions are preceded by an upper respiratory infection (30,31). The relationship of influenza infection and acute manifestations of coronary artery disease meet most of the Hill's criteria of causality: strength of association, consistency, temporal sequence, coherence, biologic plausibility, and experimental evidence. The criterion which is not met is analogy, which is the weakest criterion. Furthermore, observational studies have suggested protective effect of influenza vaccination against cardiovascular events, a 67% reduction in the risk of myocardial infarction, and a 50% reduction of risk in cardiac arrest and stroke (32). In a small randomized study by Gurfinkel and colleagues, cardiovascular death occurred in 2% of vaccinated versus 8% of the control patients (p=0.01) (33). These data need to be confirmed in large, prospective trials.

BACTERIAL INFECTIONS AND VASCULAR DISEASE

Several bacteria have been implicated with atherothrombosis and include *Chlamydia pneumoniae, Helicobacter pylori* and *Porphyromonas gingivali* (2,3,10).

CHLAMYDIA PNEUMONIAE

C. pneumonia has received a lot of attention as a putative culprit in atherothrombosis. *C. pneumoniae* is an intracellular organism responsible for upper respiratory infections, pneumonia, and sinusitis. The prevalence of infection with *C. pneumoniae* increases with age so much so that up to 80% of people 65 years of age or older have evidence of exposure (34,35). *C. pneumonia* infection introduced through the respiratory tract increases early foam-cell type atherosclerotic lesions in normocholesterolemic and mildly hypercholesterolemic rabbits (36–39). *C. pneumoniae* infection augmented and accelerated atherosclerosis only in presence of hypercholesterolemia in murine models in some (40,41), but not in other studies (42). Although azithromycin treatment was shown to reduce augmented atherosclerosis from *C. pneumoniae* infection in cholesterol-fed rabbits (38), no such benefit was observed with azithromycin in murine atherosclerosis excacerbated by *C. pneumoniae* infection (43). The ability of *C. pneumoniae* or one or more of its structural components such as the heat shock protein 60 to induce pro-atherogenic, pro-oxidant, pro-inflammatory, and pro-thrombotic reponses in cells relevant to atherothrombosis (smooth muscle cells, endothelial cells, and macrophages and T-cells) provides biological plausibility to the potential causal link between *C. pneumoniae* and vascular disease (44).

Several seroepidemiologic studies, mostly retrospective, have, in general, shown a 2-fold or more risk of coronary or cerebrovascular disease among seropositive compared to seronegative individuals (18,23,45–51), although other prospective studies have failed to demonstrate a convincing relationship (52–54). These studies used different criteria for seropositivity, different and subjective methods of antibody assay, and had statistical biases introduced by subgroup analysis. *C. pneumonia* has been detected in human atheromatous or aneurysmal tissue by immunocytochemistry in approximately 50% of specimens (range: 40–100%), by polymerase chain reaction (PCR) in 0–60% of specimens, and has been isolated from one carotid endarterectomy specimen, one coronary artery from a transplant recipient, and 16% of coronary atherosclerotic tissue removed at atherectomy (55–62). Two large retrospective case control studies have examined the relationship between prior use of antibiotics and risk of myocardial infarction. The larger of the two studies showed that the frequency of use of tetracyclines or quinolones in the three preceding years was lower among cases of myocardial infarction than controls (63), whereas the other, smaller study failed to find a relationship between the prior use of erythromycin, tetracycline, or doxycycline and first myocardial infarction (64).

Small pilot intervention trials involving anti-chlamydial antibiotics (azithromycin or roxithromycin) have been reported. Two of these studies, conducted following an index event of acute myocardial infarction or unstable angina, suggested reduction in recurrent coronary events with antibiotic therapy (65,66), but a longer term follow-up showed loss of initial benefit at 6 months in the ROXIS trial (67). The ACADEMIC randomized trial showed no clinical benefit of a 3 month course of azithromycin treatment on clinical outcomes although reduction in serum markers of inflammation was demonstrated (68). These studies used different regimens and durations of treatment, were small in size, and were not powered to provide definitive evidence for or against the hypothesis.

Another small, randomized trial showed no overall clinical event reduction in azithromycin-or amoxicillin-treated patients compared to placebo group; however, a post-hoc analysis combining the two antibiotic arms suggested a clinical benefit compared to placebo (69).

A large, randomized trial ISAR-3 involving 1100 patients undergoing angioplasty and coronary stenting (PCI) showed no prevention of restenosis with 30 mg daily of roxithromycin for 4 weeks. Post-hoc analysis suggested a significant reduction in restenosis in the subgroup with high anti-*C. pneumoniae* antibody titres (70). Similarly, 3 months treatment with doxycyline did not influence adverse clinical event and restenosis rate after PCI (71).

Three large trials using antichlamydial antibiotics, azithromycin (AZACS trial), roxithromycin (Antibio trial), and most recently PROVE IT-TIMI 22 with gatifloxacin in patients with acute coronary syndrome have been published (72–74). Although they differed in selected antibiotic, treatment regimen, and duration of follow-up from 6 months to 30 months, no effect of the active treatment arm was shown (Table 1).

Two large trials tested the effect of azithromycin in chronic coronary artery disease patients. WIZARD trial tested a 3 month course of azithromycin in patients with previous myocardial infarction and serologic evidence of *C. pneumoniae* infection. ACES trial tested weekly treatment with azithromycin for one year, with 4 years of follow-up (75,76). Both failed to show any benefit, even in several predefined subgroups of patients (Table 2). The WIZARD study suggested a transient benefit early during treatment, a finding that was not supported by other studies.

There are several potential explanations for the negative outcome of the clinical trials: (1) incorrect hypothesis, i.e., infection does not play a role either in

Table 1 Infectious Agents Implicated in Vascular Disease

1	Viruses	CMV; *Herpes simplex* 1 and 2, *Hepatitis A*, Influenza
2	Bacteria	*Chlamydia pneumoniae, Helicobacter pylori, Porphyromonas gingivalis*

Table 2 Clinical Endpoints in Trial of Antibiotics for Secondary Prevention of Coronary Artery Disease

Trial (Ref.)	Year	No. pts.	Indi-cations	Therapy	Follow-up	Endpoint (C/Rx)
ISAR (70)	2001	1020	Post PCI	Roxithromycin 1 months	D, MI 1 year	7% vs 6%, p=0.45
AZACS (72)	2003	1450	ACS	Azithromycin 5 days	D, MI, R 6 months	14% vs 15%, p=0.606
ANTIBIO (73)	2003	872	AMI	Roxithromycin 6 weeks	D 1 year	6.5% vs 6.0%, p=0.739
WIZARD (75)	2003	7724	Chr CAD	Azithromycin 3 months	D, MI, R, AP 3 years	14% vs 15%, p=0.23
PROVE-IT (75)	2005	4162	ACS	Gatifloxacin 18 months	D, MI, R, AP 2 years	23.7% vs 25.1%, p=0.41
ACES (76)	2005	4012	Chr CAD	Azithromycin 12 months	D, MI, R, AP 4 years	22.3% vs 22.4%, p=NS

Abbreviations: D, death of any cause; MI, nonfatal myocardial infarction; R, revascularization; AP, hospitalization for angina pectoris.

acute atherothrombotic events or in the chronic progression of the disease, (2) the advanced stages of the disease are not influenced by the antibiotic therapy, and least likely and (3) the selection of the antibiotic therapy and duration was inadequate. As on the other hand the observations for the role of the inflammation in the atherogenesis continue to accumulate, these findings suggest that we should rethink the strategy and not abandon the hypothesis altogether. The current conclusion, though, should be that the standard antibiotic therapy for *C. pneumoniae* does not favorably influence the outcomes related to coronary artery disease (77).

HELICOBACTER PYLORI

Seroepidemiologic data linking *H. pylori* infection to atherothrombotic vascular disease are overall not persuasive. Smaller studies suggested a positive relationship (18,78–80), while the larger studies failed to demonstrate a relationship (18,81–84). More recent studies suggested that only strains of *H. pylori*, which express the cytotoxin-associated gene A, have a link with atherosclerosis (85). Attempts to demonstrate *H. pylori* in human atherosclerotic tissue have in general proven fruitless (83). Although 1 of 39 carotid plaques was shown to contain *H. pylori* DNA, contamination could not be excluded (84). One small intervention trial reported recently showed no clinical benefit of anti-*H. pylori* drug regimen compared to placebo (69). There are no good experimental data for the relationship between *H. pylori* infection and atherosclerosis in animal models and no experimental data in vitro to demonstrate biological plausibility favoring a pro-atherogenic role. Thus, at the present time, the balance of evidence does not lend a strong support for a causal role for *H. pylori* in atherothrombosis.

PERIODONTAL DISEASE, *PORPHYROMONAS GINGIVALIS*, *STREPTOCOCCUS SANGUIS*, AND ATHEROTHROMBOSIS

Periodontitis is a common chronic inflammatory disease in the periodontal tissue leading to destruction of the bone surrounding the teeth, and is responsible for tooth loss in adults. Several studies have suggested an increased risk of coronary heart disease or stroke with periodontal disease or tooth loss (86–92), whereas others have raised questions about this link (93). Direct pathological demonstration of culprit pathogens, *Bacteroides forsythus*, *Porphyromonas gingivalis*, *Prevotella intermedia*, *Streptococcus sanguis* among others, have not been reported in human atherosclerotic tissues. Elevated levels of fibrinogen and Factor VIII have been reported with periodontal infection in small studies (89). Biological plausibility is suggested by the fact that periodontal disease may predispose to athero-thrombosis given the abundance of pathogens involved, local production of pro-inflammatory and matrix-degrading molecules, and its association with other risk factors such as fibrinogen levels and white blood cell (WBC) counts. Of the two common pathogens involved in periodontal disease, *S. sanguis* can enhance platelet aggregation and *P. gingivalis* may increase risk of thrombosis by production of platelet aggregation, associated protein, and stimulation of Factor X (87,88). A recent experimental study has shown accelerated atherosclerosis with *P. gingivalis* infection in apo E null mice (94). No intervention trials in animals or humans have been reported.

Thus the overall evidence implicating periodontal disease and athero-thrombosis remains inconclusive.

POTENTIAL ROLE OF MULTIPLE INFECTIOUS ORGANISMS

The concept of "total pathogen" burden (Fig. 1) in which instead of a single pathogen, multiple pathogens are involved in the pathogenesis of atherothrom-bosis, was recently suggested (95). This hypothesis is supported by cross-sectional studies and prospective studies wherein the risk of coronary heart disease events increased with the number of chronic infections as assessed by positive serology to specific pathogens CMV, *Hepatitis A*, *H. pylori*, *herpes simplex* 1 and 2, and *C. pneumoniae* (95,96). Increased pathogen burden was associated with increasing levels of circulating C-reactive protein believed to reflect inflammation. Similarly, the Bruneck prospective, population-based survey suggested that a history of chronic infections (respiratory, urinary, dental, and others) amplified the risk of carotid atherosclerosis independently of other known risk factors. The risk was highest in patients with a prominent inflammatory response revealed by elevated

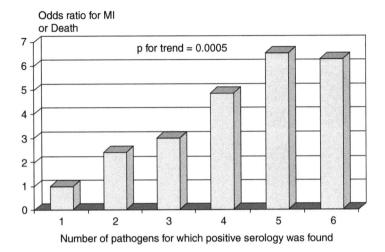

Figure 1 Relationship between pathogen burden at baseline and subsequent risk of myocardial infarction or death in a prospective cohort of 890 patients undergoing coronary angiography. Pathogen burden is defined as immunologic evidence for prior infection with one or more of the following pathogens: Cytomegalovirus, Herpes simplex virus-1, Herpes simplex virus-2, Hepatitis A virus, Chlamydia pneumoniae, Helicobacter pylori. *Source*: Adapted from Ref. 96.

circulating markers (soluble adhesion molecules, endotoxin, human heat shock protein 60, and antibodies to mycobacterial heat shock protein 65) (97). Lack of association between chronic infection with multiple agents and endothelial dysfunction suggested that these agents are not implicated as early etiologic triggers but may be involved at later stages of the atherosclerosis (98).

These studies provide support for the concept that chronic infections from a diverse group of pathogens and the consequent inflammatory response may increase the risk of atherothrombosis.

POTENTIAL MECHANISMS BY WHICH INFECTIONS MAY PREDISPOSE TO ATHEROTHROMBOSIS

Infection may be linked to atherothrombosis by at least two different mechanisms.

Direct Infection of Cells of the Vessel Wall and Pro-Atherothrombotic Effects

Infectious organisms can infect one or more types of cells relevant to atherothrombosis (monocytes-macrophages, endothelial cells, vascular smooth muscle cells) leading to a host of changes that could promote atherosclerosis, plaque

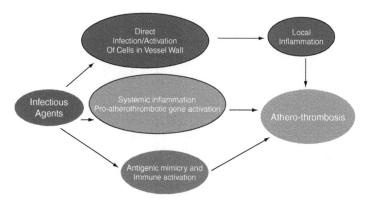

Figure 2   How chronic infections may contribute to atherothrombosis.

disruption, and thrombosis. The procoagulant effects, enhanced scavenger receptor expression and foam cell formation, enhanced expression of adhesion molecules and inflammatory cytokines, enhanced expression of metalloproteinases, and enhanced migration, survival, and proliferation of smooth muscle cells may be some of the proposed mechanisms (Fig. 2) (99–102).

Remote Effects of Infection

Antigenic Mimicry and Immune Activation

Experimental studies have suggested that breakdown of immune tolerance and development of an autoimmune response to aberrant presentation of otherwise hidden endogenous antigens may be provoked by infectious organisms carrying homologous antigens. This immune response may lead to vasculitis and myocarditis and possibly even atherosclerosis through molecular or antigenic mimicry (103). Heat shock proteins may be such antigens since bacteria contain them, viruses use them when budding from host cells, and they are highly conserved across prokaryotes and mammalian species (104–112). In this instance, an infection at a site remote from the vessel wall may be sufficient to create immune-mediated vascular injury without requiring actual infection of the vessel wall (112).

Pro-Inflammatory Effects of Remote Infections

Infections remote from the vessel wall may induce systemic inflammation by inducing pro-inflammatory circulating cytokines and/or changing the normally protective and anti-inflammatory high density lipoprotein (HDL) into a pro-atherogenic and pro-inflammatory HDL, thus contributing to atherothrombosis by an indirect mechanism also not requiring infection of the vessel wall (113–114).

SUMMARY

The hypothesis that infectious organisms may contribute to atherothrombosis, directly or indirectly through immune activation and systemic inflammation, is currently a focus of intense scrutiny. A number of recent large scale, randomized trials of antibiotics have been disappointing in terms of lack of benefits of anti-chlamydial therapy. It remains unclear as to whether negative therapeutic trials indicate: (1) lack of a significant pathophysiological role of one or more infectious organisms, (2) application of therapy too late in the course of the disease evolution ("horse being out of the barn" analogy), or (3) incorrect choice of antimicrobial therapies or other unknown factors.

REFERENCES

1. Ross R. Atherosclerosis is an inflammatory disease. Am Heart J 1999; 138:S419–S420.
2. Shah PK. Plaque disruption and thrombosis: potential role of inflammation and infection. Cardiol Rev 2000; 8:31–39.
3. Libby P, Egan D, Skarlatos S. Roles of infectious agents in atherosclerosis and restenosis: an assessment of the evidence and need for future research. Circulation 1997; 96:4095–4103.
4. Osler' W. Disease of the Arteries. Philadelphia: Lea and Febiger, 1908.
5. O Klotz MM. Fatty streaks in intima of arteries. J Pathol Bacteriol 1912; 16:211–220.
6. Frothingham C. The relationship between acute infectious diseases and arterial lesions. Arch Intern Med 1911; 8:153–162.
7. Leary T. Pathology of coronary stenosis. Am Heart J 1935; 10:423–426.
8. Saikku P, Leinonen M, Mattila K, et al. Serological evidence of an association of a novel chlanlydia, TW AR, with chronic coronary heart disease and acute myocardial infarction. Lancet 1988; 2:983–986.
9. Saikku P, Leinonen M, Tenkanen L, et al. Chronic chlamydia pneumoniae infection as a risk factor for coronary heart disease in the Helsinki Heart Study. Ann Intern Med 1992; 116:273–278.
10. Shah PK. Link between infection and atherosclerosis: who are the culprits: viruses, bacteria, both, or neither? Circulation 2001; 103:5–6.
11. Fabricant CG, Fabricant J, Litrenta MM, Minick CR. Virus-induced atherosclerosis. J Exp Med 1978; 148:335–340.
12. Minick CR, Fabricant CG, Fabricant J, Litrenta MM. Atherosclerosis induced by infection with a herpesvirus. Am J Pathol 1979; 96:673–706.
13. Lemstrom K, Sihvola R, Bruggeman C, Hayry P, Koskinen P. Cytomegalovirus infection-enhanced cardiac allograft vasculopathy is abolished by DHPG prophylaxis in the rat. Circulation 1997; 95:2614–2616.
14. Hsich E, Zhou YF, Paigen B, Johnson TM, Burnett MS, Epstein SE. Cytomegalovirus infection increases development of atherosclerosis in Apolipo-protein-E knockout mice. Atherosclerosis 2001; 156:23–28.

15. Zhou YF, Shou M, Harrell RF, Yu ZX, Unger EF, Epstein SE. Chronic non-vascular cytomegalovirus infection: effects on the neointimal response to experimental vascular injury. Cardiovasc Res 2000; 45:1019–1025.

16. Speir E, Yu ZX, Ferrans VJ. Infectious agents in coronary artery disease: viral infection, aspirin, and gene expression in human coronary smooth muscle cells. Rev Port Cardiol 1998; 17:II33–II39.

17. Jacob HS, Visser M, Key NS, Goodman JL, Moldow CF, Vercellotti GM. Herpes virus infection of endothelium: new insights into atherosclerosis. Trans Am Clin Climatol Assoc 1992; 103:95–104.

18. Danesh J, Collins R, Peto R. Chronic infections and coronary heart disease: is there a link? Lancet 1997; 350:430–436.

19. Adler SP, Hur JK, Wang JB, Vetrovec GW. Prior infection with cytomegalovirus is not a major risk factor for angiographically demonstrated coronary artery atherosclerosis. J Infect Dis 1998; 177:209–212.

20. Zhou YF, Leon MB, Waclawiw MA, et al. Association between prior cytomegalovirus infection and the risk of restenosis after coronary atherectomy. N Engl J Med 1996; 335:624–630.

21. Ridker PM, Hennekens CH, Stampfer MJ, Wang F. Prospective study of herpes simplex virus, cytomegalovirus, and the risk of future myocardial infarction and stroke. Circulation 1998; 98:2796–2799.

22. Sorlie PD, Nieto FJ, Adam E, Folsom AR, Shahar E, Massing M. A prospective study of cytomegalovirus, herpes simplex virus 1, and coronary heart disease: the atherosclerosis risk in communities (ARIC) study. Arch Intern Med 2000; 160:2027–2032.

23. Siscovick DS, Schwartz SM, Corey L, et al. Chlamydia pneumoniae, herpes simplex virus type 1, and cytomegalovirus and incident myocardial infarction and coronary heart disease death in older adults: the cardiovascular health study. Circulation 2000; 102:2335–2340.

24. Manegold C, Alwazzeh M, Jablonowski H, et al. Prior cytomegalovirus infection and the risk of restenosis after percutaneous transluminal coronary balloon angioplasty. Circulation 1999; 99:1290–1294.

25. Neumann FJ, Kastrati A, Miethke T, et al. Previous cytomegalovirus infection and restenosis after coronary stent placement. Circulation 2001; 104:1135–1139.

26. Zhu J, Quyyumi AA, Norman JE, Costello R, Csako G, Epstein SE. The possible role of hepatitis A virus in the pathogenesis of atherosclerosis. J Infect Dis 2000; 182:1583–1587.

27. Naghavi M, Barlas Z, Siadaty S, Naguib S, Madjid M, Casscells W. Association of influenza vaccination and reduced risk of recurrent myocardial infarction. Circulation 2000; 102:3039–3045.

28. Tong D-Y, Wang X-H, Xu C-F, Yang Y-Z, Xiong S-D. Hepatitis B virus infection and coronary atherosclerosis: results from a population with relatively high prevalence of hepatitis B virus. World J Gastroenterol 2005; 11:1292–1296.

29. Collins S. Excess mortality from causes other than influenza and pneumonia during influenza epidemics. Health Rep 1932; 47:2159–2179.

30. Spodick DH, Flessas AP, Johnson MM. Association of acute respiratory symptoms with onset of myocardial infarction: prospective investigation of 150 consecutive patients and matched controls patients. Am J Cardiol 1984; 53:481–482.

31. Meier CRT, Jick SS, Derby LE, Vasilakis C, Jick H. Acute respiratory-tract infection and risk of myocardial infarction. Lancet 1998; 351:1467–1471.

32. Madjid M, Aboshady I, Awan I, Cascells SW. Influenza and cardiovascular disease. Tex Heart Inst J 2004; 31:4–13.

33. Gurfinkel EP, de la Fuente RL, Mendiz O, Mautner B. Influenza vaccine pilot study in acute coronary syndromes and planned percutaneous coronary interventions: the FLU Vaccination Acute Coronary Syndromes (FLUVACS) study. Circulation 2002; 105:2143–2147.

34. Grayston JT. Infections caused by chlamydia pneumoniae strain TW AR. Clin Infect Dis 1992; 15:757–761.

35. Grayston JT, Kuo CC, Campbell LA, Benditt EP. Chlamydia pneumoniae, strain TWAR and atherosclerosis. Eur Heart J 1993; 14:66–71.

36. Fong IW, Chiu B, Viira E, Fong MW, J ang D, Mahony J. Rabbit model for chlamydia pneurnoiae infection. J Clin Microbiol 1997; 35:48–52.

37. Laitinen K, Laurila A, Pyhala L, Leinonen M, Saikku P. Chlamydia pneumoniae infection induces inflammatory changes in the aortas of rabbits. Infect Immun 1997; 65:4832–4835.

38. Muhlestein JB, Anderson JL, Hammond EH, et al. Infection with chlamydia pneumoniae accelerates the development of atherosclerosis and treatment with azithromycin prevents it in a rabbit model. Circulation 1998; 97:633–636.

39. Fong IW, Chiu B, Viira E, Jang D, Mahony JB. De novo induction of atherosclerosis by chlamydia pneumoniae in a rabbit model. Infect Immun 1999; 67:6048–6055.

40. Moazed TC, Campbell LA, Rosenfeld ME, Grayston JT, Kuo CC. Chlamydia pneumoniae infection accelerates the progression of atherosclerosis in apolipoprotein E-deficient mice. J Infect Dis 1999; 180:238–241.

41. Hu H, Pierce GN, Zhong G. The atherogenic effects of chlamydia are dependent on serum cholesterol and specific to chlamydia pneumoniae. J Clin Invest 1999; 103:747–753.

42. Caligiuri G, Rottenberg M, Nicoletti A, Wigzell H, Hansson GK. Chlamydia pneumoniae infection does not induce or modify atherosclerosis in mice. Circulation 2001; 103:2834–2838.

43. Rothstein NM, Quinn TC, Madico G, Gaydos CA, Lowenstein CJ. Effect of azithromycin on murine arteriosclerosis exacerbated by Chlamydia pneumoniae. J Infect Dis 2001; 183:232–238.

44. Kol A, Libby P. Molecular mediators of arterial inflammation: a role for microbial products? Am Heart J 1999; 138:S450–S452.

45. Ossewaarde JM, Feskens EJ, De Vries A, Vallinga CE, Kromhout D. Chlamydia pneumoniae is a risk factor for coronary heart disease in symptom-free elderly men, but Helicobacter pylori and cytomegalovirus are not. Epidemiol Infect 1998; 120:93–99.

46. Maass M, Gieffers J. Cardiovascular disease risk from prior chlamydia pneumoniae infection can be related to certain antigens recognized in the immunoblot profile. J Infect 1997; 35:171–176.

47. Fagerberg B, Gnarpe J, Gnarpe H, Agewall S, Wikstrand J. Chlamydia pneumoniae but not cytomegalovirus antibodies are associated with future risk of stroke and cardiovascular disease: a prospective study in middle-aged to elderly men with treated hypertension. Stroke 1999; 30:299–305.

48. Miyashita N, Toyota E, Sawayama T, et al. Association of chronic infection of chlamydia pneumoniae and coronary heart disease in the Japanese. Intern Med 1998; 37:913–916.

49. Thomas M, Wong Y, Thomas D, et al. Relation between direct detection of schlamydia pneumoniae DNA in human coronary arteries at postmortem examination and histological severity (Stary grading) of associated atherosclerotic plaque. Circulation 1999; 99:2733–2736.

50. Cook PJ, Honeyboume D, Lip GY, Beevers DG, Wise R, Davies P. Chlamydia pneumoniae antibody titers are significantly associated with acute stroke and transient cerebral ischemia: the West Birmingham Stroke project. Stroke 1998; 29:404–410.

51. Strachan DP, Carrington D, Mendall MA, et al. Relation of chlamydia pneumoniae serology to mortality and incidence of ischaemic heart disease over 13 years in the caerphilly prospective heart disease study. BMJ 1999; 318:1035–1039.

52. Ridker PM, Kundsin RB, Stampfer MJ, Poulin S, Hennekens CH. Prospective study of chlamydia pneumoniae IgG seropositivity and risks of future myocardial infarction. Circulation 1999; 99:1161–1164.

53. Ridker PM, Hennekens CH, Buring JE, Kundsin R, Shih J. Baseline IgG antibody titers to chlamydia pneumoniae, Helicobacter pylori, herpes simplex virus, and cytomegalovirus and the risk for cardiovascular disease in women. Ann Intern Med 1999; 131:573–577.

54. Nieto FJ, Folsom AR, Sorlie PD, Grayston JT, Wang SP, Chambless LE. Chlamydia pneumoniae infection and incident coronary heart disease: the Atherosclerosis Risk in Communities study. Am J Epidemiol 1999; 150:149–156.

55. Grayston JT, Campbell LA. The role of chlamydia pneumoniae in atherosclerosis. Clin Infect Dis 1999; 28:993–994.

56. Weiss SM, Roblin PM, Gaydos CA, et al. Failure to detect chlamydia pneumoniae in coronary atheromas of patients undergoing atherectomy. J Infect Dis 1996; 173:957–962.

57. Campbell LA, O'Brien ER, Cappuccio AL, et al. Detection of Chlamydia pneumoniae TWAR in human coronary atherectomy tissues. J Infect Vis 1995; 172:585–588.

58. Paterson DL, Hall J, Rasmussen SJ, Timms P. Failure to detect chlamydia pneumoniae in atherosclerotic plaques of Australian patients. Pathology 1998; 30:169–172.

59. Jackson LA, Campbell LA, Schmidt RA, et al. Specificity of detection of chlamydia pneumoniae in cardiovascular atheroma: evaluation of the innocent bystander hypothesis. Am J Pathol 1997; 150:1785–1790.

60. Jantos CA, Nesseler A, Waas W, Baumgartner W, Tillmanns H, Haberbosch W. Low prevalence of chlamydia pneumoniae in atherectomy specimens from patients with coronary heart disease. Clin Infect Vis 1999; 28:988–992.

61. Ramirez JA. Isolation of chlamydia pneumoniae from the coronary artery of a patient with coronary atherosclerosis. The chlamydia pneumoniae/atherosclerosis study group. Ann Intern Med 1996; 125:979–982.

62. Maass M, Bartels C, Engel PM, Mamat U, Sievers HH. Endovascular presence of viable chlamydia pneumoniae is a common phenomenon in coronary artery disease. J Am Coll Cardiol 1998; 31:827–832.

63. Meier CR, Derby LE, Jick SS, Vasilakis C, Lick H. Antibiotics and risk of subsequent first-time acute myocardial infarction. JAMA 1999; 281:427–431.
64. Jackson LA, Smith NL, Heckbert SR, Grayston JT, Siscovick DS, Psaty BM. Lack of association between first myocardial infarction and past use of erythromycin, tetracycline, or doxycycline. Emerg Infect Dis 1999; 5:281–284.
65. Gupta S, Leatham EW, Carrington D, Mendall MA, Kaski JC, Carom AJ. Elevated Chlamydia pneumoniae antibodies, cardiovascular events, and azithromycin in male survivors of myocardial infarction. Circulation 1997; 96:404–407.
66. Gurfinkel E, Bozovich G, Daroca A, Beck E, Mautner B. Randomised trial of roxithromycin in non-Q-wave coronary syndromes: ROXIS pilot study. ROXIS study group. Lancet 1997; 350:404–407.
67. Gurfinkel E, Bozovich G, Beck E, Testa E, Livellara B, Mautner B. Treatment with the antibiotic roxithromycin in patients with acute non-Q-wave coronary syndromes. The final report of the ROXIS study. Eur Heart J 1999; 20:121–127.
68. Anderson JL, Muhlestein JB, Carlquist J, et al. Randomized secondary prevention trial of azithromycin in patients with coronary artery disease and serological evidence for chlamydia pneumoniae infection: The Azithromycin in Coronary Artery Disease: Elimination of Myocardial Infection with Chlamydia (ACA-DEMIC) study. Circulation 1999; 99:1540–1547.
69. Stone AFM, Kaski J-C, Gupta S, Carom J, Northfield T. Antibiotics against chlamydia pneumoniae and helicobacter pylori reduce further cardiovascular events in patients with acute coronary syndromes. J Am Coll Cardiol 2001; 37 Supplement A:1A–648A.
70. Neumann F, Kastrati A, Miethke T, et al. Treatment of chlamydia pneumoniae infection with roxithromycin and effect on neointima proliferation after coronary stent placement (ISAR-3): a randomised, double-blind, placebo-controlled trial. Lancet 2001; 357:2085–2089.
71. Kannengiessre M, Kaltenbach M, Stille W, Reifart N, Haase J. Influence of doxycycline on clinical and angiographic outcome following percutaneous coronary intervention. J Int Cardiol 2005; 17:447–453.
72. Cercek B, Shah PK, Noc M, et al. Mahrer P for AZACS Investigators. Effect of short-term treatment with azithromycin on recurrent ischemic events in patients with acute coronary syndrome in the Azithromycin in Acute Coronary Syndrome (AZACS) trial: a randomized controlled trial. Lancet 2003; 361:809–813.
73. Zahn R, Schneider S, Frilling B, et al. Senges; working group of leading hospital cardiologists. Antibiotic therapy after acute myocardial infarction: a prospective randomized study. Circulation 2003; 107:1253–1259.
74. Cannon CP, Braunwald E, McCabe CH, et al. Antibiotic treatment of chlamydia pneumoniae after acute coronary syndrome. N Engl J Med 2005; 352:1646–1654.
75. O'Connor CM, Dunne MW, Pfeffer MA, et al. Azithromycin for the secondary prevention of coronary heart disease events: the WIZARD study: a randomized controlled trial. JAMA 2003; 290:1459–1466.
76. Graystone JT, Kronmal RA, Jackson LAS, et al. Azithromycin for secondary prevention of coronary events. N Engl J Med 2005; 352:1637–1645.
77. Anderson JL. Infection, antibiotics, and atherothrombosis-end of the road or new beginnings? N Engl J Med 2005; 352:1706–1709.

78. Ossei-Geming N, Moayyedi P, Smith S, et al. Helicobacter pylori infection is related to atheroma in patients undergoing coronary angiography. Cardiovasc Res 1997; 35:120–124.

79. Markus HS, Mendall MA. Helicobacter pylori infection: a risk factor for ischaemic cerebrovascular disease and carotid atheroma. J Neurol Neurosurg Psychiatry 1998; 64:104–107.

80. de Luis DA, Lahera M, Canton R, et al. Association of Helicobacter pylori infection with cardiovascular and cerebrovascular disease in diabetic patients. Diabetes Care 1998; 21:1129–1132.

81. Folsom AR, Nieto FJ, Sorlie P, Chambless LE, Graham DY. Helicobacter pylori seropositivity and coronary heart disease incidence. Atherosclerosis Risk In Communities (ARIC) study investigators. Circulation 1998; 98:845–850.

82. Khurshid A, Fenske T, Bajwa T, Bourgeois K, Vakil N. A prospective, controlled study of Helicobacter pylori seroprevalence in coronary artery disease. Am J Gastroenterol 1998; 93:717–720.

83. Blasi F, Denti F, Erba M, et al. Detection of chlamydia pneumoniae but not Helicobacter pylori in atherosclerotic plaques of aortic aneurysms. J Clin Microbiol 1996; 34:2766–2769.

84. Danesh J, Koreth J, Youngman L, et al. Is Helicobacter pylori a factor in coronary atherosclerosis? J Clin Microbiol 1999; 37:1651.

85. Sawayama Y, Ariyama I, Hamada M, et al. Association between chronic Helicobacter pylori infection and acute ischemic stroke: Fukuoka Harasanshin Atherosclerosis Trial (FHAT). Atherosclerosis 2005; 178:303–309.

86. Kweider M, Lowe GD, Murray GD, Kinane DF, McGowan DA. Dental disease, fibrinogen and white cell count; links with myocardial infarction? Scott Med J 1993; 38:73–74.

87. Irnamura T, Potempa J, Tanase S, Travis J. Activation of blood coagulation factor X by arginine-specific cysteine proteinases (gingipain-Rs) from Porphyromonas gingivalis. J Biol Chem 1997; 272:16062–16067.

88. Herzberg MC, Weyer MW. Dental plaque, platelets, and cardiovascular diseases. Ann Periodontol 1998; 3:151–160.

89. KJ Matilla RY, Nieminen M, et al. Yon Willebrand factor antigen and dental infection. Thromb Res 1989; 56:325–391.

90. Loesche WJ, Schork A, Terpenning MS, Chen YM, Dominguez BL, Grossman N. Assessing the relationship between dental disease and coronary heart disease in elderly U.S. veterans. J Am Dent Assoc 1998; 129:301–311.

91. Beck ill, Offenbacher S, Williams R, Gibbs P, Garcia R. Periodontitis: a risk factor for coronary heart disease? Ann Periodontoi 1998; 3:127–141.

92. Seymour RA, Steele JG. Is there a link between periodontal disease and coronary heart disease? Br Dent J 1998; 184:33–38.

93. Joshipura KJ, Douglass CW, Willett WC. Possible explanations for the tooth loss and cardiovascular disease relationship. Ann Periodontol 1998; 3:175–183.

94. Li L, Messas E, Batista EL, Jr., Levine RA, Amar S. Porphyromonas gingivalis infection accelerates the progression of atherosclerosis in a heterozygous apolipoprotein E-deficient murine model. Circulation 2002; 105:861–867.

95. Zhu J, Quyyumi AA, Nonnan JE, et al. Effects of total pathogen burden on coronary artery disease risk and C-reactive protein levels. Am J Cardiol 2000; 85:140–146.

96. Zhu J, Nieto FJ, Home BD, Anderson JL, Muhlestein JB, Epstein SE. Prospective study of pathogen burden and risk of myocardial infarction or death. Circulation 2001; 103:45–51.

97. Kiechl S, Egger G, Mayr M, et al. Chronic infections and the risk of carotid atherosclerosis: prospective results from a large population study. Circulation 2001; 103:1064–1070.

98. Khairy P, Rinfret S, Tardif J-C, et al. Absence of association between infectious agents and endothelial function in health young men. Circulation 2003; 107:1966–1971.

99. Epstein SE, Zhou YF, Zhu J. Infection and atherosclerosis: emerging mechanistic paradigms. Circulation 1999; 100:e20–e28.

100. Shah PK. Chronic infections and atherosclerosis/thrombosis. Curr Atheroscler Rep 2002; 4:113–119.

101. Medzhitov R, Janeway C, Jr. The toll receptor family and microbial recognition. Trends Microbiol 2000; 8:452–456.

102. Xu XH, Shah PK, Faure E, et al. Toll-like receptor-4 is expressed by macrophages in murine and human lipid-rich atherosclerotic plaques and upregulated by oxidized LDL. Circulation 2001; 104:3103–3108.

103. Bachmaier K, Neu N, de la Maza LM, Pal S, Hessel A, Penninger JM. Chlamydia infections and heart disease linked through antigenic mimicry. Science 1999; 283:1335–1339.

104. Xu Q, Willeit J, Marosi M, et al. Association of serum antibodies to heat-shock protein 65 with carotid atherosclerosis. Lancet 1993; 341:255–259.

105. Xu Q, Luef G, Weimann S, Gupta RS, Wolf H, Wick G. Staining of endothelial cells and macrophages in atherosclerotic lesions with human heat-shock protein-reactive antisera. Arterioscler Thromb 1993; 13:1763–1769.

106. Schett G, Xu Q, Amberger A, et al. Autoantibodies against heat shock protein 60 mediate endothelial cytotoxicity. J Clin Invest 1995; 96:2569–2577.

107. Metzler B, Mayr M, Dietrich H, et al. Inhibition of arteriosclerosis by T-cell depletion in normocholesterolemic rabbits immunized with heat shock protein 65. Arterioscler Thromb Vasc Biol 1999; 19:1905–1911.

108. Xu Q, Kiechl S, Mayr M, et al. Association of serum antibodies to heat-shock protein 65 with carotid atherosclerosis: clinical significance determined in a follow-up study. Circulation 1999; 100:1169–1174.

109. Mayr M, Metzler B, Kiechl S, et al. Endothelial cytotoxicity mediated by serum antibodies to heat shock proteins of Escherichia coli and chlamydia pneumoniae: immune reactions to heat shock proteins as a possible link between infection and atherosclerosis. Circulation 1999; 99:1560–1566.

110. Kol A, Bourcier T, Lichtman AH, Libby P. Chlamydial and human heat shock protein 60s activate human vascular endothelium, smooth muscle cells, and macrophages. J Clin Invest 1999; 103:571–577.

111. Kol A, Lichtman AH, Finberg RW, Libby P, Kurt-Iones EA. Cutting edge: heat shock protein (HSP) 60 activates the innate immune response: CD 14 is an essential receptor for HSP60 activation of mononuclear cells. J Immunol 2000; 164:13–17.

112. Epstein SE, Zhu I, Bumett MS, Zhou YF, Vercellotti G, Hajjar D. Infection and atherosclerosis: potential roles of pathogen burden and molecular mimicry. Arterioscler Thromb Vasc Biol 2000; 20:1417–1420.

113. Navab M, Berliner JA, Subbanagounder G, et al. HDL and the inflammatory response induced by LDL-derived oxidized phospholipids. Arterioscler Thromb Vasc Biol 2001; 21:481–488.

114. Van Lenten BJ, Wagner AC, Nayak DP, Hama S, Navab M, Fogelman AM. High-density lipoprotein loses its anti-inflammatory properties during acute influenza infection. Circulation 2001; 103:2283–2288.

7

Novel Psychosocial Factors and Cardiovascular Disease

Donna M. Polk

Division of Cardiology, Department of Medicine, Cedars-Sinai Research Institute, Cedars-Sinai Medical Center, and Department of Medicine, University of California at Los Angeles School of Medicine, Los Angeles, California, U.S.A.

Cheryl K. Nordstrom and James Dwyer[‡]

Department of Preventive Medicine, University of Southern California School of Medicine, Los Angeles, California, U.S.A.

Willem J. Kop and David S. Krantz

Uniformed Services University of the Health Sciences, Bethesda, Maryland, U.S.A.

C. Noel Bairey Merz

Preventive and Rehabilitative Cardiac Center, Cedars-Sinai Medical Center, Los Angeles, California, U.S.A.

INTRODUCTION

Cardiovascular disease remains the largest contributor to morbidity and mortality in developed countries (1). Advances in prevention and treatment of cardiovascular disease in the last 40 years resulted in an approximate 40% decline in cardiovascular disease mortality (1). Despite this remarkable success, it is sobering to note that this decline appears to have abated in recent years (2), paradoxically despite continued improvement in risk factor modification (3).

[‡] Deceased.

Similarly, it has also become increasingly clear that up to 50% of patients with established coronary artery disease (CAD) will have recurrent cardiac events such as myocardial infarction and cardiac death despite aggressive management of traditional risk factors (4). Both these lines of evidence suggest that development of a better understanding of novel risk factors and newer therapies aimed at these nontraditional risk factors are needed.

Multiple studies have demonstrated that psychosocial factors are associated with elevated risk of cardiovascular disease in both patients with established disease (5,6) as well as non-diseased subjects (7,8). The spectrum of psychosocial factors is diverse, ranging from acute, such as outbursts of anger and mental stress which can trigger pathophysiologic responses and an acute event, to chronic psychologic risk factors such as hostility, depression, or exhaustion that correlate with higher rates of CAD (9,10). Psychosocial factors such as work stress, financial stress, and stressful life events have been shown to be associated with myocardial infarction in the large INTERHEART study which included male and female patients from a wide range of countries and ethnicities (11). While it appears clear from these data that there is a simple and direct relationship between psychosocial factors and cardiovascular disease, not all studies have demonstrated such positive findings (12,13), and the magnitude of risk is variable between studies (5–8). Given the complex nature of human behavior, it is likely that the relationship between psychosocial factors and cardiovascular disease are mediated at multiple levels along the pathophysiologic mechanisms responsible for cardiovascular disease events (Fig. 1). These interactions may explain some of the lack of consistency between studies, and point to the need for continued mechanistic understanding as an aid to designing effective psychosocial intervention strategies.

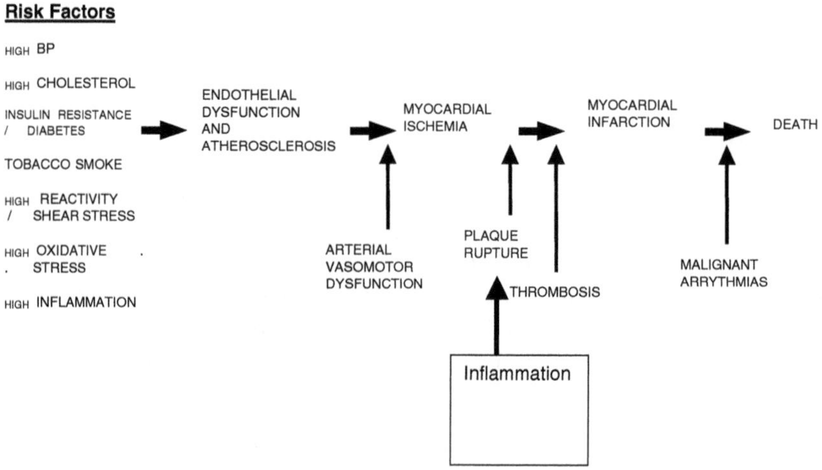

Figure 1 Pathophysiologic mechanisms of cardiovascular disease.

DEPRESSION AND CARDIOVASCULAR DISEASE

The lifetime prevalence of major depression in the general population is 15% (14), while among coronary disease patients the prevalence is even higher (17–27%), particularly among the elderly (14–18). The presence of depressive symptoms or major depressive episode has been prospectively linked to fatal and nonfatal cerebral and cardiovascular events (15,17–28) in both populations, with (15,23–26) and without diagnosed coronary disease (18–22). This increased risk holds true in individuals with a remote history (>10 years) of depression before onset of coronary artery disease and appears to be independent of other coronary risk factors (20). Not all studies have demonstrated linkage between depression and cardiovascular events, however (27). The majority of studies show an elevated risk of CAD endpoints with risk ratios ranging from 1.5 to 4.5 over a minimum of 4.5 years (17–23).

Studies that have specifically examined depression and the outcomes of recurrent cardiovascular events, revascularization procedures, and death in patients with established coronary disease demonstrated relative risks as high as 7.8 (CI: 4,9–12). In a 6-month post-infarct follow-up, Frasure-Smith showed depression (Diagnostic and Statistical Manual of Mental Disorders-III diagnosis) was an independent risk factor for mortality (relative risk 4.29, CI: 3.14–5.44) (17) and depression remained an independent mortality predictor at 18-month follow-up (relative risk 1.5, CI:1.3–10.1) (23). The Cardiac Arrest in the Cardiac Arrhythmia Pilot Study (CAPS) involving coronary patients with significant ventricular arrhythmias showed elevated all-cause and cardiovascular mortality at one year among those patients with evidence of depressive symptoms on the Beck Depression Inventory (24). Longer term outcomes utilizing self-reporting of depressive symptoms in 1250 post-infarct patients showed significantly increased cardiovascular mortality over 15.2 years in those with higher Zung Self-Rating Depression scores (25).

While the methodology and measurement tools in the previous studies are quite variable, there is a consensus of evidence that depressive symptomology is associated with increased cardiovascular morbidity and mortality. Mechanisms to explain this increased risk may be due to an increase in the incidence of sudden cardiac death in patients with depression (23), mediated by alterations in the autonomic nervous system as indicated by decreased heart rate variability (29,30), consistent with impaired vagal tone and increased sympathetic tone (30,31). Additional mechanisms may include depression-related alterations in platelet function and reactivity (32,33). Prior work has demonstrated significantly increased binding at the IIb/IIIa complex, indicating increased platelet reactivity among depressed patients compared to controls (34). Other work has shown that chemotactic factors including PF4 and ß-TG are significantly higher in patients with coronary disease and depression, as compared to those with coronary disease alone or control (35). Preliminary data, including results from the

Sertraline Antidepressant and Heart Attack Randomized Trial (SADHART), suggest that some of these platelet effects may be reversible with selective serotonin reuptake inhibitor treatment (36–38). Increased conversion of prothrombin to thrombin is noted in depressed patients (34). Finally, the poorer outcomes of depressed patients may be due to poorer compliance with medications and/or healthier lifestyles.

While recognition and treatment of depression is important in and of itself, ongoing work is testing the hypothesis that treatment of depression reduces cardiovascular morbidity and mortality. The safety of treatment of recurrent depression with sertraline in 369 patients with unstable angina and recent myocardial infarction (MI) has been established in the SADHART trial (35). The Enhancing Recovery in Coronary Heart Disease Patients (ENRICHD) randomized 1165 post-infarct patients with depression or perceived low social support to treatment with psychotherapy and pharmacotherapy for non-responders (39). While there was not a statistically significant reduction in mortality in those randomized to treatment, those with improved symptoms had increased survival as compared to non-responders (21.2% vs 10.4%) (39).

SOCIAL SUPPORT

Social isolation or lack of a social support system is associated with an increase in all-cause mortality, with relative risks ranging from 1.46–3.80 (6,40–42) Among male survivors of acute MI in the Beta-Blocker Heart Attack Trial (6), the risk was further enhanced in patients with increased measures of life stress. Prior work has demonstrated that the elevated risk associated with lack of social support is independent of left ventricular function and coronary anatomy (43), enhanced among those with diminished economic resources (43), relevant in the elderly (42), and linked with emotional support (42). Mechanisms behind the link between social support and cardiovascular disease are likely multifactorial, and may include limited access to and utilization of healthcare, poor compliance to healthy lifestyles, associated adverse pathophysiology, or combinations of these.

PSYCHOSOCIAL FACTORS AND TRADITIONAL CARDIOVASCULAR RISK FACTOR CLUSTERING

Traditional cardiovascular risk factors, as outlined in the Framingham Study, include cigarette smoking, hypertension, diabetes mellitus, dyslipidemia, family history of premature coronary disease, and sedentary lifestyle (12). It is clear that psychosocial factors directly correlate with a higher prevalence and clustering of traditional cardiovascular risk factors. Psychosocial stress may result from and contribute to high-risk behaviors that then result in the clustering of smoking, inactivity, and obesity. Mortality, for example, correlates with higher blood pressure, cardiac reactivity, blood cholesterol, and cigarette smoking, as well as poor diet and exercise habits (44). Despite the strong correlation between the hostile personality trait and traditional risk factors, the lack of evidence supporting this as an independent risk factor is probably accounted for by incompleteness and inaccuracy of traditional risk factor data collection and statistical covariance analyses. Similar clustering results have been found using psychosocial factors measures such as hostility (45), depression (46), and low socioeconomic status/social support (43). Indeed, adverse psychosocial factors likely both cluster together (e.g., hostility-depression-lack of social support), and are identifiers of clusters of traditional cardiovascular risk factors (39).

PSYCHOSOCIAL FACTORS AND ATHEROSCLEROSIS

Not surprisingly, most of the above-mentioned psychosocial factors have also been demonstrated to correlate with measures of atherosclerosis. Carefully controlled animal primate studies using cynomolgus monkeys have clearly demonstrated the roles of psychosocial stress (47) and social isolation (48), created by varying cage rotations/restrictions, in atherosclerosis measured at necropsy. Notably, it is the dominant male monkeys that appear most susceptible to the stress-induced atherosclerosis (49), in some ways parallel to the human Type A behavior and hostility work. Type A behavior personality (47), hostility (50), depression/hopelessness (51), and job stress (52) have been shown to correlate with atherosclerosis in humans using measures such as coronary angiography or carotid artery intima-media thickness. In general, these human studies have adjusted for the traditional cardiovascular risk factors, suggesting that the psychosocial factors provide additional independent risk. Pathophysiologic links between pyschosocial factors and atherosclerosis independent of traditional cardiovascular risk factors may include inflammation-induced LDL-cholesterol oxidation, elevated shear stress and adverse catecholamine, and reproductive hormonal changes which result in increased endothelial damage leading to atherosclerosis (53).

PSYCHOSOCIAL FACTORS AND ENDOTHELIAL FUNCTION

There is evidence that endothelial dysfunction is one of the earliest signs of atherosclerosis, such that the balance of local arterial mediators results in a loss of functional dilation (54). Recent evidence also suggests that arterial vasomotor dysfunction plays an important role in acute cardiac events and death. Inappropriate vasoconstriction, or lack of coronary artery dilation in response to an increased demand, is present in stable coronary heart disease (55–57). This is related to dysfunctional endothelium due to the underlying atherosclerosis and contributes to the genesis of myocardial ischemia. Arterial vasomotor function is mediated by both endothelial function and other local regulators as well as systemic autonomic nervous system activity.

Preliminary work in animals and humans suggests that psychosocial factors influence endothelial function. Psychosocial stress created by frequent cage rotation produced endothelial dysfunction in a primate model, even in the absence of diet-induced atherosclerosis (57). Notably, a gender difference was noted, in that the dominant male monkeys had the greatest endothelial dysfunction (58), whereas female subordinates demonstrated the greatest abnormalities (58), suggesting that behavioral and physiological gender differences may have implications for cardiovascular disease. One human angiographic study has demonstrated a relationship between reported anger and coronary endothelial dysfunction (59). Previous work evaluating a possible surrogate of endothelial function, peripheral vascular reactivity, has demonstrated links to psychosocial stress in monkeys (57) and hostility in humans (60), as well as progression of atherosclerosis in humans (61). Pathophysiologic links between psychosocial factors and endothelial function may involve direct endothelial damage due to catecholamine and blood pressure surges, resulting in intimal damage, inflammatory-induced free radicals blocking nitric oxide synthesis, and activated platelet-triggered endothelial reactivity (62).

PSYCHOSOCIAL FACTORS AND MYOCARDIAL ISCHEMIA

Myocardial ischemia results in the setting of atherosclerotic cardiovascular disease when myocardial blood flow demand outstrips the supply. Mechan-istically, this is triggered by both increases in demand mediated dominantly by increases in heart rate and blood pressure, and reduced supply mediated by coronary artery vasoconstriction, typically during physical and/or mental exertions (63). Prolonged myocardial ischemia results in myocardial infarction, most typically as a consequence of obstructive thrombus formation. It is well documented now that laboratory mental stress triggers increased blood pressure demand (64), coronary artery vasoconstriction, and reduced blood flow (65), with resultant myocardial ischemia (63). Parallel ambulatory studies in coronary artery disease patients in daily life show similar results (66), and have been extended to demonstrate that both intensity of mental effort and negative mood correlates with myocardial ischemia. Patients with documented mental stress ischemia had more exaggerated hemodynamic rest and stress responses to mental stress (67). Both ambulatory (68) and laboratory (69) studies have demonstrated that hostility correlates with ischemia in humans.

PSYCHOSOCIAL FACTORS AND PLAQUE RUPTURE

Current pathophysiological understanding suggests that acute cardiovascular events such as myocardial infarction and unstable angina are precipitated by atherosclerotic plaque rupture, where the cholesterol crystals and cellular debris are extruded into the coronary artery lumen and the subendothelial collagen components are exposed to circulating blood, promoting intracoronary throm-bus (70). While it is possible that plaque rupture is serendipitous, increasing lines of evidence suggest that it is more likely triggered by both internal and external events (71). Specifically, it has long been noted that these acute cardiovascular events occur in a circadian rhythm, reflecting sympathetic nervous system activity (72). Moreover, anger, and mentally stressful triggers were identified as triggers in a carefully designed study of myocardial infarction antecedent behaviors (71). Pathophysiologic links between psychosocial stress and plaque rupture may include surges in heart rate, blood pressure, and sympathetic nervous system activity, as well as weakening of the collagenous plaque cap from inflammatory processes, all of which may contribute to plaque instability (73).

PSYCHOSOCIAL FACTORS AND THROMBOSIS

It is likely that atherosclerotic plaques rupture relatively frequently and that a determining factor to progression to an acute cardiovascular event is the propensity for thrombus formation and the balance between pro- and anti-thrombic factors. Traditional risk factors clearly play a role in promoting thrombus. Data demonstrate that dyslipidemia (74), diabetes (75), and cigarette smoking (76) promote thrombus formation, via platelet- and non-platelet-mediated mechanisms. Preliminary data suggest that psychosocial factors also play a role in thrombus promotion. Pathophysiologic links appear to include a relationship between hostility and increased platelet reactivity (77), Type A/hostility, and reduced bleeding time and prostacyclin formation (78), elevated PAI-1 levels, and depressive symptoms (32), as well as enhanced platelet aggregation by mental stress related to increases in catecholamines and sympathetic nervous system activity (79).

PSYCHOSOCIAL FACTORS AND LETHAL ARRHYTHMIAS

Approximately half of the cardiovascular deaths experienced in the U.S. annually occur suddenly, due to a malignant ventricular arrhythmia (ventricular fibrillation) as the culmination of atherosclerotic plaque rupture/ischemia/infarction (Fig. 1) (1). We currently have no treatment for these patients other than the autonomic defibrillators implanted in the few who survive. Electrical stability and ventricular fibrillation threshold are influenced by many factors, including the autonomic nervous system. It is clear that lowered levels of parasympathetic nervous system tone and increased levels of sympathetic nervous system tone promote ventricular fibrillation in myocardial substrate at risk. Animal work in dogs demonstrates that anger, produced by restraining the dog, lowers ventricular fibrillatory thresholds measured directly by electrophysiological testing (80). More indirect measures are needed for human work. Heart rate variability, obtained from electrocardiographic recordings (81) and baroreflex testing (82), are noninvasive estimates of autonomic nervous system tone that are responsive to both acute (83) and chronic (29) conditions. Multiple lines of evidence indicate that psychosocial factors influence the autonomic nervous system measured by heart rate variability or baroreflex testing, including mental stress (83), depression (84), and anxiety (85). Because both heart rate variability and baroreflex measures have been demonstrated to predict future cardiovascular events (86,87), these tools provide particularly rich insight into the interplay between psychosocial factors and cardiovascular disease.

PSYCHOSOCIAL FACTORS AND INFLAMMATION

The progression of coronary artery disease can be viewed as a "response to injury" (88) that is promoted by inflammatory processes. At present, little is known about the interaction between psychosocial factors and inflammatory processes in progressive atherosclerosis. Several lines of evidence indicate that inflammatory processes play a crucial role in plaque formation (89). Both acute and chronic psychological factors may promote the expression of adhesion molecules (90). These adhesion molecules (e.g., intracellular adhesion molecule-1) may cause monocytes and T-cells to adhere to the vascular endothelium, followed by monocyte infiltration and conversion to macrophages. Two main responses emerge from the penetration of macrophages and T-cells into the vascular wall: (1) activation of the cytokine cascade, and (2) release of growth factors (e.g., insulin-like and platelet-derived growth factor). Cytokines and growth factors will accelerate smooth muscle cell proliferation from the intimal layers of the vessel wall and promote progression of atherosclerosis. It is of interest that both episodic (91–93) and acute psychological risk factors for coronary syndromes are reported to affect circulating levels of T-cell, B-cells, and aspects of the cytokine cascade. A major challenge in this area of research relates to documenting the clinical significance of elevated levels of the inflammatory measures. Furthermore, the relationship between inflammatory processes and the progression of coronary artery disease is not fully understood, and it is not clear to what extent circulating inflammatory measures reflect the processes occurring at local atherosclerotic plaques. Nonetheless, the relationship between psychosocial factors, measures of inflammation, and cardiovascular disease may reveal new insights and opportunities for intervention.

PSYCHOSOCIAL INTERVENTION TRIALS

Psychosocial interventions that have been designed to address psychosocial factors could lower recurrent coronary artery disease events. At least 23 psychosocial intervention trials have evaluated the alteration of cardiac events following behavioral interventions in patients with established coronary artery disease (93–114). Small sample sizes, resulting in low statistical power, have often been a problem among these trials. Other problems include the lack of a uniform definition of "psychosocial stress," a wide divergence of clinical approaches toward psychosocial intervention among the trials, and, in some trials, a lack of true randomization due to the behavioral study design. Nevertheless, three meta-analyses of 12 (115), 23 (116), and 11(117) controlled stress-management intervention trials involving 1484, 3180, and 3485 patients, respectively, demonstrate that psychosocial stress intervention has a beneficial impact on reducing recurrent cardiac events/death by 50–70%.

When only fully randomized trials which report recurrent cardiac events such as myocardial infarction and death as outcome variables are included, a summarized odds ratio demonstrates a significant 50% reduction in cardiac events among the intervention patients (118). One of the largest randomized trials performed in post-infarct patients, also demonstrated a statistically significant 51% one-year reduction in cardiac death (95). This trial employed simple stress management techniques performed by general nurses, and the overall mortality reduction was due primarily to a 61% reduction in out-of-hospital sudden cardiac death. Long-term follow-up of the patients in this trial has further demonstrated that withdrawal of the stress management at the end of the trial resulted in a disappearance of the beneficial mortality reduction (118). A more recent trial, from the same investigators using a similar environmental stress intervention, demonstrated no significant effect on cardiovascular events in the total group, and evidence of an adverse effect in women randomized to the intervention (119). These trials used stress-reduction interventions which included nurse visits and home help if indicated at the time of increased stress as evaluated at monthly phone checks. Another recent large trial (106), which used psychologic counseling and stress management training sessions for seven weeks following a cardiac event, demonstrated a reduction in recurrent events that was evident at six-month follow-up, but not persistent at 12-months follow-up. These later studies represent considerably larger studies with improved trial design features compared to the previous literature, and therefore cannot be easily discounted. Future trials might consider equipping patients with skills or tools to utilize during times of stress to test if this would result in better long-term outcomes.

At present, it is unknown if all patients or just those with high psychosocial stress might benefit from psychosocial stress interventions. Although essentially all patients with established coronary disease experience some psychosocial distress related to their disease, some suffer more seriously (119), and one intervention study has suggested that patients with high psychosocial stress appear to benefit the most, in terms of mortality reduction, from stress management (120). Specific stress management techniques, such as group support, yoga, biofeedback, and meditation, have not been tested in randomized clinical trials with adequate sample sizes to assess cardiovascular events. In planning these and other future psychosocial intervention trials, consideration should be given to these prior clinical trial results for optimization of successful and valid results.

SUMMARY

Psychosocial factors appear to be risk factors for cardiovascular disease morbidity and mortality. Multiple studies have demonstrated that psychosocial factors are risk factors for cardiovascular disease in both patients with established disease (5,6) and non-diseased subjects (8). Current literature also suggests that psychosocial factors contribute to coronary artery disease via complex interactions along a pathophysiological chain of events, including adverse effects on traditional risk factor clustering (45), atherosclerosis (50), endothelial function (59,65), myocardial ischemia (63,66), plaque rupture (72), thrombosis (76,77), and lethal arrhythmias (29,84).

It is clear that psychosocial factors contribute to coronary artery disease morbidity and mortality via complex interactions. Continued efforts designed at understanding the behavioral and physiologic associations between psychosocial factors and cardiovascular disease are needed. Current psychosocial factor intervention trials suggest that the magnitude of risk reduction associated with intervention may be similar to that of other proven therapies for coronary artery disease, such as lipid-lowering (120), antiplatelet therapy (121), beta-blocker medication (122), and bypass surgery (123). Continued efforts are aimed at designing effective psychosocial interventions offer, promise for further reductions in cardiovascular disease morbidity and mortality.

ACKNOWLEDGMENTS

This work was funded in part by grants from the John D. and Catherine T. MacArthur Foundation and the National Heart, Lung, and Blood Institutes Grant No. 232HL07380 and Grant No. HL49910. The opinions and assertions espressed herein are those of the authors and are not to be construed as reflecting the views of the United States Uniformed Health Services or the U.S. Department of Defense.

REFERENCES

1. Sytkowski PA, Kannel WB, Agostino RB. Changes in risk factors and the decline in mortality from cardiovascular disease. The Framingham Heart Study. N Engl J Med 1990; 322:1635–1641.
2. Rosamond WD, Chambless LE, Folsom AR, et al. Trends in the incidence of myocardial infarction and in mortality due to coronary heart disease, 1987–1994. N Engl J Med 1998; 339:861–867.
3. Levy D, Thom TJ. Death rates from coronary disease—progress and a puzzling paradox. N Engl J Med 1998; 229:915–917.
4. Haskell WL, Alderman EL, Fair JM, et al. Effects of intensive multiple risk factor reduction on coronary atherosclerosis and clinical cardiac events in men and women with coronary artery disease: the Stanford Coronary Risk Intervention Project (SCRIP). Circulation 1994; 89:975–990.

5. Frasure-Smith N. Hospital symptoms of psychological stress as predictors of longterm outcome after acute myocardial infarction in men. Am J Cardiol 1991; 67:121–127.
6. Ruberman W, Weinblatt E, Goldberg JD, et al. Psychosocial influences on mortality after myocardial infarction. N Engl J Med 1984; 311:552–559.
7. Rosengren A, Tibblin G, Wilhelmsen L. Self-perceived psychological stress and incidence of coronary artery disease in middle-aged men. Am J Cardiol 1991; 68:1171–1175.
8. Johnson JV, Stewart W, Hall EM, Fredlund P, Theorell T. Long-term psychosocial work environment and cardiovascular mortality among swedish men. Am J Public Health 1996; 86:324–331.
9. Kop WJ. Chronic and acute psychological risk factors for clinical manifestations of coronary artery disease. Psychosom Med 1999; 61:476–487.
10. Krantz DS, Kop WJ, Santiago HT, et al. Mental stress as a trigger of myocardial ischemia and infarction. Cardiol Clin 1996; 14:271–287.
11. Rosengren A, Hawken S, Ounpuu S, et al. Association of psychosocial risk factors with risk of acute myocardial infarction in 11,119 cases and 13,648 controls from 52 countries (the INTERHEART study): case-control study. Lancet 2004; 364:953–962.
12. Reed DM, LaCroix, Karasek RA, Miller D, MacLean CA. Occupational strain and the incidence of coronary heart disease. Am J Epidem 1989; 129:495–502.
13. Hlatky MA, Lam LC, Lee KL, et al. Job strain and the prevalence and outcome of coronary artery disease. Circulation 1995; 92:327–333.
14. Kessler RC, McGonagle KA, Zhao S, et al. Lifetime and 12-month prevalence of DSM-III-R psychiatric disorders in the United States: results from the National Comorbidity Survey. Arch Gen Psychiatry 1994; 51:8–19.
15. Carney RM, Rich MW, Freedland KE, et al. Major depressive disorder predicts cardiac events in patients with coronary artery disease. Psychosom Med 1988; 50:627–633.
16. Schleifer SJ, Macari-Hinson MM, Coyle DA, et al. The nature and course of depression following myocardial infarction. Arch Intern Med 1989; 149:1785–1789.
17. Frasure-Smith N, Lesperance F, Talajic M. Depression following myocardial infraction: impact on 6-month survival. JAMA 1993; 270:1819–1825.
18. Schultz R, Beach SR, Ives DG, Martire LM, Airyo AA, Kop WJ. Association between depression and mortality in older adults: the cardiovascular health study. Arch Intern Med 2000; 160:1761–1768.
19. Ford DE, Mead LA, Chang PP, et al. Depression is a risk factor for coronary artery disease in men. Arch Intern Med 1998; 158:1422–1426.
20. Pratt LA, Ford DE, Crum FM, et al. Depression, psychotropic medication, and risk of myocardial infarction: prospective data from the Baltimore ECA follow-up. Circulation 1996; 94:3123–3129.
21. Everson SA, Roberts RE, Goldberg DE, et al. Depressive symptoms and increased risk of stroke mortality over a 29-year period. Arch Intern Med 1998; 158:1113–1138.
22. Anda RF, Williamson DF, Jones D, et al. Depressed affect, hopelessness, and the risk of ischemic heart disease in a cohort of U.S. adults. Epidemiology 1993; 4:285–294.

23. Frasure-Smith N, Lesperance F, Talajic M. Depression and 18-month prognosis after myocardial infarction. Circulation 1995; 91:999–1005.
24. Ahern DK, Gorkin L, Anderson JL, et al. Biobehavioral variables and mortality or cardiac arrest in the cardiac arrhythmia pilot study (CAPS). Am J Card 1990; 66:59–62.
25. Barefoot JC, Schroll M. Symptoms of depression, acute myocardial infarction, and total mortality in a community sample. Circulation 1996; 93:1976–1980.
26. Frasure-Smith N, Lesperance F, Juneau M, et al. Gender, depression, and one-year prognosis after myocardial infarction. Psychosom Med 1999; 61:26–37.
27. Vogt T, Pope C, Mullooly J, et al. Mental health status as a predictor of morbididty and mortality: a 15-year follow-up of members of a health maintenance organization. Am J Public Health 1994; 84:227–231.
28. Gorman JM, Sloan RP. Heart rate variability in depressive and anxiety disorders. Am Heart J 2000; 140:S77–S83.
29. Carney RM, Saunders RD, Freedland KE, et al. Association of depression with reduced heart rate variability in coronary artery disease. Am J Cardiol 1995; 76:526–564.
30. Watkins LL, Grossman P. Association of depressive symptoms with reduced baroreflex cardiac control in coronary artery disease. Am Heart J 1999; 137:453–457.
31. Esler M, Turbott J, Schwartz R, et al. The peripheral kinetics of norepinephrine in depressive illness. Arch Gen Psychiatry 1982; 39:285–300.
32. Nemeroff CB, Musselman DL. Are platelets the link between depression and ischemic heart disease? Am Heart J 2000; 140:S57–S62.
33. Laghrissi-Thode F, Wagner WR, Pollock BG, et al. Elevated platelet factor 4 and ß-thromboglobulin plasma levels in depressed patients with ischemic heart disease. Biol Psychiatry 1997; 42:290–295.
34. Musselman DI, Tomer A, Manatunga AK, et al. Exaggerated platelet reactivity in major depression. Am J Psychiatry 1996; 153:1313–1317.
35. Glassman AH, O'Connor CM, Califf RM, et al. Sertraline treatment of major depression in patients with acute MI or unstable angina. JAMA 2002; 288:701–709.
36. Musselman Dl, Knight BT, Baron A, et al. Effects of paroxetine treatment on platelet reactivity in patients with major depression (abstract 86). Presented at the 37th annual meeting of the American College of Neuropsychopharmacology Pureto Rico, December 1998.
37. Pollock BG, Laghrissi-Thode F, Wagner WR. Evaluation of platelt activation in depressed patients with ischemic heart disease after paroxetine or nortriptyline treatment. J Clin Psychopharmacol 2000; 20:137–140.
38. Serebruany VL, Glassman AH, Malinin AI, et al. Platelet/Endothelial biomarkers in depressed patients treated with the selective serotonin reuptake inhibitor sertraline after acute coronary events: the Sertraline Antidepressant Heart Attack Randomized Trial (SADHART) Platelet Substudy. Circulation 2003; 180:939–944.
39. Carney RM, Blumenthal JA, Freedland KE, et al. Depression and late mortality after myocardial infarction in the Enhancing Recovery in Coronary Heart Disease (ENRICHD) study. Psych Med 2004; 66:466–474.
40. Orth-Gomer K, Rosengren A, Wilhelmsen L. Lack of social support and incidence of coronary heart disease in middle-aged Swedish men. Psychosom Med 1993; 55:37–43.
41. Gorkin L, Schron EB, Brooks MM, et al. Psychosocial predictors of mortality in the cardiac arrhythmia suppression trial-1 (CAST-1). Am J Cardiol 1993; 71:263–267.

42. Berkman LF, Leo-Summers L, Horwitz RI. Emotional support and survival after myocardial infarction. Ann Int Med 1992; 117:1003–1009.

43. Williams RB, Barefoot JC, Califf RM, et al. Prognostic importance of social and economicresources among medically treated patients with angiographically documented coronary artery disease. JAMA 1992; 267:520–524.

44. Rosanski A, Blumenthal JA, Kaplan J. Impact of psychological factors on the pathogenesis of cardiovascular disease and implications for therapy. Circulation 1999; 99:2192–2217.

45. Siegler IC, Peterson BL, Barefoot JC. Hostility during late adolescence predicts coronary risk factors at mid-life. Am J Epidemiol 1992; 136:146–154.

46. Anda RF, Williamson DF, Escobdedo LG, et al. Depression and the dynamics of smoking. JAMA 1990; 264:1541–1546.

47. Kaplan JR, Manuck SB, Clarkson TB, Lusso FM, Taub DM. Social status, environment, and atherosclerosis in cynomolgus monkeys. Arteriosclerosis 1982; 2:359–368.

48. Shively CA, Clarkson TB, Kaplan JR. Social deprivation and coronary artery atherosclerosis in female cynomolgus monkeys. Atherosclerosis 1989; 77:69–76.

49. Williams RB, Barefoot JC, Haney TL, et al. Type A behavior and angiographically documented coronary atherosclerosis in a sample of 2289 patietns. Psychosom Med 1988; 50:139–152.

50. Julkunen J, Salonen R, Kaplan GA, et al. Hostility and the progression of carotid atherosclerosis. Psychosom Med 1994; 56:519–525.

51. Everson S, Kaplan G, Goldberg D, Salonen R, Salonen J. Hopelessness and the 4-year progression of carotid atherosclerosis. The Kuopio Heart Disease Risk Factor Study. Arterioscler Thromb Vasc Biol 1997; 17:1490–1495.

52. Lynch J, Krause N, Kaplan GA, Salonen R, Salonen JT. Workplace demands, economic reward, and progression of carotid atherosclerosis. Circulation 1997; 96:302–307.

53. Davies MJ. A macro and micro view of coronary vascular insult in ischemic heart disease. Circulation 1990; 82:II38–II46.

54. Furchgott RF, Zawadski D. The obligatory role of endothelial cells in the relaxation of arterial smooth muscle by acetylcholine. Nature 1980; 288:373–378.

55. Maseri A, L'Abbate A, Baroldi G, et al. Coronary vasospasm as a possible cause of myocardial infarction. A conclusion derived from the study of preinfarction angina. N Engl J Med 1978; 99:1271–1277.

56. Maseri A. Coronary vasoconstriction: visible and invisible (editorial). N Engl J Med 1991; 325:1579–1580.

57. Williams JK, Vita JA, Manuck SB, Selwyn AP, Kaplan JR. Psychosocial factors impair vascular responses of coronary arteries. Circulation 1991; 84:2146–2153.

58. Williams JK, Shively CA, Clarkson TB. Determinants of coronary artery eactivity in premenopausal female cynomolgus monkeys with diet-induced atherosclerosis. Circulation 1994; 90:983–987.

59. Boltwood MD, Taylor CB, Burke MD, et al. Anger report predicts coronary artery vasomotor response to mental stress in atherosclerotic segments. Am J Cardiol 1993; 72:1361–1365.

60. Helmers KF, Krantz DS, Bairey Merz CN, et al. Defensive hostility: relationships to multiple markers of cardiac ischemia is patients with coronary disease. Health Psych 1995; 14:202–209.
61. Kamarck TW, Jennings JR, Manuck SB, et al. Cardiovascular reactivity is associated with carotid artery atherosclerosis in Finnish men. Ann Behav Med 1997; 19:S073.
62. Glasser SP, Selwyn AP, Ganz P. Atherosclerosis: risk factors and the vascular endothelium. Am Heart J 1996; 131:379–384.
63. Rozanski AR, Bairey CN, Krantz DS, et al. Mental stress and silent myocardial ischemia in coronary artery disease patients. N Engl J Med 1988; 318:1005–1012.
64. Krantz DS, Helmers KF, Bairey CN, Nebel LE, Hedges SM, Rozanski A. Psychophysiologic reactivity and determinants of myocardial oxygen demand in mental stress induced myocardial ischemia. Psychosomatic Med 1990; 53:1–12.
65. Yeung A, Vekshtein VI, Krantz DS, et al. The effect of atherosclerosis on the vasomotor response of coronary arteries to mental stress. N Engl J Med 1991; 325:1551–1556.
66. Gabbay FH, Krantz DS, Kop WJ, et al. Triggers of myocardial ischemia during daily life in patients with coronary artery disease: physical and mental activities, anger and smoking. J Am Coll Cardiol 1996; 27:585–592.
67. Stone PH, Krantz DS, McMahon RP, et al. Relationship among mental stress-induced ischemia and ischemia during daily life and during exercise: the Psychophysiologic Investigations of Myocardial Ischemia (PIMI) Study. J Am Coll Cardiol 1999; 33:1476–1484.
68. Helmers KF, Krantz DS, Howell RH, Klein J, Bairey CN, Rozanski A. Hostility and myocardial ischemia in coronary artery disease patients: evaluation by gender and ischemic index. Psychosom Med 1993; 55:29–36.
69. Constantinides P. Plaque hemorrhages, their genesis and their role in supraplaque thrombosis and atherogenesis. In: Glagov S, Newman WP, Schaffer SA, eds. Pathobiology of the Human Atherosclerotic Plaque. New York: Springer-Verlag, 1990:393–411.
70. Bairey CN, Krantz DS, Rozanski A. Mental stress as an acute trigger of left ventricular dysfunction and blood pressure elevation in coronary patients. Am J Card 1991; 66:28G–31G.
71. Muller JE, Stone PH, Turi SZ, et al. Circadian variation in the frequency of onset of acute myocardial infarction. N Engl J Med 1985; 313:1315–1322.
72. Mittleman MA, Maclure M, Sherwood JB, et al. Triggering of acute myocardial infarction onset by episodes of anger. Circulation 1995; 92:1720–1725.
73. Shechter M, Bairey Merz CN, Paul-Labrador M, Shah PK, Kaul S. Plasma apolipoprotein B levels predict platelet-dependent thrombosis in patients with coronary artery disease. Cardiology 1999; 92:151–155.
74. Shechter M, Bairey Merz CN, Paul-Labrador M, Kaul S. Blood glucose and platelet-dependent thrombosis in coronary artery disease patients. J Am Coll Cardiol 2000; 35:300–307.
75. Ockene JK, Kuller LH, Svendsen KH, Meilahn E. The relationship of smoking cessation to coronary heart disease and lung cancer in the Multiple Risk Factor Intervention Trial (MRFIT). Am J Public Health 1990; 80:954–958.

76. Markovitz JH, Matthews KA, Kiss J, Smitherman TC. Effects of hostility on platelet reactivity to psychological stress in coronary heart disease patients and in healthy controls. Psychosom Med 1996; 58:143–149.

77. Schonwetter DF, Dion PR, Ready AE, Dyck DG, Gerrard JM. The interactive effect of type a behavior and hostility on bleeding time thromboxane and prostacyclin formation. J Psychosom Res 1991; 35:645–650.

78. Levine SP, Towell BL, Surarez AM, Knieriem LK, Harris MM, George JN. Platelet activation and secretion associated with emotional stress. Circulation 1985; 71:1129–1134.

79. Verrier RL. Mechanisms of behaviorally induced arrhythmias. Circulation 1987; 76:148–156.

80. Akselrod S, Gordon D, Ubel FA, et al. Power spectral analysis of heart rate fluctuation: a quantitative probe of beat-to-beat cardiovascular control. Science 1981; 213:220–222.

81. La Rovere MT, Specchia G, Mortara A, et al. Baroreflex sensitivity, clinical correlates, and cardiovascular mortality among patients with a first myocardial infarction: a prospective study. Circulation 1988; 78:816–824.

82. Sloan RP, Korten JB, Myers MM. Components of heart rate reactivity during mental arithmetic with and without speaking. Physiol Behav 1991; 50:1039–1045.

83. Pardo J, Bairey Merz CN, Paul-Labrador M, et al. Reproducibility and stability of 24 hour heart rate variability variability in coronary artery disease patients with daily life ischemia. Am J Cardiol 1996; 78:866–870.

84. Kawachi I, Sparrow D, Vokonas PS, Weiss ST. Decreased heart rate variability in men with phobic anxiety (data from the Normative Aging Study). Am J Cardiol 1995; 75:882–885.

85. La Rovere MT, Bigger JT, Marcus FI, et al. Baroreflex sensitivity and heart-rate variability in prediction of total cardiac mortality after myocardial infarction. Lancet 1998;478–484.

86. Tsuji H, Larson MG, Venditti FJ, et al. Impact of reduced heart rate variability on risk for cardiac events: the Framingham Heart Study. Circulation 1996; 94:2850–2855.

87. Ross R. The pathogenesis of atherosclerosis: a perspective for the 1990s. Nature 1993; 70:801–809.

88. Kop WJ, Cohen N. Immune system involvement in cardiovascular disease. In: Ader R, Felten DL, Cohen N, eds. Psychoneuroimmunology. 3rd ed. San Diego: Academic Press, (in press).

89. Mills PJ, Ziegler MG, Rehman J, Maisel AS. Catecholamines, catecholamine receptors, cell adhesion molecules, and acute stressorrelated changes in cellular immunity. Adv Pharmacol 1998; 42:587–590.

90. Caldwell CL, Irwin M, Lohr J. Reduced natural killer cell cytotoxicity in depression but not in schizophrenia. Biol Psychiatry 1991; 30:1131–1138.

91. Maes M. Evidence for an immune response in major depression: a review and hypothesis. Prog Neuropsychopharmacol Biol Psychiatry 1995; 19:11–38.

92. Zakowski SG, McAllister CG, Deal M, Baum A. Stress, reactivity, and immune function in healthy men. Health Psychol 1992; 11:223–232.

93. Ibrahim MA, Feldman JG, Sultz HA, Staiman MG, Young LJ, Dean D. Management after myocardial infarction: a controlled trial of the effect of group psychotherapy. Int J Psychiatry Med 1974; 5:253–268.

94. Rahe RM, Ward HW, Hayes V. Brief group therapy in myocardial infarction rehabilitation: three to four year follow-up of a controlled trial. Psychosom Med 1979; 41:224–229.
95. Frasure-Smith N, Prince R. The ischemic heart disease life stress monitoring program: impact on mortality. Psychosom Med 1985; 47:431–445.
96. Fielding R. A note on behavioral treatment in the rehabilitation of myocardial infarction patients. Br J Soc Clin Psychol 1980; 19:157–161.
97. Adsett CA, Bruhn JG. Short-term group psychotherapy for post-myocardial patients and their wives. Can Med Assoc J 1968; 99:577.
98. Salonea JT, Pusha P. A community for rehabilitation and secondary revention for patients with acute myocardial infarction as part of a comprehensive community programme for control of cardiovascular diseases (North Karelia Project). Scand J Rehabil Med 1980; 12:33–41.
99. Gruen W. Effects of brief psychotherapy during the hospitalization period on the recovery process in heart attacks. J Consult Clin Psychol 1975; 43:223–232.
100. Ornish D, Scherwitz LW, Doody RS, et al. Effects of stress management training and dietary changes in treating heart disease. JAMA 1983; 249:54–59.
101. Friedman M, Thoresen CE, Gill JJ, et al. Alteration of type a behavior and reduction in cardiac recurrences in postmyocardial infarction patients. Am Heart J 1984; 108:237–248.
102. Langosch W, Seer P, Brodner G, Kalinke D, Kulick B, Heim F. Behavior therapy with coronary heart disease patients: results of a comparative study. J Psychosom Res 1982; 26:475–484.
103. Jenni MA, Wollersheim JP. Cognitive therapy, stress management training, and the Type A behavior pattern. Cogn Ther Res 1979; 3:61–73.
104. Wallace N, Wallace DC. Group education after myocardial infarction: is it effective? Med J Aust 1977; 20:245–247.
105. Stern MJ, Gorman PA, Kaslow L. The group counselling vs. exercise therapy study: a controlled intervention with subjects following myocardial infarction. Arch Intern Med 1983; 143:1719–1725.
106. Jones DA, West RR. Psychological rehabilitation after myocardial infarction: multicentre randomized controlled trial. Brit Med J 1996; 313:1517–1521.
107. Tulpule TH, Tulpule AT. Yoga, a method of relaxation for rehabilitation after myocardial infarction. Indian Heart J 1980; 32:1–7.
108. Burgess AW, Lerner DJ, D'Agostino RB, Vokonas PS, Hartman CR, Gaccione P. A randomized control trial of cardiac rehabilitation. Soc Sci Med 1987; 24:359–370.
109. Blumenthal JA, Jiang W, Babyak MA, et al. Stress management with exercise training in cardiac patients with myocardial ischemia: effects on prognosis and evaluation of mechanisms. Arch Intern Med 1997; 157:2213–2223.
110. Guzetta CE. Effects of relaxation and music therapy on patients in a coronary care unit with presumptive acute myocardial infarction. Heart Lung 1989; 18:609–616.
111. Horlick L, Cameron R, firor W, Bhalerao U, Baltzan R. The effects of education and group discussion in the postmyocardial infarction patient. J Psychosom Res 1984; 28:485–492.
112. Thompson DR, Meddis R. A prospective evaluation of in-hospital counselling for first-time myocardial infarction men. J Psychosom Res 1990; 34:237–248.

113. Van Dixhoorn J, Duivenvoorden HJ, Staal HA, Pool J, Verhage F. Cardiac events after myocardial infarction: possible effects of relaxation therapy. Eur Heart J 1987; 8:1210–1214.
114. Rahe RH, O'Neill T, Hagan A, Arthur RJ. Brief group therapy following myocardial infarction: eighteen-month follow-up of a controlled trial. Int J Psychiatry Med 1975; 6:349–358.
115. Nunes EV, Frank KA, Kornfeld DS. Psychologic treatment for type a behavior pattern and for coronary artery disease: a meta-analysis of the literature. Psychom Med 1987; 49:159–173.
116. Linden W, Stossel C, Maurice J. Psychosocial interventions for patients with coronary artery disease: a meta-analysis. Arch Intern Med 1996; 156:745–752.
117. Bairey Merz CN, Subramanian R. Efficacy of psychosocial interventions and stress management for reduction of coronary artery disease events. Prev Cardiol 1999; 1:1–6.
118. Frasure-Smith N, Prince R. Long-term follow-up of the ischemic heart disease life stress monitoring program. Psychosom Med 1984; 51:485–513.
119. Frasure-Smith N, Lesperance F, Prince RH, et al. Randomized trial of home-based psychosocial nursing intervention for patients recovering from myocardial infarction. Lancet 1997; 350:473–479. arney RM, Rich MW, Tevelde A, Saini J, Clark K, Jaffe AS. Major depressive disorder in coronary artery disease. Am J Cardiol 1987; 60:1273–1275.
120. Randomized trial of cholesterol lowering in 4444 patients with coronary heart disease: the Scandanavian Simvastatin Survival Study (4S). Lancet 1994; 344:1383–1389.
121. Antiplatelet Trialist's Collaboration. Secondary prevention of vascular disease by prolonged antiplatelet treatment. BMJ 1983; 296:320–331.
122. The Beta-Blocker Pooling Project Research Group. The Beta-Blockers Pooling Project (BBPP): subgroup findings from randomized trials in post infarction patients. Eur Heart J 1988; 9:8–16.
123. Yusuf S, Zucker D, Peduzzi P, et al. Effect of coronary artery bypass graft surgery on survival: overview of 10-year results from randomised trials by the Coronary Artery Bypass Graft Surgery Trialists Collaboration. Lancet 1994; 334:563–570.

8

Genetic Risk Assessment Strategies for Coronary Artery Disease

Maren T. Scheuner

*UCLA School of Public Health, Department of Health Services,
RAND Corporation, Santa Monica, California, U.S.A.*

INTRODUCTION

Coronary artery disease (CAD) remains the leading cause of death and premature disability in the United States and other industrialized countries (1). Individuals with genetic predisposition to atherosclerosis have substantial risk for developing CAD, especially at early ages (2). As a result, they may have the most to gain from preventive interventions (3). This chapter will review the role of genetics in the development and progression of CAD, the available genetic risk assessment strategies for CAD, and clinical application of genetic risk information for CAD prevention including recommendations for risk factor modification and early detection, and the role of genetic counseling and education.

ROLE OF GENETICS IN DEVELOPMENT AND PROGRESSION OF CAD

The accumulation of atherosclerotic plaque in an artery wall is a chronic disease that begins early in life (4). This process appears to be initiated and/or facilitated by chronic injury to the endothelium (5). Plaques may become symptomatic when they are large enough to restrict blood flow leading to tissue ischemia. Acute coronary syndromes such as unstable angina, myocardial infarction (MI), and sudden death occur when thrombus forms on a thrombogenic plaque or when unstable plaques rupture or ulcerate, leading to thrombus formation and possible vessel occlusion (6,7).

CAD is a complex disorder due to many risk factors. Multiple biochemical processes are involved, including lipid and apolipoprotein metabolism, inflammatory response, endothelial function, platelet function, thrombosis, fibrinolysis, homocysteine metabolism, insulin sensitivity, and blood pressure regulation (2). Each of the biochemical processes associated with CAD is comprised of enzymes, receptors, and ligands, which are encoded by our genes. Variations in these genes can alter the function of the constituents within a metabolic pathway. These genetic variations interact with each other and with non-genetic factors, resulting in variable susceptibility to the development and progression of atherosclerosis and thrombosis (2). Non-genetic risk factors for CAD include exposures, such as tobacco smoke, and behaviors (e.g., exercise, and dietary patterns), many of which may be culturally determined. Like genetic factors, environmental and behavioral risk factors often aggregate in families.

Dozens of candidate genes have been associated with CAD or MI (8), although some associations have conflicting results [e.g., angiotensin converting enzyme, methylenetetrahydrofolate reductase (MTHFR), platelet glycoprotein receptor IIIa, and factor VII] (9–18). The variable results may be due to chance, to errors in estimating the frequency of polymorphisms in the case or control group, to not matching the race/ethnicity of cases and controls, or to studying related but distinct phenotypes such as the presence of atherosclerosis versus the occurrence of MI. Investigations utilizing genome scan approaches have found novel genetic loci associated with CAD, which might provide additional insight to genetic factors contributing to atherosclerosis and coronary events (19–23). There are also numerous studies that have found genetic associations or linkage with related disorders such as hypertension (24–29), obesity (30–38) diabetes (39–49), lipids (50–53), and oxidative stress (54).

GENETIC RISK ASSESSMENT STRATEGIES TO ASSESS CAD AND MI SUSCEPTIBILITY

CAD is a complex disorder. This generally means that the manifestations of CAD arise from the interaction of several predisposing genetic and/or environmental factors (Fig. 1). Therefore, global risk assessment has been recognized as an effective approach in preventing CAD and its manifestations (55). Through global risk assessment a more accurate estimation of absolute risk can be determined based on the summation of risks contributed by each risk factor. Subsequently, the intensity of managing modifiable risk factors can be adjusted by the severity of the overall risk.

Most people will be served well by existing global risk assessment methods and prevention guidelines. However, genetic susceptibility to CAD is not adequately addressed by these methods, and underestimation of risk and missed opportunities for prevention can result for people who are genetically

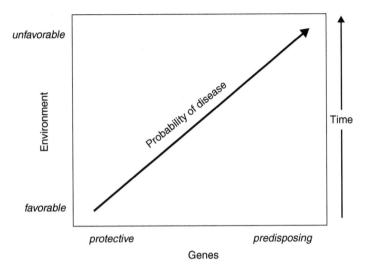

Figure 1 Characteristics of genetic susceptibility to coronary artery disease. Consultation for genetic risk assessment and specialized risk reduction should be considered for individuals with at least one of the above characteristics. CAD, coronary artery disease; close relative, first and/or second degree relative from the same lineage.

predisposed to CAD. The Framingham Risk Score is a widely used risk assessment method for prediction of CAD risk (56). It considers the established risk factors of gender, age, smoking, total cholesterol, LDL cholesterol, HDL cholesterol, and diabetes, but not family history of CAD or related disorders. The National Cholesterol Education Program Expert Panel (57) provides algorithms for treatment of lipid disorders in adults. The established risk factors of hypertension, diabetes, smoking, gender, age, and minimal family history information (parental history of MI before age 55) are used to determine risk and recommend lipid-lowering treatment. However, the risk associated with additional family history of CAD or related disorders is not included.

Family History Collection and Interpretation

The systematic collection and interpretation of family history information is currently the most appropriate screening approach to identify individuals with genetic susceptibility to CAD and MI. Family history of CAD and related conditions reflect the interactions of genetic, environmental, cultural, and behavioral risk factors shared among family members.

Family history of CAD is a significant risk factor for CAD. On average, there is a 2 to 3-fold increase in risk for CAD in first-degree relatives of affected individuals (58–62). Having two or more first-degree relatives with CAD is associated with a 3 to 6-fold increase in risk (63,64). The earlier the age of onset the greater is the risk of CAD to relatives (63–66). In addition, the risk of disease is typically greater in relatives of female cases compared to male cases, suggesting greater genetic burden in female cases (61,66–68).

Much of the familial aggregation of CAD might be explained by the familial aggregation of established risk factors such as elevated LDL cholesterol, low HDL cholesterol, and diabetes (66). In a recent analysis of the Third National Health and Nutrition Survey, adults with a parental history of CAD were more likely to have multiple risk factors (OR for four or five risk factors compared with none was 2.9, 95% CI, 1.4–6.3) (66). Yet even after adjusting for these established risk factors, family history remains a significant independent risk factor for CAD (65,66,68–75). An explanation for this remaining risk may be familial aggregation of emerging CAD risk factors including hyperhomocysteinemia (76), C-reactive protein (CRP) (77), elevated fibrin D-dimer, tissue plasminogen activator, fibrinogen (78), and insulin resistance (79). In addition, the interactions of the genetic, environmental, cultural, and behavioral risk factors shared by family members may be too complex to assess with usual statistical methods.

The estimated accuracy and prevalence of a family history of CAD and related disorders are high enough to justify using family history for risk stratification and targeting screening and prevention to the level of familial risk. Several studies have shown that family history reports of CAD in first-degree relatives are generally accurate with sensitivity estimates from 67% to 85% (63,80,81). The relatively high sensitivity values indicate that family history can be used with some confidence to stratify risk above average. The specificity estimates for family history reports are more than 90% (63,80,81), indicating a lack of over-reporting disease in relatives. Similar sensitivity and specificity estimates are seen for diabetes and hypertension (81). Prevalence rates of a positive family history of CAD are substantial, with estimates ranging from 14% among high school students (82) to 29% among healthy adults in their mid-thirties (11% having high familial risk and 18% having an intermediate familial risk) (83).

Individuals with familial risk for CAD can be identified by asking targeted family history questions, including the number of relatives affected with CAD, their age at diagnosis, gender, degree of relationship to each other and the patient, and the presence of other conditions in the family such as stroke, hypertension, lipid abnormalities, and diabetes (83). With this information, stratification into different familial risk groups is possible, which can inform prevention activities (Fig. 2) (83). Pedigree analysis, which involves collection and interpretation of more comprehensive family medical history, is performed in the setting of a genetic evaluation for individuals with high familial risk of CAD or for those who may have Mendelian forms of cardiovascular disease.

Biochemical Testing to Assess CAD and MI Susceptibility

Tests to assess genetic risk for CAD are primarily biochemical analyses that measure the different pathways involved in development and progression of

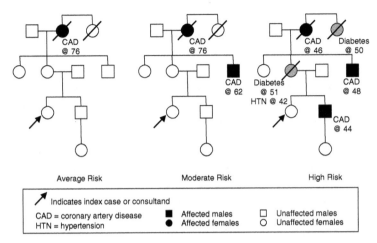

Figure 2 Examples of risk stratification with pedigree analysis. Average risk is associated with environmental risk factors with a small contribution of susceptibility genes. Moderate risk is most likely due to several susceptibility genes of small effect interacting with environmental risk factors. High risk is associated with many susceptibility alleles of small effect interacting with environmental risk factors, or rarely, single gene disorders associated with high risk.

coronary atherosclerosis. Several of these identify established risk factors, such as increased LDL cholesterol, decreased HDL cholesterol, and diabetes, which are known to be causally related to CAD (55). Many others are considered emerging risk factors that are strongly associated with CAD (84–93), but for most, a causal relationship with CAD has not been determined. Examples of emerging risk factors for CAD include small dense LDL particles, hyperhomocysteinemia, CRP, interleukin-6, and factors involved in fibrinolysis such as plasminogen activating factor inhibitor-1 and fibrinogen. Although treatment strategies exist for many emerging risk factors (see below), treatment for most of them has not so far been associated with primary prevention of CAD events. Nonetheless, measuring these risk factors can result in more accurate risk stratification. Currently, recognizing a higher level of CAD risk because of emerging risk factors allows patients and clinicians the opportunity to intensify the treatments that have been proven effective for CAD prevention.

Hyperhomocysteinemia

Extreme elevations in plasma homocysteine (>200 µmol/L), owing to deficiency of cystathione beta synthase or other key enzymes involved in homocysteine metabolism, cause premature cardiovascular disease. More modest elevations of homocysteine (>10 to 15 µmol/L) are associated with increased risk for cardiovascular disease (93). Homocysteine may increase the risk for cardiovascular disease by decreasing endothelium-dependent vasodilation, increasing platelet adhesiveness, activating certain clotting factors, and inhibiting fibrinolysis by promoting lipoprotein(a) binding to fibrin (94). Homocysteine levels are increased by deficiency of the B vitamins that are cofactors for enzymes involved in homocysteine metabolism, including folic acid and vitamins B6 and B12. Homocysteine also increases with declining renal function, pernicious anemia, thyroid dysfunction, psoriasis, certain malignancies, anticonvulsant therapies, certain oral contraceptives, methotrexate, niacin, fibrates, and metformin (95,96). Homocysteine levels can often be lowered to a desirable range with folic acid and vitamins B6 and B12 (97–99). Lowering homocysteine with B vitamins has been shown to decrease the incidence of major cardiovascular events in a double-blind placebo-controlled trial in 533 subjects with coronary stenosis (100). However, another trial comparing high versus low-dose B vitamins in 3680 patients with ischemic stroke (101), and a controlled trial of folate alone for patients with CAD (102) showed no effect of vitamin supplementation on subsequent coronary events or stroke, even though baseline homocysteine levels were associated with increased risk in these prospective studies. The preventive effect of vitamins *before* development of symptomatic atherosclerosis is unknown.

Lipoprotein(a)

Lipoprotein(a) is a lipoprotein particle composed of an apolipoprotein B-100 particle covalently linked to an apolipoprotein(a) particle. Apolipoprotein(a) is homologous to plasminogen and may compete with plasminogen, thereby limiting fibrinolysis (103). Lipoprotein(a) has also been implicated in foam cell formation, endothelium-dependent vasodilation reduction, and LDL cholesterol oxidation promotion (104). Levels of lipoprotein(a) are strongly genetically determined (105,106). Lipoprotein(a) increases slightly with age and at the time of acute illness; also, females have greater values than males, with values increasing after menopause (107). The distribution of levels varies widely among racial and ethnic groups (107). Most of the associations with CAD have been found in Caucasians. Levels >20 to 30 mg/dL are considered high. Lipoprotein(a) levels can be reduced with niacin (108). Diet and exercise have no effect on lipoprotein(a) levels (109,110). In post-menopausal women, estrogen replacement therapy can lower levels (111), and in men, testosterone can lower levels (112). Reduction in lipoprotein(a) attributed to estrogen has been associated with a reduction in cardiovascular events in women (113). However, hormone replacement therapy with either estrogen for women or testosterone for men is not the standard of care for reducing CAD risk. Aggressive LDL cholesterol lowering appears to abolish the CAD risk associated with elevated lipoprotein(a), even with unchanged lipoprotein(a) levels (114). Thus this should be the treatment goal for high-risk individuals with elevated lipoprotein(a).

Atherogenic Lipoprotein Phenotype

Atherogenic, small, dense LDL cholesterol particles, reduced fraction of HDL2b, low HDL cholesterol, elevated triglycerides, and excess apolipoprotein B are characteristic of the atherogenic lipoprotein phenotype (ALP). ALP occurs in up to 25% of middle-aged men (115) and is associated with a 3-fold increase in CAD risk (116,117). ALP can be improved with regular exercise, loss of body fat, restricted intake of simple carbohydrates and alcohol (118), medical therapy including niacin and fibrates (119,120), and avoidance of β-blockers if possible (121). Fish oil supplementation also improves the lipid profile associated with ALP (122). Modifying ALP with the above measures, particularly niacin alone or in combination with other lipid-lowering therapy, has resulted in regression or prevention of progression of coronary atherosclerotic lesions, and reduced coronary risk (123).

Insulin Resistance

Insulin resistance is associated with many traditional and emerging risk factors (hypertension, hypertriglyceridemia, small LDL cholesterol particles, decreased HDL cholesterol, elevated PAI-1, fibrinogen, and CRP). It can be considered a risk factor predisposing to CAD (55). An estimated 24% of adults in the United States have the metabolic syndrome associated with insulin resistance (124). The third report of the National Cholesterol Education Program Expert Panel on Detection, Evaluation, and Treatment of High Blood Cholesterol in Adults (ATPIII) (57) highlights the importance of treating patients with the metabolic syndrome to prevent cardiovascular disease. Insulin resistance can be effectively treated with lifestyle changes and metformin (125).

C-Reactive Protein

Many studies have shown a strong association between CRP and future cardiovascular events (126,127). Measurement of high sensitivity CRP is a useful clinical marker of inflammation related to atherosclerosis (127). Statin drugs used for cholesterol lowering have been associated with reduction in high sensitivity CRP (128). This may be due in part to the anti-inflammatory effects of these drugs. A recent report has shown that HRT increases CRP levels (92), suggesting a possible mechanism for increased CAD risk due to HRT. Thus, high sensitivy CRP (hs-CRP) could become a target of therapy for reducing CAD risk. However, at this time, measurement of hs-CRP is used primarily to stratify risk and guide recommendations for modification of other risk factors.

Thrombophilia

Several factors involved in promotion of thrombosis and inhibition of fibrinolysis are associated with CAD. Among this group of CAD risk factors, fibrinogen is one of the most important. Fibrinogen levels are modifiable through smoking cessation, aerobic exercise, weight loss, fibric acid medications, and omega-3 fish oils (129,130). Antiplatelet medications such as aspirin and other forms of anticoagulants might also reduce the thrombotic risk associated with elevated fibrinogen.

DNA-Based Testing to Assess Susceptibility to CAD and MI

There are over 30 Mendelian disorders (single gene disorders) that feature CAD or MI (Table 1) (131,132). Genetic tests for many of these Mendelian disorders are available and include DNA-based tests and biochemical analyses (131). These conditions are generally associated with a substantial risk for CAD and MI at young ages. For most of these Mendelian disorders, personal and family history characteristics are crucial for identifying individuals at risk. Specifically, early-onset CAD is usually present in multiple family members, and family members may have associated conditions such as stroke, diabetes, thrombophilia, or cholesterol abnormalities. Thus, collection and interpretation of family medical history is central to providing access to genetic testing services that are available for diagnosis of Mendelian forms of CAD and MI.

Despite the success of identifying susceptibility genes for multifactorial, non-Mendelian forms of CAD and associated conditions, the risk associated with any one of these gene variants is generally of small magnitude and by itself has little clinical significance (133). Before testing for low-risk susceptibility genes has widespread clinical application, additional studies are needed to assess the prevalence and penetrance of these genotypes, as well as the effect of other genes and environmental factors on their expression. Furthermore, the clinical utility of DNA-based testing for CAD susceptibility compared to other risk assessment strategies, including familial risk assessment and assessment of biochemical risk factors, must be proven. Nonetheless, testing for many CAD susceptibility genotypes is available. Examples below describe the potential benefit and limitations of DNA-based testing for CAD susceptibility in the clinical setting.

Cholesterol Ester Transfer Protein

Kuivenhoven and co-workers (134) found a significant association between variation at the cholesterol ester transfer protein (CETP) locus and angiographic progression of coronary atherosclerosis in men with CAD. Furthermore, there was a dose-dependent relation between one specific CETP gene polymorphism (TaqIB) and the efficacy of pravastatin in slowing the progression of atherosclerosis. Although this CETP association with CAD progression was significant, the finding has limited clinical utility. Although individuals with the B1B1 genotype derived the greatest benefit, treatment with pravastatin improved the outcome for all study subjects, abolishing any differences based on CETP genotype.

Table 1 Mendelian Disorders Featuring Coronary Artery Disease and Myocardial Infarction

Disorder	Mode of inheritance	OMIM entry
Abdominal obesity-metabolic syndrome	MF	605552
Apolipoprotein(a) polymorphism/ LPA excess	AD	152200.0001
Apolipoprotein A-I deficiency	AD, AR	107680.0011
		107680.0012
		107680.0013
		107680.0015
		107680.0017
		107680.0022
Atherosclerosis susceptibility/ atherogenic lipoprotein phenotype (ALP)	AD, MF	108725
Coronary artery dissection, spontaneous	AD	122455
Cerebrotendinous xanthomatosis	AR	213700
Fabry disease	XLR	301500
Familial combined hyperlipidemia	AD, MF	144250
Familial defective apo B	AD	144010
Familial hypercholesterolemia	AD	143890
Familial hypercholesterolemia, autosomal recessive	AR	603813
Familial partial lipodystrophy	AD	151660
Familial pseudohyperkalemia due to red cell leak	AD, AR	177720
Fibromuscular dysplasia of arteries	AD	135580
Heparin cofactor II deficiency	AD	142360
Homocystienemia	AD, MF	603174
Homocystinuria	AR	236200
Homocysteinemia/homocystinuria due to $N(5,10)$-methylenetetrahydrofolate reductase deficiency	AR	236250
Hyperlipoproteinemia, type III	AR with pseudo- dominance	107741
Methylcobalmin deficiency, cbl G type	AR	250940
Niemann-Pick disease, type E	AR	257200
Progeria	AD	176670
Protein C deficiency	AD	176860
Pseudoxanthoma elasticum	AR	264800
Pseudoxanthoma elasticum, autosomal dominant	AD	177850
Sitosterolemia	AR	210250

(Continued)

Table 1 Mendelian Disorders Featuring Coronary Artery Disease and Myocardial Infarction (*Continued*)

Disorder	Mode of inheritance	OMIM entry
Spontaneous coronary dissection	AD	122455
Tangier disease	AR	205400
Vitamin B12 metabolic defect, type 2	AR	277410
Vitamin B12 metabolic defect with methylmalonic acidemia and homocystinuria	AR	277400
Werner syndrome	AR	277700
Williams syndrome	AD	194050

Abbreviations: OMIM, On-line Mendelian Inheritance in Man (131), a periodically-updated reference to inherited disorders associated with alterations in single genes; AD, autosomal dominant; AR, autosomal recessive; MF, multifactorial; XLR, X-linked recessive.
Source: From Ref. 8.

Apo E

The ApoE4 allele has been associated with CAD in several populations (135–137). ApoE2/E2 homozygous individuals are at risk for type III hyperlipoproteinemia, which is associated with an increased risk for atherosclerosis. In addition, apoE genotyping could come to play a role in recommending lipid-lowering diets (122,138–141). Forty percent of the individual variation in response of LDL cholesterol levels to a low-saturated fat diet is familial (142). This might be due in part to the apoE locus. Several studies have shown that carriers of the apoE4 allele tend to be more responsive to the LDL-lowering effects of low-fat dietary interventions compared to non-carriers (138–141). Carriers of the apoE2 allele may be particularly susceptible to unfavorable changes in lipids and to coronary heart disease when they are exposed to diets high in saturated fat (141).

The apoE genotype influences the responsiveness to fish oil supplementation in subjects with an ALP (122). Individuals with an apoE2 allele displayed favorable changes when given fish oil, including a marked reduction in the postprandial rise in triglycerides and a trend toward increased lipoprotein lipase activity compared to non-E2 carriers (143). ApoE4 carriers had an unfavorable response compared to E3/E3 homozygotes with a significant increase in total cholesterol and a trend toward a reduction in HDL cholesterol (122).

Despite these important associations relating response to diet and the apoE genotype, clinicians must proceed with caution when considering this particular genetic test as a means to assess CAD risk. The apoE4 genotype is also associated with increased risk for Alzheimer disease (144). The American College of

Medical Genetics (ACMG) and the American Society of Human Genetics (ASHG) have not endorsed apoE testing for diagnosis or prediction of Alzheimer's disease (145). Therefore, patients should be informed of the association of apoE genotype with Alzheimer's disease if considering apoE genotyping for cardiovascular risk assessment.

Methylenetetrahydrofolate Reductase

Homozygosity for the MTHFR C677T mutation has been associated with elevated levels of homocysteine (146); homocysteine levels are associated with CAD risk (93). A recent meta-analysis of case-control studies demonstrated a significantly higher risk of CAD associated with the MTHFR C677T genotype, especially in the setting of low folate status (147). The ASHG/ACMG statement regarding measurement and use of total plasma homocysteine recommends that the basis for elevated homocysteine levels (greater than 15 μM) be determined before treatment, because inappropriate supplementation of folate, Vitamin B12, and pyridoxine has some possibility of causing harm (148).

Prothrombin G20210A

In a study of postmenopausal women, risk of MI was significantly increased (OR = 10.9, 95% CI, 2.15–55.2) in those with the prothrombin G20210A mutation who also had hypertension and were taking hormone replacement therapy (HRT) (149). Women with the prothrombin mutation had only a mildly increased risk of MI if they did not use HRT. Those without the prothrombin G20210A mutation were not at substantially increased risk for MI even if they used HRT. These findings suggest a potential benefit of prothrombin G20210A mutation testing in women at high risk for MI who are considering use of HRT. However, decision-making regarding HRT use is complex and it is uncertain how much value such testing would add in the clinical setting.

Platelet Glycoprotein Ia/IIa Receptor

Smoking is a significant risk factor for CAD and MI. However, individuals with specific genotypes have greater risks for MI associated with smoking. One example is the Gln-Arg192 polymorphism of the human paraoxonase gene (150). Another is the 807T allele of the platelet glycoprotein Ia/IIa receptor (151). Homozygosity for the platelet glycoprotein Ia/IIa receptor 807T by itself is associated with about a 3-fold increase in risk for MI, smoking alone with a 4-fold increase in risk (151). These two risk factors interact with a greater than multiplicative effect, yielding an odds ratio of 25 for MI among individuals who were homozygous for the 807T allele and also smoked (151). Although knowledge of increased risk due to high-risk alleles might be expected to improve smoking cessation efforts, this has not been demonstrated. Furthermore, the absence of these risk alleles does not allow one to smoke with impunity, since smoking very likely increases risk for MI through other mechanisms and it is associated with other hazardous health effects.

Platelet Glycoprotein IIIa Receptor

Several studies have identified a strong association between the platelet glycoprotein receptor IIIa (GPIIIa) A2 allele and extensive CAD or occurrence of coronary thrombosis (12–14). However, other studies have failed to demonstrate an association with CAD or MI (15–17). Cooke and colleagues (18) argue that differences in aspirin use might account for some of the discrepancies in studies investigating this polymorphism, because aspirin has been shown to inhibit the increased platelet aggregation observed with this polymorphism. Aspirin very likely has other beneficial effects in the prevention of CAD and acute coronary syndromes. Its use is recommended for both primary and secondary prevention of CAD (152). Thus, the clinical utility of genotyping GPIIIa would be limited since it seems unlikely that this test alone will distinguish who will benefit from chemoprevention with aspirin.

5-Lipoxygenase Polymorphisms

5-lipoxygenase converts dietary fatty acids to leukotrienes, potential inflammatory mediators of atherosclerosis. In a cross-sectional study of 470 healthy, middle-aged people, carotid artery intima-media thickness (measured as a marker of atherosclerosis) was increased in the 6% of people with a variant genotype (either of 2 polymorphisms) in the promoter region of the 5-lipoxygenased gene (153). The increased thickening, adjusted for other risk factors, was comparable to the increase seen with diabetes. Those with these polymorphisms also had doubled levels of CRP. Higher dietary intake of polyunsaturated n-6 fatty acid increased the effect of the gene variant, whereas higher intake of n-3 fatty acids (e.g., from fish oils) lessened the effect (153). Although this observation suggests a genotype-diet interaction that could identify people more likely to respond to fish oils for prevention of atherosclerosis, clinical use of 5-lipoxygenase genotyping would have to await prospective studies showing that individualized treatment prevents CAD.

α-Adducin Variant

A population-based case-control study of patients treated for hypertension found a significant interaction between the α-adducin gene variant, Trp460, and diuretic therapy on the risk of MI or stroke (154). The α-adducin gene variant was identified in more than one third of the participants. The risk of MI or stroke in individuals with the wild-type genotype did not depend on the type of antihypertensive therapy. However, in carriers of the α-adducin variant, diuretic therapy was associated with a lower risk of MI and stroke than other antihypertensive therapies (odds ratio, 0.49; 95% CI, 0.32–0.77). Other traditional cardiovascular disease risk factors did not influence this interaction. These results suggest a role for genotyping hypertensive individuals for the α-adducin variant allele, Trp460, to determine benefit from diuretic therapy.

However, these findings need to be confirmed in other studies, and other benefits and risks of diuretic therapy need to be considered before such testing translates to clinical practice.

Alcohol Dehydrogenase Type 3

Alcohol consumption has been associated with reduced risk of CHD. People with an alcohol dehydrogenase type 3 (ADH3) allele metabolize alcohol more slowly. This genetic variant in men is also associated with a lower risk of MI (RR=0.65; 95% CI, 0.43–0.99) (155). A significant interaction between this allele and alcohol intake has been found. Those who are homozygous for this allele and drink at least one drink a day have the greatest reduction in risk for MI (RR=0.14; 95% CI, 0.04–0.45) and the highest HDL cholesterol levels (for interaction P=0.05). Again, this finding has limited clinical utility since all men in this study appeared to benefit from consuming at least one drink per day regardless of their genotype. In addition, many other variables need consideration when counseling about alcohol intake.

Estrogen Receptor-α Gene

Herrington and colleagues (156) have shown that sequence variation of the estrogen receptor-α gene (IVS1-401 C/C genotype) is associated with the magnitude of increase in HDL cholesterol levels when estrogen or combination HRT is administered to women with CAD. However, this response has not yet been linked to variation in the risk of cardiovascular disease.

APPROACH TO INDIVIDUALS WITH HIGH FAMILIAL RISK

The following paragraphs will review the process of genetic evaluation for an individual referred because of personal or family history characteristics suggestive of a strong genetic susceptibility to CAD or MI (Table 2). The process includes: (1) genetic counseling and education, (2) risk assessment using personal and family medical history, physical examination, laboratory testing,

Table 2 Characteristics of Genetic Predisposition to Coronary Artery Disease (CAD)

- Early onset CAD: men age <55 and women age <65 years
- More than one close relative[a] with CAD, especially female relatives
- Multiple atherosclerotic vessels (e.g., coronary, carotid, aorta) with multifocal involvement (i.e., angiographic severity)
- Presence of multiple CAD risk factors in family members with CAD
- Presence of related disorders in close relatives (e.g., diabetes, stroke, hypertension, peripheral vascular disease)

[a] Close relative, first- or second-degree relatives.

and screening for early detection of CAD, and (3) recommendations for risk factor modification.

Genetic Counseling and Education Regarding CAD Susceptibility

An important goal of genetic evaluation for CAD is the development of individualized preventive strategies based on the genetic risk assessment, and the patient's personal medical history, lifestyle, and preferences. Genetic counseling is critical for delineating a patient's motivation and likely responses to learning of a genetic risk. Through genetic consultation patients will be educated about the role of behavioral and genetic risk factors for CAD, their mode of inheritance, and the options for prevention and risk factor modification. This communication process ensures the opportunity to provide informed consent, including discussion of the potential benefits, risks, and limitations of genetic risk assessment, and options for prevention (157).

Although family history of CAD has been shown to be a significant predictor of CAD risk, a recent report has shown that this familial risk does not translate to spontaneous improvement in lifestyles of at-risk relatives (158). In the Coronary Artery Risk Development in Young Adults study, CAD risk factors were assessed over two consecutive 5-year follow-up periods among 3950 participants aged 18 to 30 years. Kip and colleagues (158) found that the occurrence of a heart attack or stroke in a young adult's immediate family member did not lead to self-initiated, sustained change in modifiable risk factors. These results argue that primary care clinicians may need to actively intervene in people with a family history of CAD, where the opportunities for prevention are substantial (3).

Because most of the established and emerging risk factors for CAD aggregate in families, a family-based approach to risk factor modification ought to be an effective strategy, and this has been demonstrated in a few studies (159–161). Lifestyle changes, such as dietary modification, weight control, and smoking cessation, are likely to be more effective when delivered to the family than to an individual because family members can influence each other and provide ongoing support to one another.

Risk Assessment

Review of the personal medical history should include diagnoses of CAD, MI, peripheral vascular disease, stroke (including transient ischemic attacks), thrombosis, arrhythmia, heart failure, pulmonary disease, diabetes, and hypertension. Medical records, particularly procedure reports, are reviewed for confirmation. The Review of Systems will focus on cardio-respiratory function, including questions regarding angina, shortness of breath, dyspnea on exertion, paroxysmal nocturnal dyspnea, pedal edema, claudication, and exercise tolerance. Inquiry regarding tobacco exposure, history of alcohol use, exercise, and diet should also be performed.

During genetic consultation, a pedigree is constructed by obtaining demographic and medical information for all first and second-degree relatives, including current age or age at death, cause of death if deceased, history of CAD, other forms of heart disease, and related conditions such as stroke, peripheral vascular disease, aortic aneurysm, hypertension, diabetes, and lipid abnormalities, and associated risk factors such as smoking. Additional questioning can be helpful regarding procedures that might have been performed such as coronary artery bypass surgery, angioplasty, echocardiogram, or pacemaker placement. When available, medical records and autopsy reports of family members are reviewed to verify diagnoses and document test results. The family history should include ethnicity and country of origin since certain conditions might be more prevalent in certain ethnic groups. For example, the prevalence of insulin resistance is high among individuals of Native American admixture (162,163).

Once this information is collected, pedigree analysis is performed to determine the most likely mode of inheritance (i.e., Mendelian versus multifactorial) and the risk of disease to the patient and to unaffected relatives. If a Mendelian disorder is suspected, this analysis helps to elucidate the differential diagnosis. This process can inform recommendations for appropriate diagnostic tests as well as individualized management and prevention strategies. For example, an inherited susceptibility to thrombosis may be suspected in a pedigree that features multiple affected relatives with early onset of CAD, stroke, and other thromboembolic events (164). Testing of thrombotic markers might reveal important risk factors in the family. Recommendations can be made to avoid factors that may aggravate that risk such as use of oral contraceptives, HRT, and prolonged periods of immobility, and for prophylactic use of anticoagulants in high-risk situations.

A physical examination focused on CAD risk should include blood pressure in the arms and the ankles. In addition to identifying hypertension, these measurements can be used to calculate the ankle/brachial blood pressure index (ABI). Values <0.9 are correlated with atherosclerosis. In addition, a blood pressure of 130/85 or greater is a criterion for the metabolic syndrome (57). Weight and height should be obtained and body mass index should be calculated. This can be helpful in identifying a need for achieving an ideal weight and monitoring diet and exercise interventions. Waist circumference should be obtained, as it can be a factor in identifying the metabolic syndrome (57). Evaluation of lipid disorders should include examination of the eyes, assessing corneal arcus and lipemia retinalis. Examination of the skin should include assessment for xanthelasma and tendonous xanthomas. The cardiovascular exam should include careful assessment of the heart and lungs, as well as listening for bruits at major vessels in the neck, abdomen, and groin, and palpation of the aorta and distal pulses. Any abnormalities can be followed up with additional studies, such as ultrasound. Physical signs of Mendelian disorders that feature cardiovascular disease, for example, Marfan syndrome, Ehlers-Danlos syndrome type IV, pseudoxanthoma elasticum, and Fabry disease, should also be sought.

Laboratory testing to detect traditional and emerging risk factors for CAD includes fasting lipid panel, lipoprotein(a), LDL cholesterol particle size, HDL cholesterol fractionation, apolipoprotein B, hs-CRP, glucose, and homocysteine measurements. The ALP can be identified if there is a preponderance of small, dense LDL cholesterol, decreased fraction of HDL2b ($<15\%$), elevated triglycerides, and elevated apolipoprotein B. ALP can be effectively treated with lifestyle changes and/or medications (niacin or fibrates) as reviewed above (118–120). Fasting insulin can be checked if there is evidence of impaired glucose tolerance. The metabolic syndrome can be identified if at least three of the following criteria are met: blood pressure $> 130/85$ mm Hg, waist circumference > 102 cm in men and > 88 cm in women, HDL cholesterol <40 mg/dL in men and <50 mg/dL in women, triglycerides of 150 mg/dL or greater (57). If the metabolic syndrome is present, or if there are signs of insulin resistance or impaired glucose tolerance, oral glucose tolerance testing should be considered for detection of diabetes (Fig. 2).

DNA-based testing may be considered in specific situations for high-risk individuals. MTHFR mutation analysis for the C677T allele can be performed if hyperhomocysteinemia is detected. Factor V Leiden (FVL) mutation analysis can be performed for premenopausal women with other high-risk factors for MI who are considering use of oral contraceptives. If the FVL mutation is identified, oral contraceptives may be avoided because of an associated risk for MI in premenopausal women (164). Prothrombin G20210A mutation analysis can be considered for high-risk, postmenopausal women considering HRT. The combination of HRT and the G20210A mutation are associated with risk for MI (149). ApoE genotyping can be considered if there is a question about the diagnosis of type III hyperlipoproteinemia, or if the apoE genotype would significantly influence dietary recommendations.

Early detection strategies for CAD might be useful to further stratify risk in asymptomatic individuals at increased risk for CAD (55), especially if the identification of subclinical atherosclerosis will alter recommendations regarding risk factor modification or adherence to risk-reducing strategies. Noninvasive tests such as carotid artery duplex scanning to measure intima-media thickness, ABI, electron beam CT (EBCT) to detect coronary artery calcification, ultrasound-based endothelial function studies, magnetic resonance imaging techniques, and testing for hs-CRP offer the potential for measuring and monitoring atherosclerosis in asymptomatic people. Several of these methods are highly valid and predictive of CAD events (e.g., ABI, carotid intima-media thickness, and EBCT) (55). Once a higher risk is confirmed with these methods, aggressive medical therapies for primary prevention can be recommended.

The EBCT is the most popular of these early detection methods. There is consistent evidence that coronary calcification correlates with the presence and degree of plaque at autopsy, by intravascular ultrasound (165), and by angiography (166,167). Coronary calcification is also correlated with nonfatal infarction and need for subsequent coronary revascularization in both asymptomatic individuals (168–170), and patients undergoing coronary angiography (171). A prospective study has shown that EBCT identifies a high-risk group of asymptomatic subjects with clinically important silent ischemia as demonstrated by stress myocardial perfusion tomography (SPECT) (172). Abnormal SPECT was seen in 11.3% of patients with coronary calcium scores of 101–399, and 46% with scores of 400 or greater. Until recently, however, the added value of the coronary calcium score beyond the usual risk assessment methods had not been demonstrated. In a recent study of sibships at high risk for hypertension, a coronary artery calcium score above the 70th percentile was significantly associated with occurrence of coronary events, over an average of five years, after adjusting for Framingham risk scores (OR = 2.8; 95% CI, 1.2 to 6.4) (173). Thus, for individuals with a greater than average CAD risk (for example, those with a significant family history), the coronary calcium score obtained with EBCT has potential to detect advanced but asymptomatic coronary atherosclerosis, leading to recommendations for aggressive risk factor modification. At least one study has shown that knowledge of coronary calcium scores positively influenced behavior in self-referred subjects (174), although additional outcomes research regarding the utility of this approach is necessary. In addition, low coronary calcium scores may be valuable in defining a lower CAD risk (55), which could provide some reassurance to individuals assigned a high risk because of their family history. Risk factor modification could be relaxed somewhat for them, on the basis of this imaging.

Risk Factor Modification

Genetic information about CAD risk has value in guiding decision-making regarding lifestyle and other disease management and prevention strategies. Individuals with a strong genetic susceptibility to CAD, as determined by family history and the presence of established and emerging risk factors, may derive the greatest benefit from traditional preventive strategies such as smoking cessation and screening and treatment for elevated cholesterol and blood pressure. Individuals with CAD might also benefit from targeting emerging risk factors with specific interventions and lifestyle changes. However, for the most part, evidence regarding primary prevention of clinical cardiovascular events in individuals who have effectively modified emerging risk factors is lacking and prospective clinical trials are necessary. Therefore, it is crucial to discuss these potential benefits and limitations with any patient undergoing assessment of emerging CAD risk factors.

   Cholesterol lowering is an important clinical strategy in both primary and secondary prevention of CAD (57). Use of cholesterol-lowering agents has been effective in reducing atherosclerosis incidence, disease progression, and CAD mortality (174–180). In high-risk individuals, hypercholesterolemia should be treated initially with lifestyle changes, and if necessary, with lipid-lowering medications to achieve a risk-appropriate LDL cholesterol value. However, even when there is effective lipid lowering, a substantial proportion of individuals will develop CAD or have progression of their disease (181). Therefore, considering treatment of additional biochemical risk factors in high-risk individuals is a reasonable approach.

If there are small LDL cholesterol particles, then niacin should be considered in doses of up to 3 to 4 g a day (119,120). This can be used in combination with a statin drug if LDL cholesterol is elevated. Niacin can also be prescribed in similar doses to treat elevated lipoprotein(a) levels (108), or if estrogen replacement therapy is an option, this can be considered (111). Niacin can also raise HDL cholesterol (182), as do exercise (183) and moderate alcohol intake (184). With niacin therapy, monitoring of transaminases, uric acid, and blood glucose should be performed, as abnormalities can arise (185). Transaminases and creatinine kinase levels can also increase with statin drugs, although the usefulness of routine measurement is questionable (186). If there is evidence of hyperhomocysteinemia, then assessment of non-genetic factors should be performed (e.g., measurement of B vitamins, renal function, thyroid function, and review of medications) and B vitamin supplementation should be considered, titrating the amount of folic acid to the fasting homocysteine level (97–100). Homocysteine levels can become abnormal with niacin, fibric acid derivatives, and metformin (96), drugs that are often used in individuals at risk for CAD. Insulin resistance can be effectively treated with lifestyle changes or metformin (125).

SYNOPSIS

Individuals with genetic predisposition to atherosclerosis are at the greatest risk for developing CAD, especially at early ages. They may derive the greatest benefit from traditional preventive strategies as well as those targeting novel, emerging risk factors. Because CAD is a complex, multifactorial disorder, global risk assessment has been recognized as an effective approach in preventing CAD and its manifestations. However, genetic susceptibility to CAD is not adequately addressed by widely-used risk models such as the Framingham risk score, and underestimation of risk and missed opportunities for prevention can result for people who are genetically predisposed. The systematic collection and interpretation of family history information is currently the most appropriate screening approach to identify individuals with genetic susceptibility to CAD. Much of the familial aggregation of CAD might be explained by familial aggregation of established risk factors, such as elevated LDL cholesterol, low HDL cholesterol, and diabetes, and emerging CAD risk factors including hyperhomocysteinemia, CRP, elevated fibrin D-dimer, tissue plasminogen activator, fibrinogen, and insulin resistance. Tests to assess genetic risk for CAD are primarily biochemical analyses that measure the different pathways involved in development and progression of disease. Some of these can guide and explain responses to treatment. Clinical applications for DNA-based testing of CAD susceptibility genes are minimal.

SUMMARY

Several lines of evidence support the contribution of genetic variations to the development and progression of CAD, and to response to risk factor modification and lifestyle choices. Genetically predisposed individuals generally have the highest risk for CAD and develop disease at an earlier age. Collection and interpretation of the family history is the best method to identify and stratify genetic risk for CAD. Additional information from the medical history, physical examination, biochemical, and DNA testing, interpreted in the context of the family history, can further refine the genetic risk assessment. Knowledge of genetic susceptibility to CAD has value in providing risk information and can influence lifestyle choices and management options. Genetically susceptible individuals might benefit the most from aggressive treatment of established CAD risk factors. In addition, many emerging risk factors are modifiable and targeting these risk factors with specific therapies may result in improved CAD prevention. Family-based prevention might be most effective for genetically predisposed individuals, since many established and emerging risk factors aggregate in families, and most are amenable to lifestyle changes. Early detection of CAD may be appropriate for genetically susceptible individuals to guide decision-making about risk factor modification. Studies are needed to generate evidence regarding the feasibility, validity, and utility of using familial risk assessment to inform CAD prevention strategies, as well as the ethical, legal, and social issues that may arise.

ACKNOWLEDGMENTS

This work was supported in part by a Career Development Award sponsored by the Centers for Disease Control and Prevention and the Association of Teachers of Preventive Medicine.

REFERENCES

1. American Heart Association. Heart and Stroke Statistics: 2003 Update. Dallas, Texas: American Heart Association, 2002.
2. Scheuner MT. Genetic predisposition to coronary artery disease. Curr Opin Cardiol 2001; 16:251–260.
3. Tavani A, Augustin L, Bosetti C, et al. Influence of selected lifestyle factors on risk of acute myocardial infarction in subjects with familial predisposition for the disease. Prev Med 2004; 38:468–472.

4. Berenson GS, Srinivasan SR, Bao W, Newman WP, III, Tracy RE, Wattigney WA. Association between multiple cardiovascular risk factors and atherosclerosis in children and young adults. N Engl J Med 1998; 338:1650–1656.

5. Lefkowitz RJ, Willerson JT. Prospects for cardiovascular research. JAMA 2001; 285:581–587.

6. Weissberg PL. Atherogenesis: current understanding of the causes of atheroma. Heart 2000; 83:247.

7. Rauch U, Osende JI, Fuster V, Badimon JJ, Fayad Z, Chesebro JH. Thrombus formation on atherosclerotic plaques: pathogenesis and clinical consequences. Ann Intern Med 2001; 134:224–238.

8. Scheuner MT. Genetic evaluation for coronary artery disease. Genet Med 2003; 5:269–285.

9. Ridker PM, Stampfer MJ. Assessment of genetic markers for coronary thrombosis: promise and precaution. Lancet 1999; 353:687–688.

10. Girelli D, Russo C, Ferraresi P, et al. Polymorphisms in the factor VII gene and the risk of myocardial infarction in patients with coronary artery disease. N Engl J Med 2000; 343:774–780.

11. Folsom AR, Wu KK, Rosamond WD, Sharrett AR, Chambless LE. Prospective study of the hemostatic factors and incidence of coronary heart disease: the Atherosclerosis Risk in Communities (ARIC) study. Circulation 1997; 96:1102–1108.

12. Weiss EJ, Bray PF, Tayback M, et al. A polymorphism of a platelet glycoprotein receptor as an inherited risk factor for coronary thrombosis. N Engl J Med 1996; 334:1090–1094.

13. Carter AM, Ossei-Gerning N, Grant PJ. Platelet glycoprotein IIIa Pl^A polymorphism in young men with myocardial infarction. Lancet 1996; 348:485–486.

14. Carter AM, Ossei-Gerning N, Wilson IJ, Grant PJ. Association of the platelet Pl^A polymorphism of glycoprotein IIb/IIIa and fibrinogen beta 448 polymorphism with myocardial infarction and extent of coronary artery disease. Circulation 1997; 96:1424–1431.

15. Ridker PM, Hennekens CH, Schmitz C, Stampfer MJ, Lindpaintner K. Pl$^{A1/A2}$ polymorphism of platelet glycoprotein IIIa and risks of myocardial infarction, stroke, and venous thrombosis. Lancet 1997; 349:385–388.

16. Herrmann SM, Poirier O, Marques-Vidal P, et al. The Leu^{33}/Pro polymorphism (PlA1/A2) of the glycoprotein IIIa (GPIIIa) receptor is not related to myocardial infarction in the ECTIM study. Thromb Haemost 1997; 77:1170–1181.

17. Laule M, Cascorbi I, Stangl V, et al. A1/A2 polymorphism of glycoprotein IIIa and association with excess procedural risk for coronary catheter interventions: a case-control study. Lancet 1999; 353:708–712.

18. Cooke GE, Bray PF, Hamlington JD, Pham DM, Goldschmidt-Clermont PJ. Pl^{A2} polymorphism and efficacy of aspirin. Lancet 1998; 351:1253.

19. Pujukanta P, Cargill M, Viitanen L, et al. Two loci on chromosomes 2 and X for premature coronary heart disease identified in early- and late-settlement populations of Finland. Am J Hum Genet 2000; 67:1481–1493.

20. Hein L, Barsh GS, Pratt RE, Dzau VJ, Kobilka BK. Behavioural and cardiovascular effects of disrupting the angiotensin II type-2 receptor in mice. Nature 1995; 377:744–747.

21. Harrap SB, Zammit KS, Wong ZYH, et al. Genome-wide linkage analysis of the acute coronary syndrome suggests a locus on chromosome 2. Arterioscler Thromb Vasc Biol 2002; 22:874–878.

22. Lange LA, Lange EM, Bielak LF, et al. Autosomal genome-wide scan for coronary artery calcification loci in sibships at high risk for hypertension. Arterioscler Thromb Vasc Biol 2002; 22:418–422.

23. Gudmundsson G, Matthiasson SE, Arason H, et al. Localization of a gene for peripheral arterial occlusive disease to chromosome 1p31. Am J Hum Genet 2002; 70:586–592.

24. Bray MS, Krushkal J, Li L, et al. Positional genomic analysis identifies the beta-adrenergic receptor gene as a susceptibility locus for human hypertension. Circulation 2000; 101:2877–2882.

25. Krushkal J, Xiong M, Ferrell R, Sing CF, Turner ST, Boerwinkle E. Linkage and association of adrenergic and dopamine receptor genes in the distal portion of the long arm of chromosome 5 with systolic blood pressure variation. Hum Mol Genet 1998; 7:1379–1383.

26. Krushkal J, Ferrell R, Mockrin SC, Turner ST, Sing CF, Boerwinkle E. Genome-wide linkage analyses of systolic blood pressure using highly discordant siblings. Circulation 1999; 99:1407–1410.

27. Williams RR, Hunt SC, Hopkins PN, Wu LL, Lalouel JM. Evidence for single gene contributions to hypertension and lipid disturbances: definition, genetics, and clinical significance. Clin Genet 1994; 46:80–87.

28. Geller DS, Farhi A, Pinkerton N, et al. Activating mineralocorticoid receptor mutation in hypertension exacerbated by pregnancy. Science 2000; 289:119–123.

29. Frossard PM, Lestringant GG, Malloy MJ, Kane JP. Human renin gene BglI dimorphism associated with hypertension in two independent populations. Clin Genet 1999; 56:428–433.

30. Deng H-W, Deng H, Liu Y-J, et al. A genomewide linkage scan for quantitative-trait loci for obesity phenotypes. Am J Hum Genet 2002; 70:1138–1151.

31. Lee JH, Reed DR, Li W-D, et al. Genome scan for human obesity and linkage to markers in 20q13. Am J Hum Genet 1999; 64:196–209.

32. Heinonen P, Koulu M, Pesonen U, et al. Identification of a three-amino acid deletion in the alpha-2B-adrenergic receptor that is associated with reduced basal metabolic rate in obese subjects. J Clin Endocrinol Metab 1999; 84:2429–2433.

33. Large V, Hellstrom L, Reynisdottir S, et al. Human beta-2 adrenoceptor gene polymorphisms are highly frequent in obesity and associate with altered adipocyte beta-2 adrenoceptor function. J Clin Invest 1997; 100:3005–3013.

34. Nagase T, Aoki A, Yamamoto M, et al. Lack of association between the trp64arg mutation in the beta-3-adrenergic receptor gene and obesity in Japanese men: a longitudinal analysis. J Clin Endocrinol Metab 1997; 82:1284–1287.

35. Mitchell BD, Blangero J, Comuzzie AG, et al. A paired sibling analysis of the beta-3 adrenergic receptor and obesity in Mexican Americans. J Clin Invest 1998; 101:584–587.

36. Sina M, Hinney A, Ziegler A, et al. Phenotypes in three pedigrees with autosomal dominant obesity caused by haploinsufficiency mutations in the melanocortin-4 receptor gene. Am J Hum Genet 1999; 65:1501–1507.

37. Ristow M, Müller-Wieland D, Pfeiffer A, Krone W, Kahn CR. Obesity associated with a mutation in a genetic regulator of adipocyte differentiation. N Engl J Med 1998; 339:953–959.
38. Walder K, Norman RA, Hanson RL, et al. Association between uncoupling protein polymorphisms (UCP2-UCP3) and energy metabolism/obesity in Pima Indians. Hum Mol Genet 1998; 7:1431–1435.
39. Busfield F, Duffy DL, Kesting JB, et al. A genomewide search for type 2 diabetes-susceptibility genes in indigenous Australians. Am J Hum Genet 2002; 70:349–357.
40. Di Paola R, Frittitta L, Miscio G, et al. A variation in 3'UTR of hPTP1B increases specific gene expression and associates with insulin resistance. Am J Hum Genet 2002; 70:806–812.
41. Lindgren CM, Mahtani MM, Widén E, et al. Genomewide search for type 2 diabetes mellitus susceptibility loci in Finnish families: the Botnia study. Am J Hum Genet 2002; 70:509–516.
42. Horikawa Y, Oda N, Cox NJ, et al. Genetic variation in the gene encoding calpain-10 is associated with type 2 diabetes mellitus. Nature Genet 2000; 26:163–175.
43. Vionnet N, Hani EH, Dupont S, et al. Genomewide search for type 2 diabetes-susceptibility genes in French Whites: Evidence for a novel susceptibility locus for early-onset diabetes on chromosome 3q27-qter and independent replication of a type 2-diabetes locus on chromosome 1q21-q24. Am J Hum Genet 2000; 67:1470–1480.
44. Ghosh S, Watanabe RM, Valle TT, et al. The Finland-United States investigation of non-insulin dependent diabetes mellitus genetics (FUSION) study, I. An autosomal genome scan for genes that predispose to type 2 diabetes. Am J Hum Genet 2000; 67:1174–1185.
45. Watanabe RM, Ghosh S, Langefeld CD, et al. The Finland-United States Investigation of non-insulin-dependent diabetes mellitus genetics (FUSION) study, II. An autosomal genome scan for diabetes-related quantitative-trait loci. Am J Hum Genet 2000; 67:1186–1200.
46. Stone LM, Kahn SE, Fujimoto WY, Deeb SS, Porte D, Jr. A variation at position -30 of the beta-cell glucokinase gene promoter is associated with reduced beta-cell function in middle-aged Japanese-American men. Diabetes 1996; 45:422–428.
47. Hart LM, Stolk RP, Dekker JM, et al. Prevalence of variants in candidate genes for type 2 diabetes mellitus in the Netherlands: the Rotterdam study and the Hoorn study. J Clin Endocrinol Metab 1999; 84:1002–1006.
48. Reis AF, Ye W-Z, Dubois-Laforgue D, Bellanne-Chantelot C, Timsit J, Velho G. Association of a variant in exon 31 of the sulfonylurea receptor 1 (SUR1) gene with type 2 diabetes mellitus in French Caucasians. Hum Genet 2000; 107:138–144.
49. Altshuler D, Hirschhorn JN, Klannemark M, et al. The common PPAR gamma Pro12Ala polymorphism is associated with decreased risk of type 2 diabetes. Nat Genet 2000; 26:76–80.
50. Soro A, Pajukanta P, Lilja HE, et al. Genome scans provide evidence for low-HDL-C loci on chromosomes 8q23, 16q24.1-24.2, and 20q13.11 in Finnish families. Am J Hum Genet 2002; 70:1333–1340.

51. Arya R, Duggirala R, Almasy L, et al. Linkage of high-density lipoprotein-cholesterol concentrations to a locus on chromosome 9p in Mexican Americans. Nat Genet 2002; 30:102–105.

52. Peacock JM, Arnett DK, Atwood LD, et al. Genome scan for quantitative trait loci linked to high-density lipoprotein cholesterol. The NHLBI family heart study. Arterioscler Thromb Vasc Biol 2001; 21:1823–1828.

53. Klos KL, Kardia SLR, Ferrell RE, Turner ST, Boerwinkle E, Sing CF. Genome-wide linkage analysis reveals evidence of multiple regions that influence variation in plasma lipid and apolipoprotein levels associated with risk of coronary heart disease. Arterioscler Thromb Vasc Biol 2001; 21:971–978.

54. Wang XL, Rainwater DL, VandeBerg JF, Mitchell BD, Mahaney MC. Genetic contributions to plasma total antioxidant activity. Arterioscler Thromb Vasc Biol 2001;1190–1195.

55. Smith SC, Greenland P, Grundy SM. AHA Conference Proceedings. Prevention Conference V. Beyond secondary prevention: Identifying the high-risk patient for primary prevention. Executive Summary. Circulation 2000; 101:111–116.

56. Wilson PWF, D'Agostino RB, Levy D, Belanger AM, Silbershatz H, Kannel WB. Prediction of coronary heart disease using risk factor categories. Circulation 1998; 97:1837–1847.

57. Expert Panel on Detection, Evaluation, and Treatment of High Blood Cholesterol in Adults. Executuve summary of the third report of the national cholesterol education program (NCEP) expert panel on detection, evaluation, and treatment of high blood cholesterol in adults (adult treatment panel III). JAMA 2001; 285:2486–2497.

58. Gertler MM, White PD. Coronary Heart Disease in Young Adults: A Multi-disciplinary Study. Cambridge, Massachusetts: Harvard University Press, 1954.

59. Thomas CB, Cohen BH. The familial occurrence of hypertension and coronary artery disease with observations concerning obesity and diabetes. Ann Intern Med 1955; 42:90–127.

60. Rose G. Familial patterns in ischaemic heart disease. Br J Prev Soc Med 1964; 18:75–80.

61. Slack J, Evans KA. The increased risk of death from ischaemic heart disease in first-degree relatives of 121 men and 96 women with ischaemic heart disease. J Med Genet 1966; 3:239–257.

62. Rissanen AM. Familial occurrence of coronary heart disease: effect of age at diagnosis. Am J Cardiol 1979; 44:60–66.

63. Hunt SC, Williams RR, Barlow GK. A comparison of positive family history definitions for defining risk of future disease. J Chron Dis 1986; 39:809–821.

64. Silberberg JS, Wlodarczyk J, Fryer J, Robertson R, Hensley MJ. Risk associated with various definitions of family history of coronary heart disease. The Newcastle family history study II. Am J Epidemiol 1998; 147:1133–1139.

65. Nora JJ, Lortscher RH, Spangler RD, Nora AH, Komberling WJ. Genetic-epidemiologic study of early-onset ischemic heart disease. Circulation 1980; 61:503–508.

66. Brown DW, Giles WH, Burke W, Greenlund KJ, Croft JB. Familial aggregation of early-onset myocardial infarction. Community Genet 2002; 5:232–238.

67. Frielander Y, Kark JD, Stein Y. Family history of myocardial infarction as an independent risk factor for coronary heart disease. Br Heart J 1985; 53:382–387.
68. Sesso HD, Lee IM, Gaziano JM, Rexrode KM, Glynn RJ, Buring JE. Maternal and paternal history of myocardial infarction and risk of cardiovascular disease in men and women. Circulation 2001; 104:393–398.
69. Sholtz RI, Rosenman RH, Brand RJ. The relationship of reported parental history to the incidence of coronary heart disease in the Western Collaborative Group Study. Am J Epidemiol 1975; 102:350–356.
70. Colditz GA, Stampfer MJ, Willett WC, Rosner B, Speizer FE, Hennekens CH. A prospective study of parental history of myocardial infarction and coronary heart disease in women. Am J Epidemiol 1986; 123:48–58.
71. Khaw KT, Barrett-Connor E. Family history of heart attack: a modifiable risk factor? Circulation 1986; 74:239–244.
72. Schildkraut JM, Myers RH, Cupples LA, Kiely DK, Kannel WB. Coronary risk associated with age and sex of parental heart disease in the Framingham Study. Am J Cardiol 1989; 64:555–559.
73. Phillips AN, Shaper AG, Pocock SJ, Walker M. Parental death from heart disease and the risk of heart attack. Eur Heart J 1988; 9:243–251.
74. Hopkins PN, Williams RR, Kuida H, et al. Family history as an independent risk factor for incident coronary artery disease in a high-risk cohort in Utah. Am J Cardiol 1988; 62:703–707.
75. Colditz GA, Rimm EB, Giovannucci E, Stampfer MJ, Rosner B, Willett WC. A prospective study of parental history of myocardial infarction and coronary artery disease in men. Am J Cardiol 1991; 67:933–938.
76. De Jong SC, Stehouwer CDA, Mackaay AJC, et al. High prevalence of hyperhomocysteinemia and asymptomatic vascular disease in siblings of young patients with vascular disease and hyperhomocysteinemia. Arterioscler Thromb Vasc Biol 1997; 17:2655–2662.
77. Margaglione M, Cappucci G, Colaizzo D, Vecchione G, Grandone E, Di Minno G. C-reactive protein in offspring is associated with the occurrence of myocardial infarction in first-degree relatives. Arterioscler Thromb Vasc Biol 2000; 20:198–203.
78. Mills JD, Mansfield MW, Grant PJ. Tissue plasminogen activator, fibrin D-dimer, and insulin resistance in the relatives of patients with premature coronary artery disease. Arterioscler Thromb Vasc Biol 2002; 22:704–709.
79. Kareinen A, Viitanen L, Halonen P, Lehto S, Laakso M. Cardiovascular risk factors associated with insulin resistance cluster in families with early-onset coronary heart disease. Arterioscler Throm Vasc Biol 2001; 21:1346–1352.
80. Kee F, Tiret L, Robo JY, et al. Reliability of reported family history of myocardial infarction. Br Med J 1993; 307:1528–1530.
81. Bensen JT, Liese AD, Rushing JT, et al. Accuracy of proband reported family history: the NHLBI Family Heart Study (FHS). Genet Epidemiol 1999; 17:141–150.
82. Williams RR, Hunt SC, Heiss G, et al. Usefulness of cardiovascular family history data for population-based preventive medicine and medical research (the Health Family Tree Study and the NHLBI Family Heart Study). Am J Cardiol 2001; 87:129–135.

83. Scheuner MT, Wang S-J, Raffel LJ, Larabell SK, Rotter JI. Family history: a comprehensive genetic risk assessment method for the chronic conditions of adulthood. Am J Med Genet 1997; 71:315–324.

84. Lamarche B, Lemieux I, Després JP. The small, dense LDL phenotype and the risk of coronary heart disease: epidemiology, pathophysiology and therapeutic aspects. Diabetes Metab 1999; 25:199–211.

85. Gardner CD, Fortmann SP, Krauss RM. Association of small low-density lipoprotein particles with the incidence of coronary artery disease in men and women. JAMA 1996; 276:875–881.

86. Lamarche B, Tchernof A, Moorjani S, et al. Small, dense LDL particles and the risk of ischemic heart disease: prospective results from the Québec Cardiovascular Study. Circulation 1997; 95:69–75.

87. Stampfer MJ, Krauss RM, Ma J, et al. A prospective study of triglyceride level, low-density lipoprotein particle diameter, and risk of myocardial infarction. JAMA 1996; 276:882–888.

88. St-Pierre AC, Ruel IL, Cantin B, et al. Comparison of various electrophoretic characteristics of LDL particles and their relationship to the risk of ischemic heart disease. Circulation 2001; 104:2295–2299.

89. Superko HR. Small, dense LDL subclass phenotype B: issues for clinicians. Curr Atheroslcerosis Rep 1999; 1:50–57.

90. Ridker PM, Rifai N, Rose L, Buring JE, Cook NR. Comparison of C-reactive protein and low-density lipoprotein cholesterol levels in the prediction of first cardiovascular events. N Engl J Med 2002; 347:1557–1565.

91. Ridker PM, Stampfer MJ, Rifai N. Novel risk factors for systemic atherosclerosis. A comparison of C-reactive protein, fibrinogen, homocysteine, lipoprotein(a), and standard cholesterol screening as predictors of peripheral arterial disease. JAMA 2001; 285:2481–2485.

92. Pradhan AD, Manson JE, Rossouw JE, et al. Inflammatory biomarkers, hormone replacement therapy, and incident coronary heart disease. Prospective analysis from the Women's Health Initiative Observational Study. JAMA 2002; 288:980–987.

93. Danesh J, Lewington S. Plasma homocysteine and coronary heart disease: systematic review of published epidemiological studies. J Cardiovasc Risk 1998; 5:229–232.

94. Tawacol A, Omland T, Gerhard M, Wu JT, Creager MA. Hyperhomocysteinemia is associated with impaired endothelial-dependent vasodilation in humans. Circulation 1997; 95:1191–1211.

95. Mangoni AA, Jackson SH. Homocysteine and cardiovascular disease: current evidence and future prospects. Am J Med 2002; 112:556–565.

96. Desouza C, Keebler M, McNamara DB, Fonseca V. Drugs affecting homocysteine metabolism: impact on cardiovascular risk. Drugs 2002; 62:605–616.

97. Ubbink JB. The role of vitamins in the pathogenesis and treatment of hyperhomocysteinemia. J Inherit Metab Dis 1997; 20:315–325.

98. Malinow MR, Bostrom AG, Krauss RM. Homocyst(e)ine, diet, and cardiovascular diseases. A statement for healthcare professionals from the nutrition committee. Am Heart Assoc Circ 1999; 99:178–182.

99. Brattstrom LE, Israelsson B, Norrving B, et al. Impaired homocysteine metabolism in early-onset cerebral and peripheral occlusive arterial disease. Effects of pyridoxine and folic acid treatment. Atherosclerosis 1990; 81:51–60.

100. Schnyder G, Roffi M, Flammer Y, Pin R, Hess OM. Effect of homocysteine-lowering therapy with folic acid, vitamin B12, and vitamin B6 on clinical outcome after percutaneous coronary intervention: the Swiss heart study: a randomized controlled trial. JAMA 2002; 288:973–979.

101. Toole JF, Malinow MR, Chambless LE, et al. Lowering homocysteine in patients with ischemic stroke to prevent recurrent stroke, myocardial infarction, and death. The Vitamin Intervention for Stroke (VISP) randomized controlled trial. JAMA 2004; 291:565–575.

102. Baker F, Picton D, Blackwood S, et al. Blinded comparison of folic acid and placebo in patients with ischemic heart disease: an outcome trial. Circulation 2002; 106:741S.

103. Stein JH, Rosenson RS. Lipoprotein Lp(a) excess and coronary heart disease. Arch Intern Med 1997; 157:1170–1176.

104. Jenner JL, Ordovas I, Lamon-Fava S, et al. Effects of age, sex and menopausal status on plasma lipoprotein(a) levels: the Framingham Offspring Study. Circulation 1993; 87:1135–1141.

105. Berg k. Lp(a) lipoprotein: a monogenic risk factor for cardiovascular disease. In: Goldbourt U, de Faire U, Berg K, eds. Genetic Factors in Coronary Heart Disease. Boston: Kluwer Academic Publishers, 1994:275–287.

106. Kraft HG, Lingenhel A, Kochl S, et al. Apolipoprotein(a) kringle IV repeat number predicts risk for coronary heart disease. Arterioscler Thromb Vasc Biol 1996; 16:713–719.

107. Marcovina SM, Kochinsky ML. Lipoprotein(a) concentration and apolipoprotein(a) size: a synergistic role in advanced atherosclerosis? Circulation 1999; 100:1151–1153.

108. Gurakar A, Hoeg JM, Kostner G, Papadopoulos NM, Brewer HB, Jr. Levels of lipoprotein(a) decline with neomycin and niacin treatment. Atherosclerosis 1985; 57:293–301.

109. Temme EH, Mensink RP, Hornstra G. Comparison of the effects of diets enriched in lauric, palmitic, or oleic acids on serum lipids and lipoproteins in healthy women and men. Am J Clin Nutr 1996; 63:897–903.

110. Thomas TR, Ziogas G, Harris WS. Influence of fitness status on very-low density lipoproteins subfractions and lipoprotein(a) in men and women. Metabolism 1997; 46:1178–1183.

111. Espeland MA, Marcovina SM, Miller V, et al. Effect of postmenopausal hormone therapy on lipoprotein(a) concentration, PEPI Investigators. Postmenopausal Estrogen/Progestin Interventions. Circulation 1998; 97:979–986.

112. Zmuda JM, Thompson PD, Dickenson R, Bausserman LL. Testosterone decreases lipoprotein(a) in men. Am J Cardiol 1996; 77:1244–1247.

113. Shlipak MG, Simon JA, Vittinghoff E, et al. Estrogen and progestin, lipoprotein(a), and the risk of recurrent coronary heart disease events after menopause. JAMA 2000; 283:1845–1852.

114. Maher VM, Brown BG, Marcovina SM, Hillger LA, Zhao XQ, Albers JJ. Effects of lowering elevated LDL cholesterol on the cardiovascular risk of lipoprotein(a). JAMA 1995; 274:1771–1774.

115. Krauss RM. Dense low-density lipoproteins and coronary artery disease. Am J Cardiol 1995; 75:53B–57B.
116. Austin MA, Breslow JL, Hennekens CH, Buring JE, Willett WC, Krauss RM. Low density lipoprotein subclass patterns and risk of myocardial infarction. JAMA 1988; 260:917–921.
117. Griffin BA, Freeman DJ, Tait GW, et al. Role of plasma triglyceride in the regulation of plasma low density lipoprotein (LDL) subfractions: relative contribution of small, dense LDL to coronary heart disease risk. Atherosclerosis 1994; 106:241–253.
118. Dreon DM, Fernstrom HA, Williams PT, Krauss RM. LDL subclass phenotypes and lipoprotein response to a low-fat, high-carbohydrate diet in women. Arterioscler Thromb Vasc Biol 1997; 17:707–714.
119. Superko HR, Krauss RM. Differential effects of nicotinic acid in subjects with different LDL subclass phenotypes. Atherosclerosis 1992; 95:69–76.
120. Sakai T, Kamanna VS, Kashyap ML. Niacin, but not gemfibrozil, selectively increases LP-AI, a cardioprotective subfraction of HDL, in patients with low HDL cholesterol. Arterioscler Thromb Vasc Biol 2001; 21:1783–1789.
121. Superko HR, Haskell WL, Krauss RM. Association of lipoprotein subclass distribution with use of selective and non-selective beta-blocker medications in patients with coronary heart disease. Atherosclerosis 1993; 101:1–8.
122. Minihane AM, Khan S, Leigh-Firbank EC, et al. ApoE polymorphism and fish oil supplementation in subjects with atherogenic lipoprotein phenotype. Arterioscler Thromb Vasc Biol 2000; 20:117–128.
123. Ito MK. Niacin-based therapy for dyslipidemia: past evidence and future advances. Am J Manag Care 2002; 8:S315–S322.
124. Ford ES, Giles WH, Dietz WH. Prevalence of the metabolic syndrome among U.S. adults. JAMA 2002; 287:356–359.
125. Diabetes Prevention Program Research Group. Reduction in the incidence of type 2 diabetes with lifestyle intervention or metformin. N Engl J Med 2002; 346:393–403.
126. Backes JM, Howard PA, Moriarty PM. Role of C-reactive protein in cardiovascular disease. Ann Pharmacother 2004; 38:110–118.
127. Ridker PM, Morrow DA. C-reactive protein, inflammation, and coronary risk. Cardiol Clin 2003; 21:315–325.
128. Ridker PM, Rifai N, Pfeffer MA, Sacks F, Braunwald E. Long-term effects of pravastatin on plasma concentration of C-reactive protein. Circultation 1999; 100:230–235.
129. Maison P, Mennen L, Sapinho D, et al. A pharmacoepidemiological assessment of the effect of statins and fibrates on fibrinogen concentration. Atherosclerosis 2002; 160:155–160.
130. Harper CR, Jacobson TA. The fats of life: the role of omega-3 fatty acids in the prevention of coronary heart disease. Arch Intern Med 2001; 161:2185–2192.
131. Scheuner MT, Yoon P, Khoury MJ. Contribution of Mendelian disorders to common chronic disease: opportunities for recognition, intervention and prevention. Am J Med Genet 2004; 125C:50–65.

132. Online Mendelian Inheritance in Man, OMIM™. McKusick-Nathans Institute for Genetic Medicine, Johns Hopkins University (Baltimore, MD) and National Center for Biotechnology Information, National Library of Medicine (Bethesda, MD), 2000. (Accessed April, 2003, at http://www.ncbi.nlm.nih.gov/omim/).

133. Glazier AM, Nadeau JH, Aitman TJ. Finding genes that underlie complex traits. Science 2002; 298:2345–2349.

134. Kuivenhoven JA, Jukema JW, Zwinderman AH, et al. The role of a common variant of the cholesterol ester transfer protein gene in the progression of coronary atherosclerosis. N Engl J Med 1998; 338:86–93.

135. Nieminen MS, Mattila KJ, Aalto-Setala K, et al. Lipoproteins and their genetic variation in subjects with and without angiographically verified coronary disease. Arteriosclerosis Thromb 1992; 12:58–69.

136. Eto M, Watanable K, Makino I. Increased frequencies of apolipoprotein E2 and E4 alleles in patients with ischemic heart disease. Clin Genet 1989; 39:183–189.

137. Cumming AM, Robertson F. Polymorphism at the apoE locus in relation to risk of coronary heart disease. Clin Genet 1984; 25:310–313.

138. Tikkanen MJ, Huttunen JK, Ehnholm C, Pietinen P. Apolipoprotein E4 homozygosity predisposes to serum cholesterol elevation during high fat diet. Arteriosclerosis 1990; 10:285–288.

139. Lopez-Miranda J, Ordovás JM, Mata P, et al. Effect of apolipoprotein E phenotype on diet-induced lowering of plasma low density lipoprotein cholesterol. J Lipid Res 1994; 35:1965–1975.

140. Ordovás JM, Lopez-Miranda JM, Mata P, Perez-Jimenez F, Lichtenstein AH, Schaefer EJ. Gene-diet interaction in determining plasma lipid response to dietary intervention. Atherosclerosis 1995; 118:S11–S27.

141. Campos H, D'Angostino M, Ordovás JM. Gene-diet interactions and plasma lipoproteins: role of apolipoprotein E and habitual saturated fat intake. Genet Epidemiol 2001; 20:117–128.

142. Denke MA, Adams-Huet B, Nguyen AT. Individual cholesterol variation in response to a margarine- or butter-based diet. JAMA 2000; 284:2740–2747.

143. Hokanson JE, Austin MA. Plasma triglyceride is a risk factor for cardiovascular disease independent of high-density lipoprotein cholesterol: a meta analysis of population based studies. J Cardiovasc Risk 1996; 3:213–219.

144. Roses AD. Apolipoprotein E affects the rate of Alzheimer disease expression: beta-amyloid burden is a secondary consequence dependent on APOE genotype and duration of disease. J Neuropathol Exp Neurol 1994; 53:429–437.

145. American College of Medical Genetics/American Society of Human Genetics Working Group on ApoE and Alzheimer Disease. Statement on use of apolipoprotein E testing for Alzheimer disease. JAMA 1995; 274:1627–1629.

146. Brattstrom L, Wilcken DE, Ohrvik J, Brudin L. Common methylenetetra-hydrolfolate reductase gene mutation leads to hyperhomocysteinemia but not to vascular disease: the result of a meta-analysis. Circulation 1998; 98:2520–2526.

147. Klerk M, Verhoef P, Clarke R, et al. MTHFR 677C-T polymorphism and risk of coronary heart disease. A meta-analysis. JAMA 2002; 288:2023–2031.

148. American Society of Human Genetics/American College of Medical Genetics Test and Technology Transfer Committee Working Group. ASHG/ACMG statement,

measurement and use of total plasma homocysteine. Am J Hum Genet 1998; 63:1541–1543.

149. Psaty BM, Smith NL, Lemaitre RN, et al. Hormone replacement therapy, prothrombotic mutations, and the risk of incident nonfatal myocardial infarction in postmenopausal women. JAMA 2001; 285:906–913.

150. Sen-Banerjee S, Siles X, Campos H. Tobacco smoking modifies association between Gln-Arg192 polymorphism of human paraoxonase gene and risk of myocardial infarction. Arterioscler Thromb Vasc Biol 2000; 20:2120–2126.

151. Moshfegh K, Wuillemin WA, Redondo M, et al. Association of two silent polymorphisms of platelet glycoprotein Ia/IIa receptor with risk of myocardial infarction. Lancet 1999; 353:351–354.

152. U.S. Preventive Services Task Force. Aspirin for the primary prevention of cardiovascular events: recommendation and rationale. Ann Intern Med 2002; 136:157–160.

153. Dwyer JH, Allayee H, Dwyer KM, et al. Arachidonate 5-lipoxygenase promoter genotype, dietary arachidonic acid, and atherosclerosis. N Engl J Med 2004; 350:29–37.

154. Psaty BM, Smith NL, Heckbert SR, et al. Diuretic therapy, the alpha-adducin gene variant, and the risk of myocardial infarction or stroke in persons with treated hypertension. JAMA 2002; 287:1680–1689.

155. Hines LM, Stampfer MJ, Ma J, et al. Genetic variation in alcohol dehydrogenase and the beneficial effect of moderate alcohol consumption on myocardial infarction. N Engl J Med 2001; 344:549–555.

156. Herrington DM, Howard TD, Hawkins GA, et al. Estrogen-receptor polymorphisms and effects of estrogen replacement on high-density lipoprotein cholesterol in women with coronary disease. N Engl J Med 2002; 346:967–974.

157. McKinnon WC, Baty BJ, Bennett RL, et al. Predisposition genetic testing for late-onset disorders in adults. A position paper of the National Society of Genetic Counselors. JAMA 1997; 278:1217–1220.

158. Kip KE, McCreath HE, Roseman JM, Hulley SB, Schreiner PJ. Absence of risk factor change in young adults after family heart attack or stroke. The CARDIA Study. Am J Prev Med 2002; 22:258–266.

159. Knutsen SF, Knutsen R. The Tromso Survey: the family intervention study-the effect of intervention on some coronary risk factors and dietary habits, a 6-year follow-up. Prev Med 1991; 20:197–212.

160. No authors listed. Randomised controlled trial evaluating cardiovascular screening and intervention in general practice: principal results of British family heart study. Br Med J 1997; 308:313–320.

161. Pyke SDM, Wood DA, Kinmonth AL, Thompson SG. Change in coronary risk and coronary risk factor levels in couples following lifestyle intervention. Arch Fam Med 1997; 6:354–360.

162. Arnoff SL, Bennett PH, Gorden P, Rushforth N, Miller M. Unexplained hyperinsulinemia in normal and 'prediabetic' Pima Indians compared with normal Caucasians. Diabetes 1977; 26:827–840.

163. Sharp PS, Mohan V, Levy JC, Mather HM, Kohner EM. Insulin resistance in patients of Asian Indian and European origin with non-insulin dependent diabetes. Horm Metab Res 1987; 19:84–85.

164. Rosendaal FR, Siscovick DS, Schwartz SM, et al. Factor V Leiden (resistance to activated protein C) increases the risk of myocardial infarction in young women. Blood 1997; 89:2817–2821.
165. Rumberger JA, Simons DB, Fitzpatrick LA, Sheedy PF, Schwartz RS. Coronary artery calcium area by electron-beam computed tomography and coronary atherosclerotic plaque area. A histopathologic correlative study. Circulation 1995; 92:2157–2162.
166. Bielak LF, Rumberger JA, Sheedy PF, Schwartz RS, Peyser PA. Probabilistic model for prediction of angiographically defined obstructive coronary artery disease using electron beam computed tomography calcium score strata. Circulation 2000; 102:380–385.
167. Nallamothu BK, Saint S, Rubenfire M, Fendrick AM. Electron beam computed tomography in the diagnosis of obstructive coronary artery disease. J Am Coll Cardiol 2001; 37:689–690.
168. Arad Y, Spadaro LA, Goodman K, et al. Predictive value of electron beam computed tomography of the coronary arteries. 19-month follow-up of 1173 asymptomatic subjects. Circulation 1996; 93:1951–1953.
169. Secci A, Wong N, Tang W, Wang S, Doherty T, Detrano R. Electron beam computed tomographic coronary calcium as a predictor of coronary events: comparison of two protocols. Circulation 1997; 96:1122–1129.
170. Raggi P, Callister TQ, Cooil B, et al. Identification of patients at increased risk of first unheralded acute myocardial infarction by electron-beam computed tomography. Circulation 2000; 101:850–855.
171. Detrano R, Hsiai T, Wang S, et al. Prognostic value of coronary calcification and angiographic stenoses in patients undergoing coronary angiography. J Am Coll Cardiol 1996; 27:285–290.
172. He ZX, Hedrick TD, Pratt CM, et al. Severity of coronary artery calcification by electron beam tomography predicts silent myocardial ischemia. Circulation 2000; 101:244–251.
173. Raggi P, Cooll B, Callister TQ. Use of electron beam tomography data to develop models for prediction of hard coronary events. Am Heart J 2001; 141:372–382.
174. Wong ND, Detrano RC, Diamond G, et al. Does coronary artery screening by electron beam computed tomography motivate potentially beneficial lifestyle behaviors? Am J Cardiol 1996; 78:1220–1223.
175. Blankenhorn DH, Nessim SA, Johnson R, Sanmarco ME, Azen SP, Cashin-Hemphill L. Beneficial effects of combined colestipol-niacin therapy on coronary atherosclerosis and coronary venous bypass grafts. JAMA 1987; 247:3233–3240.
176. Blankenhorn DH, Azen SP, Kramsch DM, et al. Coronary angiographic changes with lovastatin therapy: the Monitored Atherosclerosis Regression Study (MARS). Ann Intern Med 1993; 119:969–976.
177. Brown G, Albers JJ, Fisher LD, et al. Regression of coronary artery disease as a result of intensive lipid lowering therapy in men with high levels of apolipoprotein B. N Engl J Med 1990; 323:1289–1298.
178. Scandinavian Simvastatin Survival Study Group. Randomised trial of cholesterol lowering in 4444 patients with coronary heart disease: the Scandinavian Simvastatin Survival Study (4S). Lancet 1994; 344:1383–1389.

9

Oxidants and Antioxidants

Jan Nilsson

*Department of Clinical Sciences, Malmö University Hospital,
Lund University, Lund, Sweden*

Risk factors are generally first identified in epidemiological studies and the mechanisms through which they cause disease subsequently analyzed in cellular and animal models. Although this is partly true also for low levels of antioxidant vitamins as being a cardiovascular risk factor, the concept of increased oxidative stress in atherosclerosis originates mainly from experimental studies. The idea that oxidation of low density lipoprotein (LDL) in the arterial wall plays a key role in the development of atherosclerosis has gained impressive support from molecular studies in cell culture as well as from experiments performed in different animal models of atherosclerosis and subsequently also by extensive epidemiology (1,2). However, the outcome of both primary and secondary randomized intervention trials in which the effect of antioxidant vitamins on cardiovascular disease has been studied have so far largely been disappointing (3). Keeping in mind the complexity of cardiovascular disease, this may not be entirely surprising. We have for many years been well aware of the fact that smoking, diabetes, and hypertension are major risk factors for cardiovascular disease, but our knowledge of the molecular mechanism by which they cause disease remains incomplete and superficial. It may turn out to be equally difficult to identify proper treatments for specific disease mechanisms even if they are well characterized at the molecular level, such as in the case of lipid oxidation and atherosclerosis. This chapter will summarize the experimental studies on which the concept of LDL oxidation as a key mechanism in atherosclerosis is based as well as the epidemiological and intervention studies performed to assess the role of antioxidants in cardiovascular disease.

THE ANTIOXIDATIVE DEFENSE AND LIPID OXIDATION

The Antioxidative Defense

The controlled use of oxidation reactions is of course vital for all cells. The oxidation of molecular oxygen to produce energy is an extremely efficient way to produce energy but is at the same time quite hazardous as it depends on the generation and metabolism of a number of highly reactive oxygen intermediates. If these intermediates escape from the protected environment of the mitochondria they will react with and cause severe damage to cellular lipids, proteins, and DNA. A number of cellular antioxidative enzymes such as glutathione peroxidase and the cellular form of superoxide dismutase provide an effective defense against these molecules (4).

Reactive oxygen intermediates are generated also in the extracellular environment. One example is activated neutrophils that secrete oxygen radicals to kill infecting microorganisms. Other reactive radicals are produced by enzymatic reactions or through interactions with metal ions. A radical is a molecule that contains an unpaired electron. Unpaired electrons are highly reactive and will attract an electron from another molecule. The molecule that loses this electron is oxidized (oxidation is the same as loss of an electron) and becomes in turn a radical (a molecule containing an unpaired electron). If not stopped by an antioxidant this process results in an oxidative chain reaction. Lipids are particularly susceptible to oxidation. The extracellular antioxidative defense includes enzymes (such as extracellular superoxide dismutase) and vitamins. The most important antioxidative vitamins are vitamin A, C, and E and beta-carotene. Vitamin E is the main lipid-soluble antioxidant in the circulation and tissues and acts by converting the peroxyl-free radical to the less reactive hydro peroxide radical. Beta-carotene is a carotenoid that acts as a scavenger of radicals. When lipoproteins are exposed to oxidative stress, vitamin E functions as the first line of defense and beta-carotene as the second. Vitamin C is a water-soluble antioxidant that will interact with radicals primarily in non-lipid compartments. However, it also plays an important role in the regeneration of vitamin E.

Dietary Sources of Antioxidant Vitamins

The recommended daily intake of vitamin E is 10 mg. The major dietary sources of vitamin E are vegetable oils, such as olive and sunflower oil. Wheat germs and green vegetables are also good sources of vitamin E. The daily intake of vitamin E in olive oil-based Mediterranean diet is about 20 mg. Beta-carotene is present in yellow, red, and dark green vegetables such as carrots, tomatoes, yellow pumpkin, yellow chili, apricot, and beetroot. To reach a daily intake of 20 mg of beta-carotene (a supplement level commonly used in intervention trials), one should eat at least 290 g of carrots, 2496 g of tomatoes, or 2395 g of yellow chili. The recommended intake of vitamin C is 50 mg. An orange or a grapefruit per day is sufficient to meet this requirement (3).

LDL Oxidation

Oxidation of LDL is initiated by an attack of a radical on an unsaturated fatty acid. As a result of this attack a hydrogen atom is extracted from a double bond, leaving behind an unpaired electron on the carbon atom. This carbon radical becomes stabilized by rearrangement into a conjugated diene, which rapidly reacts with oxygen to produce a hydroperoxy radical. The hydroperoxy radical will subsequently abstract hydrogen atoms from other lipid molecules resulting in a chain reaction of lipid peroxidation. The oxidative modification of LDL also results in a number of compositional changes, including increased electrophoretic mobility, increased fragmentation of apolipoprotein B, formation of reactive aldehydes such as malondealdehyde, formation of oxysterols, and derivatization of lysine amino groups in the LDL binding domain. The net result of these changes is that the LDL particle loses its ability to bind to the LDL receptor and becomes highly cytotoxic (5).

LIPID OXIDATION IN ATHEROSCLEROSIS

Lipid Oxidation Induces Vascular Inflammation

The initial step in the development of atherosclerosis is the accumulation of lipoproteins in the extracellular matrix of large and medium-sized arteries. Areas exposed to low shear stress, such as branching points, are particularly susceptible to lipoprotein penetration and accumulation. Lipoproteins are normally present in the extracellular fluid of arteries and represent an important source of cholesterol and other lipids for vascular cells. At lower levels, all lipoproteins are metabolized or removed from the vascular wall, but if present in higher concentrations they begin to attach to proteoglycans in the extracellular matrix and aggregate. These lipoproteins also become oxidized. The mechanisms responsible for inducing this oxidation remains to be fully elucidated but appear to include enzymatic modifications and reactive oxygen intermediates (Fig. 1).

In hypercholesterolemic animals, accumulation of lipoproteins in the arterial wall is associated with activation of a local inflammation (6). The process is initially manifested as an endothelial expression of adhesion molecules, including VCAM, ICAM-1, and E-selectin. These adhesion molecules recruit circulating leukocytes, primarily monocytes, and T cells (Fig. 1) that migrate through the endothelium into the intima. The function of this process is probably to remove the oxidized lipoproteins that may otherwise disturb vascular function and even cause cell death. In the vessel wall, monocytes differentiate into macrophages that express scavenger receptors. These receptors effectively bind and ingest oxidized lipoproteins. Scavenger receptors are not only specific for oxidized LDL but also recognize membrane phospholipids on dying cells. Hence,

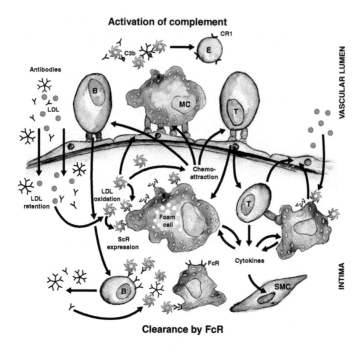

Figure 1 *The role of LDL oxidation in the initiation of atherosclerosis.* LDL particles penetrate the endothelial lining and become trapped in the extracellular matrix of the arterial wall. Some of these LDL particles become aggregated and oxidized, resulting in the release of a number of proinflammatory and toxic substances that activates endothelial expression of adhesion molecules. Monocytes (MC), T cells (T), and occasional B cells (B) attach to the endothelial surface and infiltrate the arterial intima. Monocytes differentiate into scavenger receptor (ScR), expressing macrophages that ingest oxidized LDL and become foam cells. Activation of macrophages and T cells result in release of cytokines that further enhance inflammation and stimulate smooth muscle cell (SMC) proliferation. Antibodies produced against oxidized LDL released from activated B cells may help to clear oxidized LDL from the extracellular space and the circulation.

it is likely to be part of a more general system used by the body to remove degenerated lipids and phospholipids that otherwise may cause severe damage to the surrounding tissue. When looked upon in this way, inflammation activated by oxidized lipoproteins serves a good function by limiting further injury to the vessel. However, if the accumulation of oxidized lipoprotein in vessel continues to occur at a rate exceeding their removal by macrophages, the inflammatory reaction may instead contribute to the tissue injury caused by oxidized lipids.

Macrophages that have ingested large amounts of oxidized lipids have a very characteristic morphology and are referred to as foam cells. Although they have been able to remove oxidized LDL from the extracellular matrix, they appear to have a greater difficulty in removing the oxidized lipids from the vessel itself. Instead, large numbers of foam cells accumulate and form fatty streaks that represent the earliest stage of visible atherosclerotic lesions. The reason for the inability of the macrophage foam cell to leave the vascular wall remains to be clarified, but may involve disturbances in basic cellular functions by the large amounts of ingested oxidized lipids.

In most animal models, treatment with antioxidants such as probucol, BHT, and vitamin E leads to a reduced expression of adhesion molecules and to inhibition of fatty streak formation. Notably, most animal studies using antioxidants to inhibit atherosclerosis are relatively short-term and have focused on the role of early lesion growth. More recently, the notion that oxidation of LDL is involved in atherogenesis has also been supported by experiments carried out in knockout mice. For example, a targeted disruption of the gene for 12/15 lipoxygenase, a potent inducer of LDL oxidation, profoundly inhibits atherogenesis in apoE-deficient mice. Disruption of the gene for CD 36, one of the members of the scavenger receptor family, also results in significant reduction of atherosclerosis in apoE-deficient mice.

Immune Reactions Against Oxidized LDL

In 1989 Palinski and coworkers (7) were able to produce antibodies that specifically recognized epitopes in oxidized LDL. Using these antibodies, they could demonstrate that human atherosclerotic plaques contained oxidized LDL. However, they also found that circulating antibodies against oxidized LDL was a quite common phenomenon in man. Indeed, exactly as was found to be the case for the scavenger receptors, these antibodies cross-reacted with phospholipids occurring on dying cells. Both the scavenger receptors and the oxidized LDL antibodies are thus likely to be part of an immune response involved in identifying and removing debris from dying cells, oxidatively damaged lipoproteins, and other potentially damaging phospholipid-associated degradation products (Fig. 1).

These observations suggested the interesting possibility that atherosclerosis may be caused by autoimmune reactions against our own lipoproteins once they had been oxidized in the vascular wall. Some studies also reported association between high levels of oxidized LDL antibodies and a more aggressive progression of atherosclerosis. One possibility to test this hypothesis is to immunize experimental animals with oxidized LDL and to study if this results in development of a more aggressive disease. However, somewhat surprisingly, such studies demonstrated that immune responses against oxidized LDL have a protective effect (8–11). Activation of these immune responses represents a new and promising target for prevention and treatment of cardiovascular disease (12).

Lipid Oxidation and Development of Advanced Lesions

As the process of atherosclerosis continues, fatty streaks develop into fibromuscular plaques. The initial step in this transition is the phenotypic modulation of contractile smooth muscle cells of the media into synthetically active repair cells. The mechanisms involved in activation of this modulation remain to be fully understood, but they appear to involve degradation of the extracellular matrix surrounding the smooth muscle cells by proteases released from inflammatory cells. Accordingly, inflammation has a key role in activation of the vascular fibroproliferative process. This is not surprising since inflammation is the general signal for repair after any tissue injury. Again, lipid oxidation may influence this process primarily by causing injury and inflammation.

At lower concentrations, products generated during lipoprotein oxidation may also act directly as growth factors for smooth muscle cells. However, at higher concentrations, these products generally become cytotoxic and limit the proliferative capacity of the smooth muscle cells. The latter situation may indeed be more relevant for the clinical situation. Fibromuscular plaques that cover more than 75% of the lumen may significantly compromise blood flow and give rise to angina, but they rarely cause infarction. Most infarcts are attributed to degenerative changes in plaques leading to plaque rupture and formation of occlusive thrombosis.

A necrotic core covered by a thin fibrous cap characterizes vulnerable plaques. The fibrous cap consists of smooth muscle cells, collagen, and other extracellular matrix. This matrix holds the plaque together, but it is constantly under the risk of being degraded by collagenase and other matrix proteases released by macrophages surrounding the necrotic core. If the fibrous cap contains viable smooth muscle cells, these may replace the degraded extracellular matrix. However, if the smooth muscle cells, are severely injured or killed by toxic lipid oxidation metabolites, the fibrous cap will become weakened and rupture in response to shear stress caused by the blood flow (13). In man, treatment with statins have been shown to decrease the amount of oxidize lipids and inflammatory cells and to increase collagen content and smooth muscle cell viability in atherosclerotic plaques (14).

EPIDEMIOLOGICAL STUDIES OF ANTIOXIDANTS
AND CARDIOVASCULAR DISEASE

A number of prospective observational studies have addressed whether intake of vitamin C, vitamin E, or beta-carotene affects cardiovascular risk after adjustments for known cardiovascular risk factors. Both dietary intake, as well as vitamin supplementation, have been assessed in several of these studies. The study designs used include cross-sectional studies comparing population in different countries, large epidemiological cohort studies, and case-control studies. In general, the results of these studies provide support for a protective effect of antioxidant vitamins on cardiovascular disease.

The most consistent and solid support for a protective effect of antioxidants has been obtained for vitamin E. In the Nurse's Health Study, 87,000 women were followed for an average of 8 years. Those in the highest quintile of vitamin E intake had a 34% reduction in risk of cardiovascular events as compared with the lowest quintile after adjustment for known risk factors and the intake of other antioxidant vitamins (15). Similar analyses in the Health Professional's Study (40,000 adult men followed for an average of 4 years) demonstrated a 39% reduction in coronary events for those with the highest intake of vitamin E as compared to those with the lowest intake (16). In the Iowa Women's Health Study, a study performed on almost 35,000 post-menopausal women followed for an average of 7 years, a 62% reduction in cardiovascular deaths was demonstrated in those with the highest intake of vitamin E from food (17). A meta-analysis based on studies that together included 166,774 subjects found statistically significant inverse relations between intake of vitamin E and risk of developing cardiovascular disease (OR 0.64; 95% CI 0.56–0.73) (3). Most studies suggest that a cardiovascular protection by vitamin E requires a longer period of increased intake (>2 years).

Cross-sectional studies have shown that median plasma levels of vitamin E is significantly higher in countries with a low cardiovascular mortality, such as the Mediterranean countries, than in countries with a high cardiovascular mortality, such as Finland and Scotland.

Some epidemiological studies have also reported that a high intake of beta-carotene is associated with a reduced risk for cardiovascular disease. The Health Professional's Study reported a 29% reduction (95% CI—14 to -47%) of coronary heart disease in the highest quintile of beta-carotene intake as compared to the lowest (16). However, in contrast, no beneficial effect of beta-carotene was found in the Nurse's Health Study (15) and the Iowa Women's Health Study (17). These three large studies also failed to demonstrate any association between intake of vitamin C and cardiovascular mortality.

Randomized Clinical Trials

The effects of antioxidant vitamins on cardiovascular disease have now been evaluated in several double blind, placebo-controlled, randomized clinical trials. With the exception of the Cambridge Heart Antioxidative Study (CHAOS) (18), all of these studies have failed to demonstrate any beneficial cardiovascular effect of antioxidants. In the CHAOS, 2,002 patients with angiographically documented coronary heart disease were randomized to vitamin E (400–800 IU daily) for an average of 18 months. Cardiovascular events were reduced by 53% (95% CI -17 to -66%), but there was no significant effect on cardiovascular or total mortality.

The Alpha-Tocopherol Beta Carotene Cancer Prevention Study tested daily supplementation with 20 mg of beta-carotene and 50 mg of alpha-tocopherol in 1,862 men with previous myocardial infarction (19). The study was a randomized, double blind, placebo-controlled trial with a median follow-up of 5.3 years. Beta-carotene supplementation led to a significant increase in total mortality ($+9\%$; 95% CI $+2$ to $+17\%$) and lung cancer ($+18\%$; 95%CI $+3$ to $+36\%$), and a non-significant increase in mortality from cardiovascular disease (+11%; 95% CI -1 to +23%).

In the Beta-Carotene and Retinol Efficacy Trial, the effect of 30 mg beta-carotene and 25,000 IU of vitamin A daily on lung cancer and cardiovascular disease was tested in multicenter, randomized, double-blind, placebo-controlled, primary prevention trial involving 18,314 smokers, former smokers, and workers exposed to asbestos followed for up to 4 years (20). Treatment was associated with a higher risk of lung cancer (+28%; 95% CI +4 to +57%) and had no protective effect on cardiovascular disease.

In the Physicians' Health Study, 22,071 healthy, adult U.S. male physicians were randomized to 50 mg of beta-carotene on alternate days or placebo (21). There was no effect on total mortality, cancer mortality, or cardiovascular mortality after an average follow-up of 12 years.

The Heart Outcomes Prevention Evaluation (HOPE) study used a two-by-two factorial design to test the effect of 10 mg of the angiotensin-converting enzyme inhibitor ramipril and 400 IU of vitamin E daily on cardiovascular disease (the primary outcome was a composite of myocardial infarction, stroke, or death from cardiovascular causes) in 9297 high-risk patients (22). The average age of the patients was 66 years; a little over half had had a previous myocardial infarction and about one-quarter had unstable angina. Whereas ramipril significantly reduced death, myocardial infarction, and stroke, vitamin E was without effect.

The GISSI (Gruppo Italiano per lo Studio della Sopravvivenza nell'Infarto miocardico)-Prevenzione trial also used a two-by-two factorial design to study the effect of 300 mg of vitamin E, 1 g of n-3polyunsaturated fatty acids (PUFA) or the combination of both in 11,324 patients surviving a recent (<3 months) myocardial infarction (23). Treatment with n-3 PUFA significantly reduced the risk of death by 14% (95% CI 3 to 24%) and cardiovascular death by 17% (95% CI 3 to 29%). The effect of combined treatment was the same as that for n-3 PUFA alone and vitamin E was without effect.

The Heart Protection Study analyzed the effects of 40 mg simvastatin and/or antioxidant vitamins (600 mg E, 250 mg C and 20 mg beta-carotene daily) in 20,563 individuals with or without prior cardiovascular disease. Whereas treatment with simvastatin was found to reduce risk of major cardiovascular events by more than 30%, there was no effect of treatment with antioxidant vitamins.

In the Women's Health Study conducted between 1992 and 2004, 39,876 apparently healthy U.S. women aged at least 45 years were randomly assigned to receive vitamin E (600 IU) or placebo and aspirin or placebo, using a 2 × 2 factorial design, and were followed up for an average of 10.1 years. During follow-up, there were 482 major cardiovascular events in the vitamin E group and 517 in the placebo group, a nonsignificant 7% risk reduction. There were no significant effects on the incidences of myocardial infarction or stroke, as well as ischemic or hemorrhagic stroke. For cardiovascular death, there was a significant

24% reduction (P=.03). There was no significant effect of vitamin E on total mortality (24).

Antioxidants have also been tested for a potential therapeutic role in the reduction of restenosis after angioplasty. In the Multivitamin and Probucol study, the effect of a combination of vitamins (1 g of vitamin C, 1,400 IU of vitamin E and 100 mg of beta-carotene) and probucol given separately or together on the rate of restenosis after angioplasty was investigated (25). Probucol was found to significantly reduce restenosis, whereas antioxidant vitamins were without effect. Also the Probucol Angioplasty Restenosis Trial reported a significant reduction in restenosis in response to probucol treatment (26).

In 2004, the American Heart Association Science Advisory concludes that at present the existing scientific database does not justify routine use of antioxidants for prevention and treatment of cardiovascular disease, but it recommends that research continue to clarify the discrepancy between the randomized trials and the population studies (27).

Why have so many Antioxidant Trials been Negative?

Against the background of all experimental and epidemiological data suggesting that lipid oxidation plays an important role in atherogenesis, the outcome of large intervention trials such as HOPE and GISSI are clearly disappointing. The reasons for this lack of effect have been discussed by Daniel Steinberg (28):

1. Vitamin E, while able to inhibit the early stages in atherosclerosis in animal models, has little or no effect on advanced lesions or on plaque rupture and thrombosis
2. Vitamin E is not a sufficiently potent antioxidant in humans or does not have appropriate pharmacokinetic properties
3. There is a true species difference between humans and animal models such that antioxidants will simply never have an effect on atherogenesis in humans.

If any of the first two explanations are true, we have not yet seen the results of a trial that tests the lipid oxidation hypothesis under proper conditions.

REFERENCES

1. Ross R. Atherosclerosis—an inflammatory disease. N Engl J Med 1999; 340:115–126.
2. Glass CK, Witztum JL. Atherosclerosis: the road ahead. Cell 2001; 104:503–516.
3. Marchioli R. Antioxidant vitamins and prevention of cardiovascular disease: laboratory, epidemiological and clinical trial data. Pharmacol Res 1999; 40:227–238.
4. Halliwell B, Chirico S. Lipid peroxidation: its mechanism, measurement, and significance. Am J Clin Nutr 1993; 57:715S–725S.

5. Steinberg D, Lewis A. Oxidative modification of LDL and atherogenesis. Circulation 1997; 95:1062–1071.
6. Berliner J, Navab M, Fogelman A, et al. Atherosclerosis: basic mechanisms. Oxidation, inflammation and genetics. J Clin Invest 1995; 91:2488–2496.
7. Palinski W, Rosenfeld ME, Yla-Herttuala S, et al. Low density lipoprotein undergoes oxidative modification in vivo. Proc Natl Acad Sci USA 1989; 86:1372–1376.
8. Palinski W, Miller E, Witztum JL. Immunization of low density lipoprotein (LDL) receptor-deficient rabbits with homologous malondialdehyde-modified LDL reduces atherogenesis. Proc Natl Acad Sci USA 1995; 92:821–825.
9. Ameli S, Hultgardh-Nilsson A, Regnstrom J, et al. Effect of immunization with homologous LDL and oxidized LDL on early atherosclerosis in hypercholesterolemic rabbits. Arterioscler Thromb Vasc Biol 1996; 16:1074–1079.
10. George J, Afek A, Gilburd B, et al. Hyperimmunization of apo-E-deficient mice with homologous malondialdehyde low-density lipoprotein suppresses early atherogenesis. Atherosclerosis 1998; 138:147–152.
11. Zhou X, Robertson AK, Rudling M, Parini P, Hansson GK. Lesion development and response to immunization reveal a complex role for CD4 in atherosclerosis. Circ Res 2005; 95:427–434.
12. Nilsson J, Hansson GK, Shah PK. Immunomodulation of atherosclerosis: implications for vaccine development. Arterioscler Thromb Vasc Biol 2005; 25:18–28.
13. Falk. Why do plaques rupture? Circulation 1992; 86:III30–III42.
14. Crisby M, Nordin-Fredriksson G, Shah PK, Yano J, Zhu J, Nilsson J. Pravastatin treatment increases collagen content and decreases lipid content, inflammation, metalloproteinases, and cell death in human carotid plaques: implications for plaque stabilization. Circulation 2001; 103:926–933.
15. Stampfer MJ, Hennekens CH, Manson JE, Colditz GA, Rosner B, Willett WC. Vitamin E consumption and the risk of coronary disease in women. N Engl J Med 1993; 328:1444–1449.
16. Rimm EB, Stampfer MJ, Ascherio A, Giovannucci E, Colditz GA, Willett W. Vitamin E consumption and the risk of coronary heart disease in men. N Engl J Med 1993; 328:1450–1456.
17. Kushi LH, Folsom AR, Prineas RJ, Mink PJ, Wu Y, Bostick RM. Dietary antioxidant vitamins and death from coronary heart disease in postmenopausal women. N Engl J Med 1996; 334:1156–1162.
18. Stephens NG, Parsons A, Schofield P, Kelly F, Cheeseman K, Mitchinson MJ. Randomised controlled trial of vitamin E in patients with coronary disease: Cambridge Heart Antioxidant Study (CHAOS). Lancet 1996; 347:781–786.
19. The Alpha-Tocopherol, Beta Carotene Cancer Prevention Study Group. The effect of vitamin E and beta carotene on the incidence of lung cancer and other cancers in male smokers. N Engl J Med 1994; 330:1029–1035.
20. Omenn GS, Goodman GE, Thornquist MD, et al. Effects of a combination of beta carotene and vitamin A on lung cancer and cardiovascular disease. N Engl J Med 1996; 334:1150–1155.
21. Hennekens CH, Buring JE, Manson JE, et al. Lack of effect of long-term supplementation with betacarotene on the incidence of malignant neoplasms and cardiovascular disease. N Engl J Med 1996; 334:1145–1149.

22. Yusuf S, Sleight P, Pogue J, Bosch J, Davies R, Dagenais G. Effects of an angiotensin-converting-enzyme inhibitor, ramipril, on cardiovascular events in high-risk patients. The heart outcomes prevention evaluation study investigators. N Engl J Med 2000; 342:145–153.

23. Gruppo Italiano Per Lo Studio Della Sopravvivenza Nell'Infarto miocardico. Dietary supplementation with n-3 polyunsaturated fatty acids and vitamin E after myocardial infarction: results of the GISSI-Prevenzione trial. Lancet 1999; 354:447–455.

24. Lee IM, Cook NR, Gaziano JM, et al. Vitamin E in the primary prevention of cardiovascular disease and cancer: the women's health study: a randomized controlled trial. JAMA 2005; 294:56–65.

25. Lisi DM. Probucol and multivitamins in the prevention of restenosis after coronary angioplasty. N Engl J Med 1997; 337:1919.

26. Yokoi H, Daida H, Kuwabara Y, et al. Effectiveness of an antioxidant in preventing restenosis after percutaneous transluminal coronary angioplasty: the probucol angioplasty restenosis trial. J Am Coll Cardiol 1997; 30:855–862.

27. Kris-Etherton PM, Lichtenstein AH, Howard BV, Steinberg D, Witztum JL. Antioxidant vitamin supplements and cardiovascular disease. Circulation 2004; 110:637–641.

28. Steinberg D. Is there a potential therapeutic role for vitamin E or other antioxidants in atherosclerosis? Curr Opin Lipidol 2000; 11:603–607.

Index

.

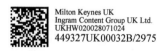